Microbiology
Guide for FMGE

Microbiology
Guide for FMGE

Apurba Sankar Sastry
MD (JIPMER), DNB, MNAMS, PDCR
Assistant Professor
Department of Microbiology
Jawaharlal Institute of
Postgraduate Medical Education and Research
Puducherry, Tamil Nadu, India

Sandhya Bhat K
MD, DNB, MNAMS, PDCR
Assistant Professor
Department of Microbiology
ESI Medical College and PGIMSR
Chennai, Tamil Nadu, India

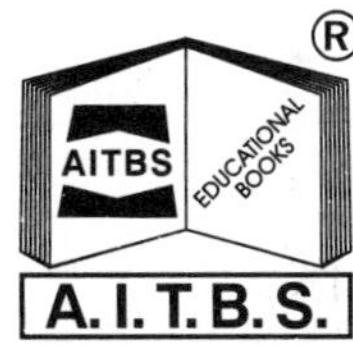

AITBS PUBLISHERS, INDIA
Medical Publishers
J-5/6, Krishan Nagar, Delhi-110051 (INDIA)
Phone: 011-40167052, 49067602
E-mail: aitbsindia@gmail.com & aitbsindia@hotmail.com

First Edition : 2013
Second Edition : 2014
Third Edition : 2016
Fourth Edition : 2018
Fifth Edition : 2020
Sixth Edition : 2026

ISBN: 978-93-7473-516-9

Published by:
Virender Kumar Arya for
AITBS Publishers, India
MEDICAL PUBLISHERS
J-5/6 Krishan Nagar, Delhi-110051 (INDIA)
Phone: 011-40167052, 49067602
E-mail: aitbsindia@gmail.com & aitbsindia@hotmail.com

Printed by AITBS, Delhi

This Book is Dedicated to

Our Beloved Parents

Mr. Anooj Kumar Sastry and Mrs. Tarini Purohit
Mr. K. Ganesh Bhat and Mrs. Shakunthala G. Bhat

Brother and Sister-in-law

Dr. Anand Sankar Sastry and Santosini Panigrahi

Sister and Brother-in-law

Dr. Santhosh Shenoy, Mrs. Gayathri Shenoy
and Nephew Pranav

Our Lovable Aunty

Ms. Usha Rani Chaudhary

Our Beloved Son

Master Adarsh Sastry

And above all, Lord Ganesha who gave us the knowledge and inspiration

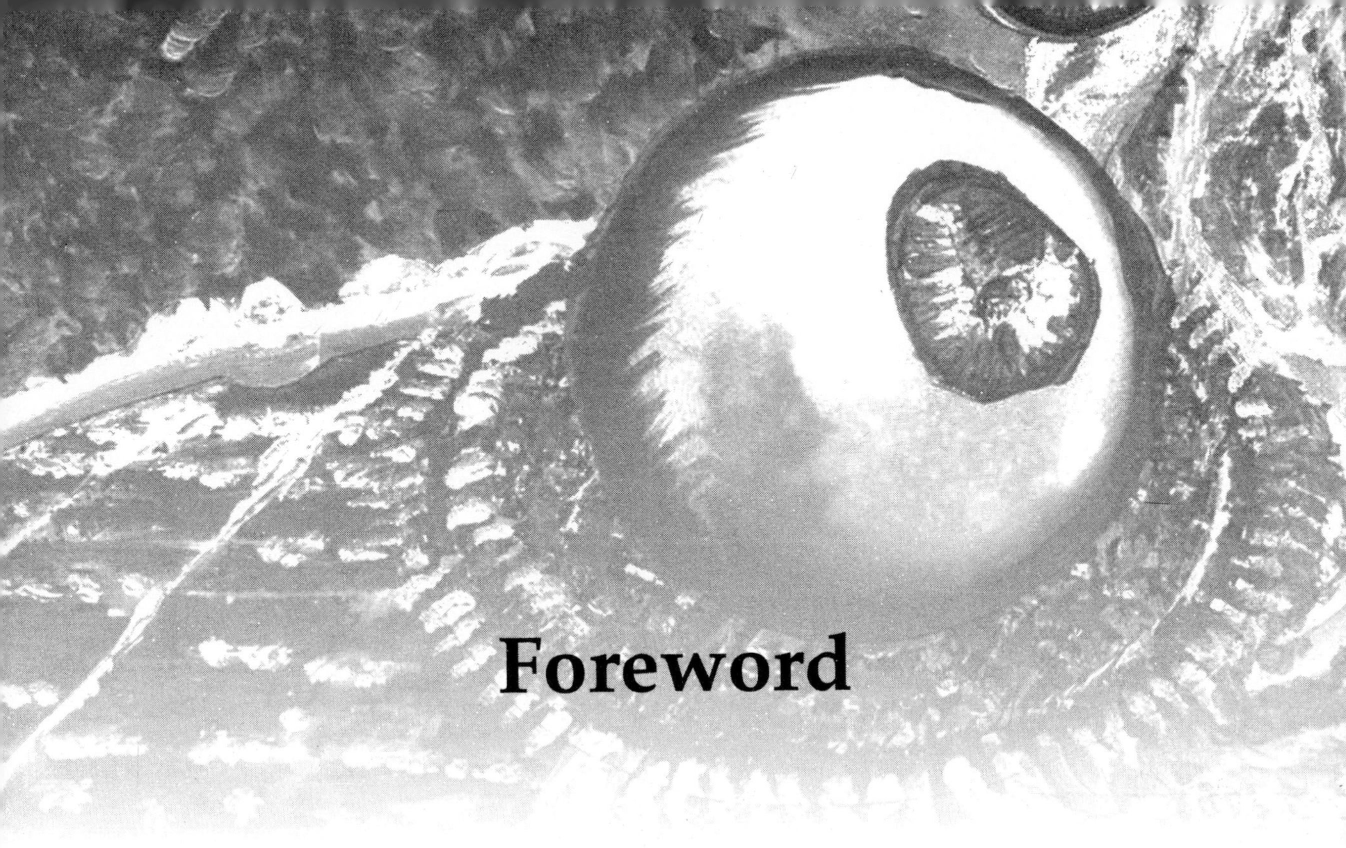

Foreword

The most awaited book by the FMGE aspirants is now in the market. The book provides all the essential facts and multiple choice questions for all FMGE aspirants. The book deals with each and every topic in an excellent way that we need not refer any other book for verification. The authors being microbiologists themselves had done extra ordinary work to bring this book for the welfare of students.

This is the first ever book written by two Microbiologists, with excellent references and data. I am sure this book will be the most loved book by all soon. All the best for the authors for their future release of many more books.

Rajesh Sharma
Managing Director
DIAMS, Delhi

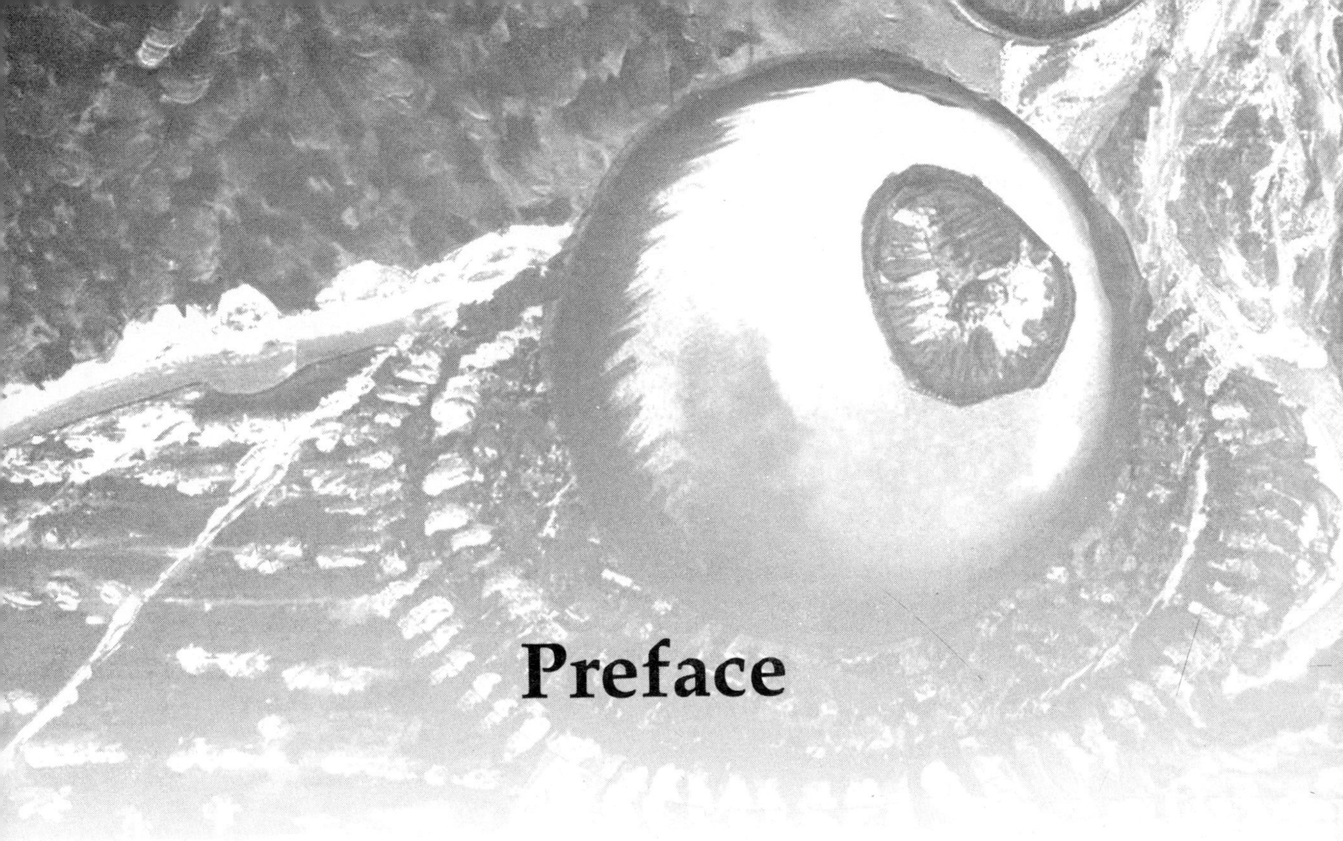

Preface

This is the first book released in **Microbiology Guide for FMGE (Foreign Medical Graduate Entrance)** examination. This book is prepared taking into account of all the parameters like:

- Importance of Microbiology for FMGE exam.
- Number of MCQs asked from Microbiology/Infection.
- MCQ prone areas from where maximum MCQs asked.
- Microbiology made simplified, easy and lucid taking into account for foreign medical students.
- More tables and mnemonics (for better remembering).
- Recent 2013 March and September papers are also included.

Importance of Microbiology for FMGE Examination

- Microbiology is one of the high scoring sections and hence is the key subject for FMGE exam.
- Though it might look tough before you start, but as you go through gradually, you will surely realize that, repeated revisions can take you to that level at which you can answer all the possible MCQs in any entrance exam.
- The beauty of this subject is, if you are thorough in Microbiology, you can solve many infection related MCQs of Medicine, PSM, Pediatrics, etc.
- Microbiology acts as opening batsman for your exam. As the FMGE paper starts with Microbiology MCQs, so your good preparation will boost you to do well in the rest of the paper. Opening batsman play the most crucial role in a match. A good start will always carry the innings well.

Entrance	Microbiology MCQ	Infection MCQ
FMGE March 2013	29/300	51/300
FMGE September 2013	11/300	31/300
FMGE March 2012	19/300	38/300
FMGE September 2012	31/300	55/300

Each Chapter Contains

- *Chapter Review* – Gives a preliminary overall idea about a chapter – can be finished fast.
- *FMGE MCQs* with fully detailed explanations – Gone to the depth covering all the important aspects in detail.
- *Practice section* (An altogether new concept) – Contains new MCQs similar to FMGE pattern. Useful for self-assessment of the students.

Tips for your Preparation

- Target oriented labour is more crucial than aimless labour.
- That means – You should know where to read and how much to read and not to waste time in reading unnecessary things which are least asked.
- **Repeated revisions** – The Most Important Crucial Factor.
- **Last 100 days** of reading is very crucial-because the students, survey has shown that 80% of what you will correct in the exam lies in last 2-3 months, reading.
- Sleeping well the previous night – increases the efficiency at least by 10%.
- Should never attempt those MCQs in which you cannot exclude any options.
- Do not forget the importance of time once lost, can never be recycled.

Do not stop your preparation after you clear your MCI Screening Test
Continue your study for PG entrances

- Please remember, FMGE preparation is not totally different from PG entrance preparation. It is a subset of the what you have to cover for PG entrances exam.
- So if you are done with FMGE preparation, then you can consider that you have finished 60% of the content required for PG entrances. You are very close to the target.
- Instead of getting frustrated, if you continue your hard labour, then it is a very easy task to click in PG entrances and many of your seniors have already proved it.
- What is required is, you should not give a long break after your FMGE exam, otherwise you will forget everything.
- Please remember, doing MBBS is nothing now a days as more than 50,000 students are graduating every year from India.
- So, joining a Post graduate course is not an optional, but a MUST thing for you if you want to be different from others.

Wish You "ALL THE BEST FOR THE SUCCESS AND THE BRIGHT FUTURE AHEAD".

–Apurba Sankar Sastry

–Sandhya Bhat K

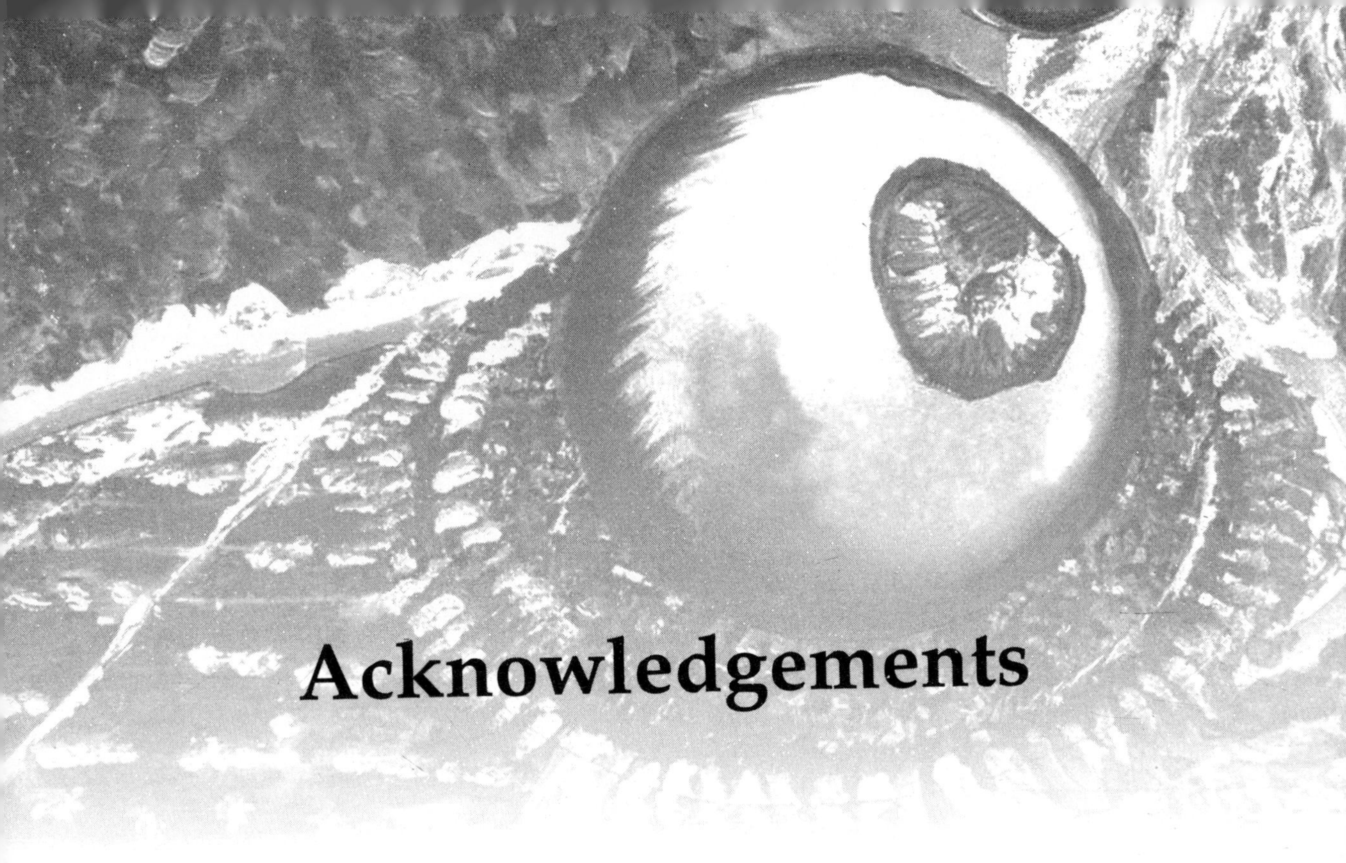

Acknowledgements

We like to express our gratitude to **Mr. Rajesh Sharma,** Director, DIAMS, Delhi for his constant support and inspiration.

We express our deep sense of reverence and gratitude to our teachers for giving us the wonderful opportunity to work under their guidance during our post graduation time and enlightened us by their knowledge without which we would not have ever thought of initiating this project.

Dr. B.N. Harish, Professor and Head Department of Microbiology, JIPMER, Puducherry

Dr. S.C. Parija, Professor, Department of Microbiology, JIPMER, Puducherry

Dr. S. Sujatha, Professor, Department of Microbiology, JIPMER, Puducherry

Dr. E.R. Nagaraj, Professor and Head, Department of Microbiology, Sri Siddhartha Medical College, Tumkur, Karnataka.

We would like to sincerely thank our beloved Director of JIPMER, Puducherry who gave us constant inspiration and support for writing this book.

We also like to express our gratitude to the Dean of ESI Medical College and PGIMSR, Chennai for her help and encouragement.

We are thankful to all the faculties, residents, PhD Scholar, MSc PGs and technical staffs of JIPMER, Puducherry our department for their help and encouragement.

We can never forget the support given by the staffs of department of Microbiology of our previous working institute – Meenakshi Medical College, Chennai.

We also like to express our gratitude to all our friends, colleagues and all other staffs and technicians of ESI Medical College and PGIMSR, Chennai.

We offer our hearty gratitude to all our paternal and maternal relatives and all our cousins.

We also thankful to Virender Kumar Arya and his team at AITBS Publishers, India, for their meticulous efforts in the direction of bringing out this book on time.

And the most important of all........ We like to express our gratitude to our beloved FMGE aspirants who have made our book successful.

–Authors

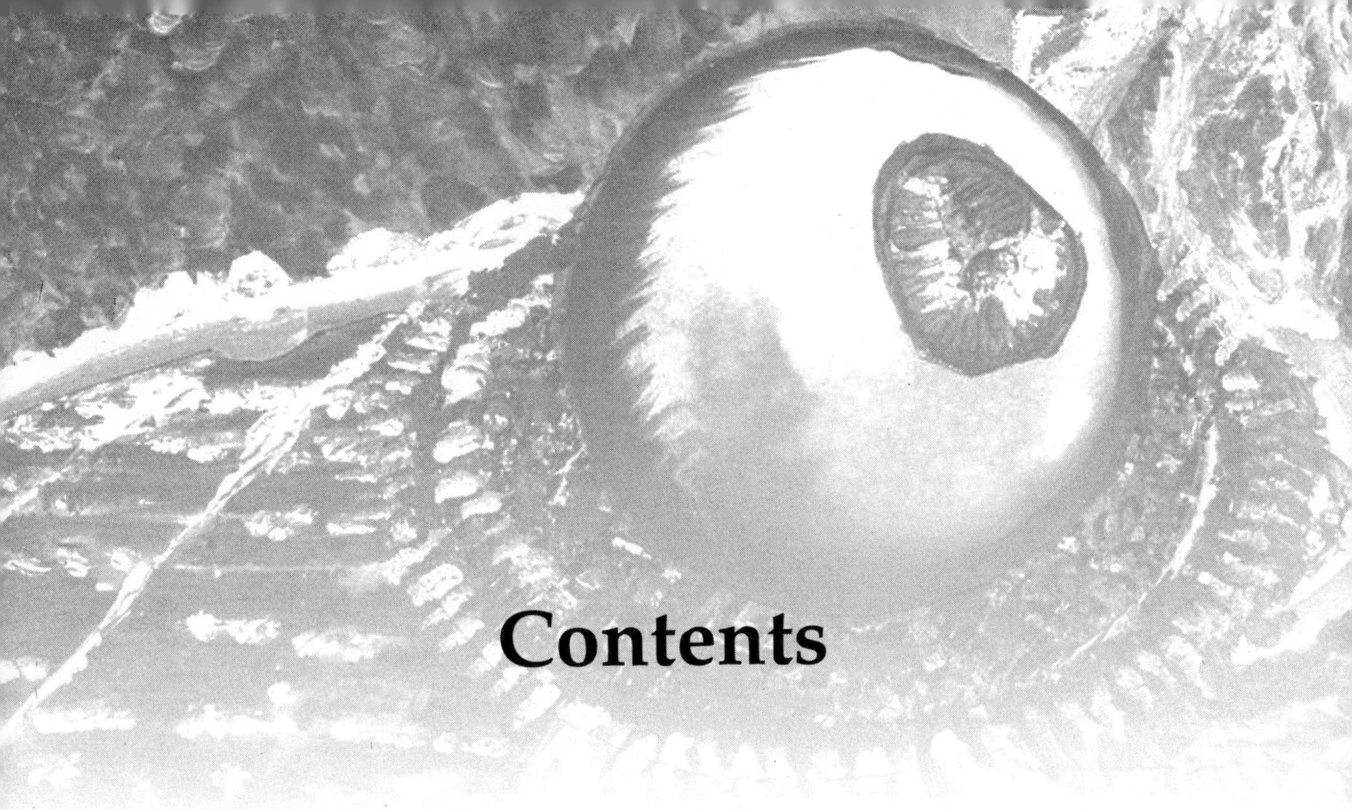

Contents

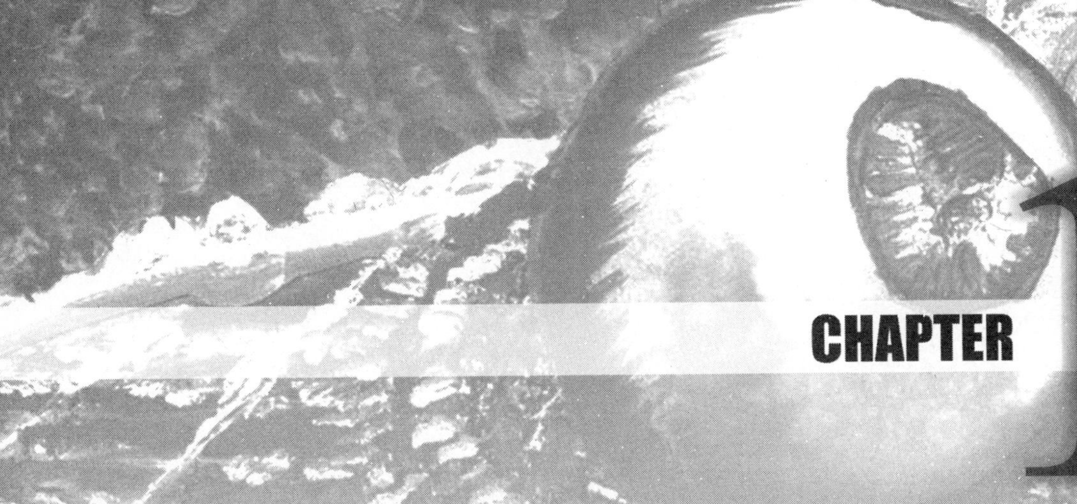

General Microbiology

(Morphology of Bacteria, Sterilization and Disinfection, Culture Media and Culture Methods, Bacterial Genetics)

HISTORY

Louis Pasteur

- Known as Father of Microbiology.
- Proposed Fermentation Principle.
- Devised – Autoclave, steam sterilizer, hot air oven and pasteurization of milk.
- Prepared the Vaccines for – Anthrax, Rabies, Cholera ***(CAR).***

Robert Koch

- Known as Father of Medical Microbiology.
- Proposed Koch Postulates.
- Discovered – TB, cholera bacilli.
- Started Aniline dye staining.
- Proposed Solid culture media concept.

Koch's Postulates

- **1st:** The microorganism must be present in every case of the disease but absent from healthy organisms.
- **2nd:** The suspected microorganism must be isolated and grown in a pure culture.
- **3rd:** The same disease must result when the isolated microorganism is inoculated into a healthy host.
- **4th:** The same microorganism must be isolated again from the diseased host.
- Additional **5th postulate:** Antibody to the causative organism usually develops during the course of the disease.

- ***Bacteria that do not fulfill Koch's postulates are Treponema pallidum, Lepra bacilli and Neisseria gonorhoeae because for the 1st two are non-cultivable and the 3rd one has no animal model.***

Paul Ehrlich

- Proposed Ehrlich Phenomena.
- Detected – Ehrlichia (Bacteria).
- Founder – Acid fast stain.
- Standardized toxin and antitoxin.
- Proposed Side Chain Theory for Ab Production.

Other Important Contributors

- Joseph Lister – Antiseptic measures to prevent surgical sepsis.
- Antony van Leeuwenhoek – Founder of Microscopy.
- Karry B. Mullis – Discovered PCR.

Discoverers

- *Kleb-Loeffler bacilli* – Corynebacterium diphtheriae.
- *Preisz Nocard bacilli* – Corynebacterium pseudotuberculosis.
- *Koch Weeks bacilli* – Haemophilus aegypticus.
- *Whitmore bacilli* – Burkholderia pseudomallei.
- *Pfeiffer's bacilli* – Haemophilus influenzae.

MORPHOLOGY

- **Microorganisms** – classified under the kingdom *Protista*.
- **Kingdom *Protista*** – Divided into following groups:
  - **Prokaryotes –** Include bacteria and blue green algae.
    - They do not have Organelles except Ribosome (70s).
    - Principal sites of ***respiratory enzymes*** in the bacteria – ***Mesosomes.***
  - **Eukaryotes** – Include fungi, algae (other than blue green), protozoa and slime moulds.

MICROSCOPY

Principle of Microscope depends on

- **Magnification:** Takes place at objective lens and eye piece (increased by using convex lens).
- **Contrast:** Increased by staining.
- **Resolution:** Ability to distinguish two points separate (improves by using immersion oil).

Resolution power of

- Human eye – 0.2 mm.
- Light microscope – 0.2 μm.
- Electron microscope – 0.2 nm.

Type of light used

- Reflected light – Used in dark field microscope.

- Polarized light – Used in differential interference contrast microscope.
- Transmitted light – Used in light microscope.

Types of Microscopy

Dark Field Microscopy – Used for:

- Visualization of live thin organism like Spirochete.
- Demonstration of flagella (hence motility of bacteria).

Phase Contrast Microscope – Used for:

- For visualization of live thin organism.
- Demonstration of motility (Spirochaete) of bacteria.
- Demonstration of endospores and inclusion bodies.

Fluorescence Microscope

- **Flourochrome dyes used as stains:**
    - Auramine O.
    - Acridine orange.
    - Fluorescent Isothiocyanate.
- **Uses:**
    - Auto fluorescence – Cyclospora.
    - Acridine orange stain (QBC) – used for détection of malarial parasites.
    - Auramine phenol stain – used for detection of Tubercle bacilli.

Electron Microscope

- Magnification >1 lakh.
- Resolution power – 0.2 nm.
- Radiation source used – electron beam.

Staining Methods

A. **Negative Staining**
- **Stains used:** India ink and Nigrosin.
- In negative staining, ***the background is stained, while the structures to be demonstrated is not stained.***
- **Uses:** Demonstration of capsule and thin bacteria such as Spirochetes.

B. **Silver Impregnation Methods:** To visualize too thin bacteria (*Treponema pallidum, Leptospira, Borrelia*) by impregnation of silver on their surface.

C. **Differential Stains**

Gram's Stain

- It differentiates bacteria into two groups: Gram-positive and Gram-negative bacteria.
- GPB appear violet – they have a relatively thick amorphous cell wall.
- Gram-negative bacteria take counter stain, appearing red.

Classification of Bacteria According to Gram's Staining

- Gram positive cocci – *Staphylococcus, Streptococcus, Enterococcus, Pneumococcus.*

- Gram negative cocci – *Meningococcus, Gonococci, Veillonella, Moraxella.*
- Gram positive bacilli – *Corynebacterium, Clostridium, Bacillus, Listeria, Rhodococcus, Actinomycetes/Nocardia, Mycobacteria, Erysipelothrix* etc.
- Gram negative bacilli – *Enterobacteriaceae, Vibrio, Pseudomonas* etc.

Acid-Fast Stain

- Ziehl-Neelsen (ZN) staining method.
- Acid-fast bacilli (AFB) – appears bright red against blue background.
- Acid fastness is due to:
  - The high content of mycolic acid and
  - Depends on integrity of the cell wall.
- Used for staining following acid-fast micro-organisms:
  - *Mycobacterium tuberculosis* (20% sulfuric acid).
  - *Mycobacterium leprae* (5% sulfuric acid).
  - *Nocardia* (1% sulfuric acid).
  - *Spores* (0.5% sulfuric acid).
  - *Rhodococcus.*
  - Parasites such as *Cryptosporidium, Cyclospora, Isospora.*

Albert's Stain:

- Used for staining the volutin granules (metachromatic granules) of *Corynebacterium diphtheriae.*

GENERAL MICROBIOLOGY

Shape of Bacteria

Classification of bacteria depending on their shape:

1. **Cocci: Oval or spherical cells, arranged in**

   Arrangement
   - Clusters, e.g., *Staphylococci.*
   - Pairs, e.g.,
     - *Pneumococci* (lanceolate shaped)
     - *Meningococcus, Gonococci* (kidney shaped)
     - *Enterococcus* (spectacle eyed shaped).
   - Tetrads, e.g., *Micrococci.*
   - Chains, e.g., *Streptococci.*
   - Octate, e.g., *Sarcina.*

2. **Bacilli: Rod shaped**

   Arrangement:
   - *Coccobacilli*, e.g., *Brucella.*
   - *Streptobacilli*: Arranged in chains, e.g., *Streptobacillus, B. anthracis* (Bamboo stick appearance).
   - *Cuneiform pattern*: Chinese letter or cuneiform pattern, e.g., *Corynebacterium.*
   - *Comma shaped*: Curved appearance, e.g., *Vibrio.*
   - *Spirally coiled*, e.g., *Spirillum and Spirochete.*

- *Pleomorphic*, e.g., *Haemophilus, Proteus.*
- Branching filamentous bacteria, e.g., Actinomycetes.

Bacterial Cell Structure

Difference between Gram Positive and Gram Negative Bacterial Cell Wall

Characters	Gram-positive cell wall	Gram-negative cell wall
Thickness	15-80 nm	2 nm
Lipid content	2- 5% only	15-20%
Teichoic acid	Present	Absent
Variety of amino acid	Few	Several
Aromatic amino acid	Absent	Present
Lipopolysaccharide in outer membrane ***(endotoxin)***	Absent	Present

Capsule and Slime Layer

The capsule has various functions:

- ❖ It contributes to invasiveness of bacteria by protecting the bacteria from phagocytosis.
- ❖ It facilitates adherence of bacteria to surfaces.
- ❖ It plays a role in formation of biofilms.
- ❖ **Demonstration of capsule:**
- ❖ Negative staining.
- ❖ M'Faydean capsule stain – used for demonstration of capsule of *Bacillus anthracis* (polychrome methylene blue stain).
- ❖ Quellung's reaction – Since capsules are antigenic they can be demonstrated by serologic methods and useful for rapid identification of capsular serotypes of *Streptococcus pneumoniae.*

Capsules of Various Bacteria

Organism	Polymer
Pneumococcus	Polysaccharide
Meningococcus	Polysaccharide
H. influenzae	Polysaccharide
Bacillus anthracis	Polypeptide (glutamate)
Streptococcus pyogenes	Hyaluronic acid

Atypical forms of bacteria

- ❖ ***Cell wall deficient forms (L-forms):***
  - Discovered by Klinberger.
  - Discovered at Lister Institute, London.
  - Streptobacillus moniliformis.

- Mycoplamsa – Unstable.
- Resistant to cell wall acting drug.
- L form organisms are ***resistant to cell wall acting drugs.***

❖ ***Involution forms:*** Swollen and aberrant form of bacteria (Gonococci and *Yersinia pestis*) in ageing culture and high salt concentration.

Flagella

❖ Thread-like appendages that confers ***motility*** to the bacteria.

❖ ***Demonstration by:***
- Tannic acid staining *(Leifson method)*
- Dark ground/phase contrast/electron microscope
- By demonstration of motility:
  - Craige tube
  - Hanging drop
  - Semisolid medium.

❖ ***Various types of motility:***
- Tumbling – *Listeria*
- Gliding – *Mycoplasma*
- Stately – *Clostridium*
- Darting – *Vibrio/Campylobacter*
- Swarming – *Proteus.*

Fimbriae or Pili

❖ Hair-like filaments that extend from cell surface.

❖ Organ of adhesion – responsible for the attachment.

❖ Sex pili helps in conjugation.

❖ They are antigenic.

❖ Form surface pellicle in liquid culture.

Sporulation

❖ Bacterial spores are a highly resistant ***resting phase.***

❖ Observed in *Bacillus* and *Clostridium.*

Growth and Multiplication of Bacteria

❖ Generation time – time required for a bacterium to give rise to two daughter cells under optimum condition.

❖ Generation time for different pathogenic bacteria:
- *Escherichia coli* – 20 minutes
- *Mycobacterium tuberculosis* – 20 hours
- *Mycobacterium leprae* – 20 days.

Phases of Bacterial Growth Curve

❖ **Lag phase:**
- Time required to make its own enzyme and metabolites.
- Bacteria increases in size (maximum at end of lag phase) but does not multiply.

GENERAL MICROBIOLOGY

❖ **Log phase:**
- Bacteria divides maximum.
- Biochemically active.
- Smaller size.
- Uniformly stained.

❖ **Stationary phase:**
- Bacteria starts dying which nullifies its multiplication.
- Appears Gram variable.
- More storage granules produced.
- Sporulation occurs in this phase.
- Produce exotoxin, antibiotics.

❖ **Decline phase:**
- Bactria only dies without multiplication.
- Involution forms are seen.

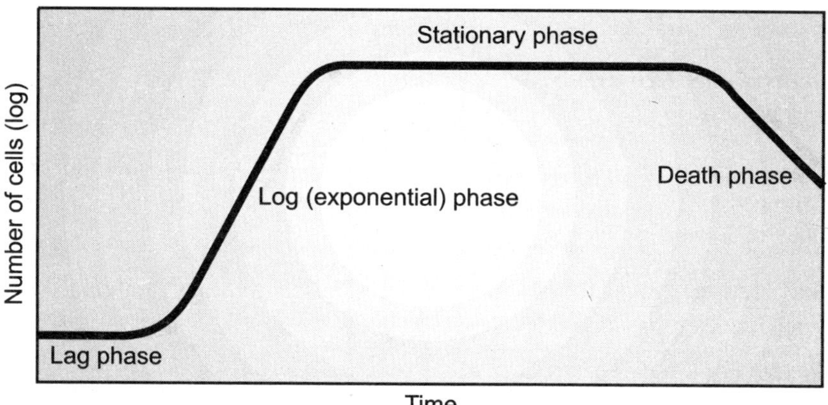

Fig. 1.1: ***Bacterial growth curve***

STERILIZATION AND DISINFECTION

Sterilization

Defined as a process by which an article, surface or medium is freed of all living microorganisms ***either in the vegetative or spore state.***

Disinfection

Physical process or a chemical agent that destroys or removes all pathogenic organisms or organisms capable of giving rise to infection, but ***not bacterial endospores.***

Methods of sterilization classified as:

❖ Physical methods of sterilization.

❖ Chemical methods of sterilization.

Physical Methods of Sterilization

❖ Heat – Dry heat and Moist heat.

- Filtration.
- Radiation.
- Sound (sonic) waves.

Dry Heat

- The dry heat kills microorganisms by ***(CODE)***
  - Charring
  - Oxidative damage
  - Denaturation of protein
  - Elevated electrolyte.
- Types of dry heat – Sun light, flaming, incineration and hot air oven.
- Hot air oven:
  - Temp. maintained – **160°C for 1 hr**.
  - Materials sterilized – glass ware, forceps, liquid paraffin, grease, fat, glycerol, dust powder.
  - Sterilization Control – spores of ***Clostridium tetani*** (non-toxigenic strain).

Moist heat

- ***Mechanism:*** *Coagulation and denaturation of protein.*
- ***Moist heat is of three kinds:***
  1. *Sterilization at a temperature below 100ºC:*
     - Pasteurization – Holder method (63ºC for 30 min), Flash method (72ºC for 20 sec) followed by rapid cooling to 13ºC.
     - Vaccine bath – 60ºC for 1 hr.
     - Inspissation – 80ºC for 30 min for three consecutive days (suitable for LJ media and Loeffler's serum slope).
  2. *Sterilization at a temperature of 100ºC:*
     - Boiling
     - Koch's or Arnold's steam sterilizer
     - ***Tyndalisation:*** Intermittent sterilization – 100ºC for 20 min for three days. Used for sugar solution, gelatin.
  3. *Sterilization at a temperature above 100ºC:*
     - Autoclaves
     - ***121°C for 15 min at 15 psi pressure***
     - Sterilization control for autoclave – spores of *B. stearothermophillus.*

Filtration

- Excellent way to reduce the microbial population in solutions of **heat-labile material like serum, sugar, vaccine, antibiotics and toxin.**
- Asbestos filters (Seitz filters).
- Sintered glass filters – Carcinogenic and inflammable, so not in use.
- *Membrane filters:*
  - Made up of cellulose acetate, cellulose nitrate, polycarbonate or other synthetic materials.
  - Average pore diameter – ***0.22µ***.

GENERAL MICROBIOLOGY

Radiation

- *Non ionizing radiation:*
  - Example: UV and infrared rays.
  - Used for sterilization of enclosed area like OT, labs.
- *Ionizing radiation:*
  - Example: α, β, γ (cobalt), X-ray.
  - Known as ***Cold sterilization*** (as temperature is not raised).
  - Used for sterilization of heat labile substances like plastic syringes and catgut suture.

Disinfection

Important Disinfectants

- **Phenolic compounds** (e.g., phenol, cresol, dettol etc.) – active in presence of organic matter.
- **Isopropyl alcohol –** Used for thermometers.
- **Formaldehyde** – Used for fumigation of wards, preserves anatomical specimen.
- **Glutaraldehyde** – Used for sterilization of bronchoscope cystoscope, anesthetic tube and rubber face mask.
- **Gaseous agents -** Ethylene oxide, formaldehyde gas and betapropiolactone.
- **Ethylene oxide:**
  - Temperature maintained as 55°C for 4 hr.
  - Explosive, inflammable, carcinogenic, sweet ether smell.
  - Used for heart lung machine, respirator, suture.

> - Prions are highest resistant structure.
> - **Decreasing order of resistance:** Prion > Cryptosporidium cyst > spore > Non-enveloped and small sized virus > MTB > fungi > vegetative bacteria + enveloped/medium-large virus.

Testing of Disinfectants:

- Phenol coefficient (Rideal Walker) test
- Chick Martin test
- Capacity (Kelsey-Sykes) test.

Sporicidal Agents:

- ***EFGH:*** Ethylene oxide, Formaldehyde, Glutaraldehyde, Hypochlorite, H_2O_2
- Autoclave, Hot air oven.

Biological Sterilization Indicator:

Hot air oven	*Clostridium tetani non-toxigenic strain*
Autoclave	*B. Stearothermophillus*

Various Methods of Sterilization

Material	Method of Sterilization
Clinical thermometer	Isopropyl alcohol
Paraffin, glass syringe, flask, slide, oil, grease, fat, glycerol	Hot air oven

OT, entryway, ward, lab fumigation	Formal dehyde > UV > BPL
Cystoscope, bronchoscope	Orthophthaldehyde and glutaraldehyde 2% (cidex)
Heart lung machine, respirator, dental equipments	Ethylene oxide
Vaccine, sera, antibiotic, sugar	Filtration
Sharp instrument	Cresol
Milk	Pasteurization
Plastic syringe, cadgut, swab, catheter	Ionizing radiation
Culture media, all instruments except glass, all suture except cadgut	Autoclave

CULTURE MEDIA

- **Basic Ingredients:**
  - Agar:
    - Made up long chain polysaccharide
    - It has no nutritive value.
  - Peptone
  - Meat extract.
- **Simple/Basal Media:**
  - Peptone water – Peptone + NaCl
  - Nutrient broth – Peptone + meat extract + NaCl
  - Nutrient agar – Nutrient broth + 2% agar.
- **Enriched media** contains – blood, serum, egg.
  - *Example:* Blood agar, Chocolate agar, Loeffler's serum slope.
- **Enrichment broth (liquid media)** – Selectively allows certain organism to grow and inhibit others
  - Tetrathionate broth – (Salmonella Typhi)
  - Alkaline peptone water (APW) – Vibrio
  - Selenite F broth – Shigella, Salmonella.
- **Selective media (solid media)** – Selectively allows certain organism to grow and inhibits others
  - Lowestein Jensen media – *Mycobacterium tuberculosis*
  - Crystal violet blood agar – *Streptococcus*
  - Mannitol salt agar – *Staphylococcus*
  - Potassium tellurite agar (PTA) – *Corynebacterium diphtheriae*
  - Wilson blair bismuth sulfite medium – *Salmonella Typhi*
  - Thiosulphate Citrate Bile salt Sucrose agar (TCBS) – *Vibrio.*

- **Transport media:** Bacteria does not multiply, only maintains viability of desired pathogenic bacteria.

Organism	Transport media
Streptococcus	Pike's media
Neisseria	Amies, Stuart's media
Vibrio	VR, Autoclaved sea water, Carry Blair
Enteric pathogen	Carry Blair medium
Shigella, typhoid bacilli	Buffered glycerol saline

- **Differential media:**
  - Mac Conkey agar.
  - Cystein Lysine Electrolyte Deficient agar (CLED).
- **Anaerobic culture methods:**
  - Obligate anaerobes are bacteria that grow only in the ***absence of oxygen.***
  - Commonly used media:
    - Robertson cooked meat broth (RCM)
    - Thioglycolate broth
    - Neomycin blood agar
    - Egg yolk agar.
  - ***McIntosh-Fildes anaerobic jar***
  - Gas pack system.

BACTERIAL GENETICS

Plasmids

- Extra chromosomal DNA substances.
- Circular and double stranded DNA molecules that encode traits that are not essential for bacterial viability.
- Plasmids are of different types:
  - F factor,
  - R factors,
  - Col factor.
- Plasmids confer new properties to recipient bacteria
  - Resistance to one or several antibiotics,
  - Production of toxins,
  - Synthesis of cell surface structures required for adherence or colonization.
- Plasmids integrated with host chromosome are known as ***episomes.***

Methods of Transfer of DNA between Bacterial Cells

- Transformation,
- Transduction and
- Conjugation.

Transformation

- Process of the transfer of free DNA from one bacterium to another.
- Griffith experiment – was done on Mice provides the evidence of transformation.

Transduction

- Transfer of a portion of the DNA from one bacterium to another mediated by a **bacteriophage.**
- Bacterophages encoded toxin:
  - Diphtheria toxin
  - Botulin toxin C and D
  - Cholera toxin
  - Streptococcal erythrogenic exotoxin A and C
  - Verocytotoxin of E.coli.
- Transduction is of two types: generalized and specialized.

Conjugation: Process of transfer of DNA from the donor bacterium to the recipient bacterium.

- Occurs between two closely related species
- It occurs mostly in Gram negative bacteria
- Donor ability of the bacteria is determined by specific conjugative plasmids called fertility (F^+) plasmids or sex plasmids.
- Pilus forms the sex pilus or conjugation tube.
- The sex pilus produces a bridge between conjugating cells in Gram-negative bacteria.
- The transfer of plasmids during conjugation is responsible for the spread of multiple drug resistance among bacteria.

Transposon/Jumping gene (Transfer of DNA within bacterial cells)

- They are extra chromosomal genes that can transfer from one site of the bacterial chromosome/ plasmid to another site in a cut and paste manner (transposition).
- They do not have self replicative power (differs from plasmid).
- They code for drug resistance enzymes, toxins or a variety of metabolic enzymes.

Blotting Methods

- **Northern blot –** used to detect RNA (Hybridization of DNA to RNA)
- **Southern blot –** used to detect DNA (Hybridization of DNA to DNA)
- **Western blot –** used to detect Protein (Antibodies).

Polymerase Chain Reaction – (PCR)

- Amplification of the DNA of the organism present in the clinical sample to such an extent that it can be detected by gel electrophoresis.
- **Modification of PCR:**
  - Reverse transcriptase PCR (RT-PCR) – used for detection of RNA (used for RNA viruses)
  - Nested PCR – two round PCR making it more specific and sensitive
  - Multiplex PCR – Uses >1 primers which can detect many organism in one reaction
  - Real-time PCR (rt-PCR) – recent development.
    - Real time visualization of amplification process
    - Takes less time
    - Less contamination rate
    - Quantification is possible.

GENERAL MICROBIOLOGY

FMGE MCQ's

Morphology of Bacteria

1. **PCR is invented by:** [*March 2011*]
   (a) Carry B Mullis (b) Pasteur
   (c) Robert Koch (d) Van Joseph.
2. **Which of the following is seen in dark field microscopy?** [*September 2009*]
   (a) Vibrio (b) Spirochaetes
   (c) Chlamydia (d) All of the above.
3. **Type of light used in dark ground microscopy:** [*September 2005*]
   (a) Dark light (b) Reflected light
   (c) Polarized light (d) Transmitted light.
4. **Peptidoglycans are found in large quantities in cell wall of:** [*March 2009*]
   (a) Virus (b) Gram-positive bacteria
   (c) Gram negative bacteria (d) All of the above.

Sterilization and Disinfection

5. **Phenol coefficient indicates:** [*FMGE, March 2011*]
   (a) Efficiency of a disinfectant (b) Dilution of a disinfectant
   (c) Quantity of a disinfectant (d) Purity of a disinfectant.
6. **Pasteurization of milk is determined by:** [*September 2005, 2007 and 2009*]
   (a) Methylene blue reduction test (b) Phosphatase test
   (c) Turbidity test (d) Resazurin test.
7. **Effective mode of sterilization is:** [*September 2005*]
   (a) Hot water (b) Steam under pressure
   (c) Steam at atmospheric pressure (d) Dry heat.
8. **Temp. for about autoclaving is:** [*March 2007*]
   (a) 115°C for 20 min (b) 121°C for 15 min
   (c) 118°C for 15 min (d) 124°C for 15 min.
9. **Surgical blades are sterilized by:** [*March 2007*]
   (a) Boiling (b) Autoclave
   (c) Hot air oven (d) Gamma rays.
10. **Operation theatres are sterilized by:** [*March 2007*]
    (a) Ethylene oxide gas (b) Formaldehyde fumigation
    (c) Washing with soap water (d) Carbolic acid spraying.
11. **Best way to sterilize all-glass syringes is:** [*September 2007*]
    (a) Boiling (b) Autoclave
    (c) Hot air oven (d) Formaldehyde.

12. Cold sterilization is done: [*September 2007*]

(a) Steam
(b) Inionizing radiation
(c) Infra red
(d) UV.

13. Incineration is done for which of the following: [*September 2008*]

(a) Liquid waste
(b) Anatomical waste
(c) Sharp waste
(d) All of the above.

14. Biological indicator for determining efficacy of autoclaving is: [*September 2009*]

(a) Pseudomonas aeruginosa
(b) Clostridium perfringens
(c) Bacillus stereothermophilus
(d) Salmonella typhi.

15. Endoscopes are best sterilized by: [*September 2007*]

(a) Boiling
(b) Autoclave
(c) Lysol solution 20%
(d) Cidex solution.

16. Moist heat (pasteurization) kills all of the following except: [*September 2009*]

(a) Coxiella burnetii
(b) Brucella
(c) Salmonella
(d) Mycobacterium.

17. Sharp instrument should be disposed in: [*September 2005*]

(a) Blue bag
(b) Red bag
(c) Black bag
(d) Yellow bag.

GENERAL MICROBIOLOGY

Culture Media

18. Blood agar is an example of: [*March 2010*]

(a) Enrichment media
(b) Enriched media
(c) Selective media
(d) Transport media.

19. Best medium to grow anaerobic bacteria exclusively is: [*March 2008*]

(a) Blood agar
(b) Robertson's cooked meat medium
(c) Thioglycollate medium
(d) Sabouraud Dextrose agar.

20. Which of the following is an enrichment media? [*September 2009*]

(a) Alkaline peptone water
(b) Monsour's taurocholate Tellurite peptone water
(c) Selenite F broth
(d) All of the above.

ANSWERS TO FMGE MCQ's

Morphology of Bacteria

1. Ans. (a) Karry B Mullis

[*Ref.:* **Ananthnarayan, 8th ed., page no. 69]**

- ❖ In 1983, Kary Mullis developed a new technique called polymerase chain reaction or PCR technique that made it possible to synthesize large quantities of a DNA fragment by amplification of the target DNA of the organism present in the sample.

Other Important Contributors

- **Joseph Lister** – Antiseptic measures to prevent surgical sepsis.
- **Antony van Leeuwenhoek** – Founder of Microscopy.
- **Robert Koch –** Proposed Koch Postulates and Discovered – TB, cholera bacilli.
- **Loius Pasteur**
  - Proposed fermentation principle
  - Devised – Autoclave, steam sterilizer, hot air oven
  - Proposed Pasteurization of milk
  - Prepared the Vaccines for – Anthrax, Rabies, Cholera.

2. Ans. (d) All of the above

[*Ref.:* L.M. Prescott, 5th ed., Chapter 2.2, page no. 24; Parija's, Microbiology 1st ed., page no. 13]

❖ **Dark – ground microscopy is useful for demonstration of very thin bacteria such as spirochetes, not visible under ordinary illumination, since the reflection of the light makes them appear larger.** *–Parija's*

❖ *The method is also useful for demonstration of motility of motile bacteria and protozoa.*

3. Ans. (b) Reflected light

[*Ref.:* L.M. Prescott, 5th ed., Chapter 2.2, page 24; Parija's, Microbiology 1st ed., page no. 12, 13]

"Dark – ground microscope uses reflected light instead of transmitted light used on the ordinary ***light microscope***" *–Parija's*

❖ It has a dark field condenser with a central circular stop, which illuminates the object with a cone of light. It prevents light to fall directly on the objective lens.

❖ Light rays falling on the object are reflected or scattered on to the objective lens with the result that the microorganisms appears brightly against a dark background.

Type of Light Used in Microscopes

- Reflected light – used in dark field
- Polarized light – used in differential interference contrast microscope
- Transmitted light – used in light microscope.

4. Ans. (b) Gram-positive bacteria

[*Ref.:* Ananthnarayan, 8th ed., page no. 17]

❖ ***"The cell wall of gram-positive cell wall has a more thick homogenous wall (~80 nm) than that of the gram-negative cell wall (2 nm) because it contains large amount of peptidoglycan present in several layers that constitutes about 40-80% of dry weight of the cell wall."***

❖ ***Gram-positive cell wall has more peptidoglycan layers and teichoic acid where as gram-negative cell wall has more aromatic amino acid and lipopolysaccharide (endotoxin).***

Characters	Gram-positive cell wall	Gram-negative cell wall
Thickness	15-80 nm	2 nm
Lipid content	2- 5% only	15-20%
Teichoic acid	Present	Absent
Aromatic amino acid	Absent	Present
Lipopolysaccharide in outer membrane ***(endotoxin)***	Absent	Present

Sterilization and Disinfection

5. Ans. (a) Efficiency of a disinfectant

[*Ref.:* Ananthnarayan, 8th ed., page no. 38]

- *Chick Martin test is a modification of Rideal and Walker test, in which, disinfectants acts in the presence of organic contaminants (e.g., dried yeast, faeces, etc.) to simulate the natural conditions.*
- **Testing the efficiency of disinfectant:**
  - ***Phenol coefficient (Rideal Walker) test:*** Compare the performance of a phelonic disinfectant with that of phenol for the ability to kill *Salmonella typhi*. The test, however, does not show the action of disinfectant in natural condition, in the presence of organic contaminants.
  - ***Chick Martin test:*** It is a modification of Rideal and Walker test, in which, disinfectants acts in the presence of organic contaminants (e.g., dried yeast, faeces, etc.) to simulate the natural conditions.
  - ***Capacity (Kelsey-Sykes) test:*** Measures the capacity of a disinfectant to retain its activity when repeatedly used in the presence of organic material.
  - ***In-use (Kelsey and Maurer) test:*** Determines whether the chosen disinfectant is effective in actual use in hospital practice.

6. Ans. (b) Phosphatase test

[*Ref.:* Ananthnarayan, 8th ed., page no. 596]

"Phosphatase test is used to check the effectiveness of pasteurization of milk."

Phosphatase test: Alkaline phosphatase is normally present in milk and is inactivated if pasteurization has been carried out effectively. Successful pasteurization which kills non-sporing pathogens also inactivates alkaline phosphatase. If the pasteurization is not proper, then alkaline phosphatase can be detected by adding disodium p-nitrophenyl phosphate which breaks down to p-nitro phenyl phosphate.

Other tests for Bacteriological examination of milk are:

- Methylene blue reduction test
- Turbidity test
- Detection of specific pathogens in milk includes – *M. tuberculosis* and *Brucella* spp.
- Viable count
- Coliform count.

7. Ans. (b) Steam under pressure

[*Ref.:* Ananthnarayan, 8th ed., page no. 33-34]

- Effective mode of sterilization means methods that kills all vegetative organism including spores.
- Among the options, steam under pressure, i.e., autoclave is the only, e.g., that can kill spores.
- **Sporicidal agents:**
  - **EFGH:** Ethylene oxide, formaldehyde, glutaral dehyde, Hypochlorite, H_2O_2
  - o-Phthalic acid, peracetic acid
  - Autoclave
  - Hot air oven.

8. Ans. (b) 121°C for 15 min.

[*Ref.:* Ananthnarayan, 8th ed., page no. 34]

Refer to previous explanation.

9. Ans. (b) Autoclave

[*Ref.:* Park, 21st ed., page no. 734-35; 20th ed., 696-699]

- ❖ ***Sharp instruments (e.g., needles, syringes, scalpels blades) should be treated by Autoclaving/ Micro waving/Chemical treatment and Destruction/Shredding.***

10. Ans. (b) Formaldehyde fumigation

[*Ref.:* Ananthnarayan, 8th ed. page no. 36]

Fumigation of Hospital Ward and Operation Theatre is done by:

- ❖ Formalin (40% **Formaldehyde)**
- ❖ Non-inionizing radiation like UV and infra red rays
- ❖ Betapropiolactone.

Formalin (40% Formaldehyde) is used:

- ❖ For preserving fresh tissue specimens
- ❖ For destroying anthrax spores in hair and wool
- ❖ To prepare toxoids from toxins
- ❖ Fumigation of hospital ward and operation theater.

11. Ans. (c) Hot air oven

[*Ref.:* Ananthnarayan, 8th ed., page no. 32]

"All glass items like glass syringes, glass flask, glass slides etc. are best sterilized by hot air oven".

✍ **Remember**

- ❖ Glass syringes are best sterilized by hot air oven.
- ❖ Disposable syringes are best sterilized by ionizing radiation.

Hot air oven

- ❖ Temp. maintained: 160°C for 1 hr
- ❖ Materials sterilized by Hot air oven
  - All Glass ware
  - Liquid paraffin
  - Grease
  - Fat
  - Glycerol
  - Dust powder
- ❖ Sterilization Control of Hot air oven – Spores of *Clostridium tetani* (non toxigenic strain).

12. Ans. (b) Inionizing radiation

[*Ref.:* Ananthnarayan, 8th ed., page no. 35]

- ❖ ***Ionizing radiations***
  - Ionizing radiations is an excellent sterilizing agent with very high penetrating power.
  - It acts by breaking the DNA of the organism.
  - Since there is no detectable increase of temperature, this method is called as ***'cold sterilization"***.

- Examples of ionizing radiations include X-rays, gamma rays and cosmic rays.
- Used for sterilization of heat labile substances like disposable syringes.

13. Ans. (b) Anatomical waste

[*Ref.:* Park, 21st ed., page no. 734-35; 20th ed., page no. 696-699]

Incineration is a process in which combustible materials are converted into non-combustible residue or ash. Incineration has traditionally been the principal method used by hospitals, medical colleges and other healthcare facilities providers to process their anatomical and non-anatomical biomedical wastes.

Incineration/deep burial is done for disposal of:

- ❖ Waste Category 1 – Human anatomical waste
- ❖ Waste Category 2 – Animal waste
- ❖ Waste Category 3 – Microbiology and biotechnology waste
- ❖ Waste Category 6 – Solid waste (*items contaminated with blood and body fluids).*

Option	Waste Category
Category No. 1	Human anatomical waste
Category No. 2	Animal waste
Category No. 3	Microbiology and biotechnology waste (wastes from laboratory cultures)
Category No. 4	Waste sharps (needles, syringes, scalpels blades, glass etc)
Category No. 5	Discarded medicines and cytotoxic drugs
Category No. 6	Solid waste (items contaminated with blood and body fluids including cotton, dressings)
Category No. 7	Solid waste (waste generated from disposable items other than *Category No. 5, 6)*
Category No. 8	Liquid waste
Category No. 9	Incineration ash (ash from incineration of any bio-medical waste).
Category No. 10	Chemical waste

Colour Coding	Waste Category	Treatment Options
Yellow	1, 2, 3, 6	Incineration/deep burial
Red	3, 6, 7	Autoclaving/Micro waving/Chemical Treatment
Blue/ White	4, 7	Autoclaving/Micro waving/Chemical treatment and Destruction/Shredding
Black	5, 9, 10 (Solid)	Disposal in secured landfill

14. Ans. (c) *Bacillus stereothermophilus*

[*Ref.:* Ananthnarayan, 8th ed., page no. 34]

- ❖ **Bacillus stereothermophilus spores are used as the indiactors of moist heat sterilization in the autoclave.**

GENERAL MICROBIOLOGY

- ❖ The efficacy of the autoclave is carried out by placing paper strips impregnated with air dried 10^6 spores of thermophilic *Bacillus stereothermophilus* in envelope and keeping those envelopes inside the autoclave.
- ❖ The strips, after sterilization are inoculated into a suitble recovering medium. Spores are destryoed if sterilizing condition of the autoclave is proper.

Biological Indicator (Sterilization Control) for determining efficacy of

- ❖ Autoclave – *Bacillus stereothermophilus.*
- ❖ Hot air oven – *Clostridium tetani* (non-toxigenic strain).

Other Indicators for determining efficacy of Sterilization by autoclave –

- ❖ Thermocouples (Brown's tube).
- ❖ Chemical indicators.
- ❖ Autoclave tapes.

15. Ans. (d) Cidex solution

[*Ref.:* Ananthnarayan, 8th ed., page no. 36]

- ❖ **Glutaraldehyde 2% (Cidex):**
  - An effective disinfectant used for cleaning cystoscopes and bronchoscopes.
  - It is less irritating and corrosive than formaldehyde but equally affective against tubercle bacilli, fungi and viruses and spores.
  - It has no deleterious effect on lenses of instruments like cystoscopes and bronchoscopes. So, it can be used safely for cleaning cystoscopes and bronchoscopes, corrugated rubber anaesthetic tubes and face masks, plastic endotracheal tubes, metal instruments and polythene tubing.
  - Other methods to sterilize Endoscopes – Orthophthaldehyde.

16. Ans. (a) Coxiella burnetii

[*Ref.:* Ananthnarayan, 8th ed., page no. 32]

- ❖ **"Coxiella burnetii is relatively heat resistant and it survives holder method of Pasteurization".** *–Ananthnarayan*
- ❖ **Pasteurization** (named after Louis Pasteur) is a method is extensively used for sterilization of milk and other liquid beverages (while at the same time retaining the liquid's flavor and food value).
- ❖ Two methods of pasteurizations are followed:
  - In the flash method, the milk is exposed to heat at 72ºC for 15-20 seconds followed by sudden cooling it to at 13ºC or lower.
  - In the holder method, the milk is exposed to a temperature of 63ºC for 30 minutes.
- ❖ The flash method is preferable for sterilization of milk compared to holder method because it is less likely to change flavor and nutrient content, and it is more effective against certain resistant pathogens such as *Coxiella* and *Mycobacterium.*

17. Ans. (a) Blue bag

[*Ref.:* Park, 21st ed., 734-35; 20th ed., 696-699]

- ❖ Sharp instruments (e.g., needles, syringes, scalpels blades) belongs to Waste Category No. 4.
- ❖ They should be disposed in Blue/White plastic bags.
- ❖ Sharp instruments should be treated by Autoclaving/Micro waving/Chemical treatment and Destruction/Shredding.

Culture Media

18. Ans. (b) Enriched media

[*Ref.:* Ananthnarayan, 8th ed., page no. 40]

"Blood agar is an enriched medium in which nutritionally rich whole blood supplements the basic nutrients".

–Ananthnarayan

- **Enriched media** are prepared by adding substances like blood, serum and egg to the basal media in order to meet the nutritional requirements of more exacting and more fastidious bacteria.
- **Examples include:**
  - Blood agar
  - Chocolate agar
  - Loeffler's serum slope
  - Brain heart infusion agar
  - Egg based media like – Dorset's egg media.

19. Ans. (b > c) Robertson's cooked meat medium > Thioglycollate medium

[*Ref.:* Ananthnarayan, 8th ed., page no. 47)

The commonly used media foı anaerobic culture are:

- Robertson cooked meat (RCM) broth
- Thioglycollate broth
- Neomycin blood agar
- Egg Yolk agar.

Robertson cooked meat (RCM) broth is the recommended media for anaerobic culture.

- It primarily contains fat-free minced and cooked meat of ox heart in the nutrient broth.
- The unsaturated fatty acids, glutathione and cysteine present in meat utilize oxygen for auto oxidation, which is catalyzed by haematin present in the meat.
- The sulphydril compounds present in the cysteine also contributes to a reduced oxidation-reduction (OR) potential in the medium.
- Sacharolytic anaerobe like *Clostridium perfringens* changes the color meat pieces into red while the proteolytic anaerobe like *Clostridium tetani* changes black color.

20. Ans. (d) All of the above

[*Ref.:* Ananthnarayan, 8th ed., page no. 40]

- Enrichment media are the liquid media that stimulate the growth of wanted (pathogenic) bacteria and suppress the growth of other commensals present in the sample.
- These medium are useful for isolation of wanted bacteria from specimens containing more than one bacterial, such as stool and sputum.
- **Examples of Enrichment Media:**
  - Selenite F broth (used for the isolation of Salmonella typhi and *Shigella)*
  - Tetrathionate broth (used for the isolation of Salmonella typhi and *Shigella)*
  - Alkaline peptone water (for Vibrio)
  - Monsour's taurocholate tellurite peptone water (for Vibrio).

PRACTICE MCQ's

Morphology of Bacteria

1. **Generation time for *M.Tuberculosis* is:**
   (a) 20 seconds (b) 20 minutes
   (c) 20 hours (d) 20 days.
2. **Anthrax bacillus is a:**
   (a) Obligate aerobe (b) Facultative aerobe
   (c) Facultative aerobe (d) Microaerophilic bacterium.
3. **All the following statements are true for bacterial DNA except:**
   (a) No nuclear membrane (b) It does not have any nucleolus
   (c) It replicates by binary fission (d) It is diploid.
4. **Bacillus stearothermophilus is a:**
   (a) Psychrophilic bacteria (b) Mesophilic bacteria
   (c) Capnophilic bacteria (d) Thermophilic bacteria.

Sterilization and Disinfection

5. **All the following statements are true for sterilization by ultraviolet (UV) radiations except:**
   (a) It acts by denaturation of bacterial protein (b) Useful for fumigation of wards
   (c) Temperature is not raised (d) Example of non-ionizing radiation.
6. **Autoclave is not useful for sterilization of:**
   (a) Plastic petri dishes (b) Surgical dressings
   (c) Culture media (d) Liquid paraffin.
7. **The test that shows the effectiveness of a disinfectant in the presence of an organic material is:**
   (a) Chick Martin test (b) Kelsey-Sykes test
   (c) Rideal Walker test (d) Phenolic coefficient test.

Culture Media

8. **The agar is used in the media primarily to:**
   (a) Selectively enhances the growth (b) Make the medium solid
   (c) Source of electrolytes (d) Source of nutrition.
9. **Selenite F broth is an example of:**
   (a) Transport medium (b) Enriched medium
   (c) Enrichment medium (d) Selective medium.
10. **Nutrient broth consists of all the following ingredients except:**
    (a) Peptone (b) Meat extract
    (c) Sodium chloride (d) Agar.
11. **All the following media are examples of selective media except:**
    (a) CLED agar (b) Wilson Blair medium

(c) Mannitol salt agar (d) TCBS medium.

12. The most useful method for obtaining discrete colonies of the bacteria is by:

(a) Lawn culture (b) Stab culture

(c) Pour plate culture (d) Streak culture.

13. The most useful method for obtaining a uniform confluent layer of bacterial growth on a solid medium is:

(a) Lawn culture (b) Stab culture

(c) Pour plate culture (d) Streak culture.

14. The most useful method to determine appropriate number of viable organisms in liquid is by:

(a) Stab culture (b) Lawn culture

(c) Pour plate culture (d) Streak culture.

15. Smith Noguchi's media is used for:

(a) Salmonella (b) Klebsiella

(c) Spirochetes (d) Bacillus.

16. The specimen not suitable for anaerobic culture is:

(a) Sputum (b) Blood

(c) Cerebrospinal fluid (d) Direct lung aspirate.

17. All the following media are used for anaerobic culture except:

(a) Egg yolk agar (b) Robertson cooked meat broth

(c) Mannitol salt agar (d) Neomycin blood agar.

ANSWERS TO PRACTICE MCQ's

Morphology of Bacteria

1. Ans. (c) 20 hours

[*Ref.:* Ananthnarayan, 8th ed., page no. 23]

❖ Refer text.

2. Ans. (a) Obligate aerobe

[*Ref.:* Ananthnarayan, 8th ed., page no. 25]

❖ Examples of Obligate aerobe (strict aerobe that die in presence of O_2) include – Bacillus, M. tuberculosis, Pseudomonas brucella and Nocardia.

3. Ans. (d) It is diploid

[*Ref.:* Ananthnarayan, 8th ed., page no. 18]

❖ Bacterial DNA is haploid in nature.

4. Ans. (d) Thermophilic bacteria

[*Ref.:* Ananthnarayan, 8th ed., page no. 26]

❖ **Thermophilic bacteria** grow at a high temperature range of 55°C – 80°C.

❖ **Example:** *Bacillus stearothermophilus.*

Sterilization and Disinfection

5. Ans. (c) Temperature is not raised

[*Ref.:* Ananthnarayan, 8th ed., page no. 35]

- Examples of non-ionizing radiations include infra red and ultraviolet radiations.
- Ultraviolet (UV) radiation acts by denaturation of bacterial protein.
- Temperature is raised hence known as "*Hot air sterilization*".
- Low penetrating power (does not penetrate glass, dirt films, water).
- It is used primarily for disinfection of closed areas in microbiology laboratory, inoculation hoods, laminar flow and operating theatres.

6. Ans. (d) Liquid paraffin

[*Ref.:* Ananthnarayan, 8th ed., page no. 32]

- *Hot air oven is the recommended method of sterilization of liquid paraffin.*
- *Glass petri dishes are sterilized by hot air oven whereas heat resistant plastic petri dishes are sterilized by autoclave.*

7. Ans. (a) Chick Martin test

[*Ref.:* Ananthnarayan, 8th ed., page no. 38]

"Chick Martin test is a modification of Rideal and Walker test, in which, disinfectants acts in the presence of organic contaminants (e.g., dried yeast, faeces, etc.) to simulate the natural conditions."

Culture Media

8. Ans. (b) Make the medium solid

[*Ref.:* Ananthnarayan, 8th ed., page no. 39]

- Agar is a solidifying agent that makes the medium solid.
- It has no nutritive power.

9. Ans. (c) Enrichment medium

[*Ref.:* Ananthnarayan, 8th ed., page no. 40]

- Refer text.

10. Ans. (d) Agar

[*Ref.:* Ananthnarayan, 8th ed., page no. 40]

- **Simple/Basal media:**
  - Peptone water – Peptone + NaCl
  - ***Nutrient broth – Peptone + NaCl + meat extract***
  - Nutrient agar – Nutrient broth + 2% agar.

11. Ans. (a) CLED agar

[*Ref.:* Ananthnarayan, 8th ed., page no. 40]

- CLED agar is a differential medium.

12. Ans. (d) Streak culture

[*Ref.*: Ananthnarayan, 8th ed., page no. 44]

Streak culture is the most useful method for obtaining discrete colonies and pure cultures. It is done on the surface of a dry agar plate using bacteriological loop and heating the loop in between the streaking.

13. Ans. (a) Lawn culture

[*Ref.*: Ananthnarayan, 8th ed., page no. 44]

- ***Lawn culture*** provides a uniform surface of growth of the bacterium on the solid medium.
- It is prepared by flooding the surface of the plate with a liquid culture and pipetting off the excess inoculum or inoculating the culture plate by a sterile swab soaked in liquid bacterial culture.
- It is used for antibiotic susceptibility testing by disc diffusion method and for bacteriophage typing.

14. Ans. (c) Pour plate culture

[*Ref.*: Ananthnarayan, 8th ed., page no. 45]

- ***Pour plate culture*** is used to determine the appropriate number of viable organisms in liquid such as water or urine. It is used to quantitate bacteria in urine cultures and also to estimate viable bacterial count in a suspension.

15. Ans. (c) Spirochetes

[*Ref.*: Ananthnarayan, 8th ed., page no. 47]

- *Smith Noguchi's media is anaerobic media used for culture of non-pathogenic Treponema like Reitter's Treponema.*

16. Ans. (a) Sputum

[*Ref.*: Ananthnarayan, 8th ed., page no. 47]

- *Direct lung aspirate* is the sample of choice for anaerobic *culture. Sputum sample is not recommended because of risk of exposure to oxygen.*
- Other specimens that are not suitable for anaerobic cultures like rectal swab, nasal or throat swab, urethral swab wound swab and voided urine.

17. Ans. (c) Mannitol salt agar

[*Ref.*: Ananthnarayan, 8th ed., page no. 198]

- Mannitol salt agar is seletive medium for Staphylococcus aureus.
- **The commonly used media for anaerobic culture are:**
  - Robertson cooked meat (RCM) broth.
  - Thioglycolate broth.
  - Willis and Hobb's media.
  - Neomycin blood agar.
  - Egg Yolk agar.

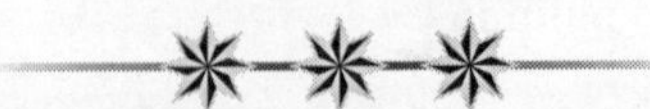

GENERAL MICROBIOLOGY

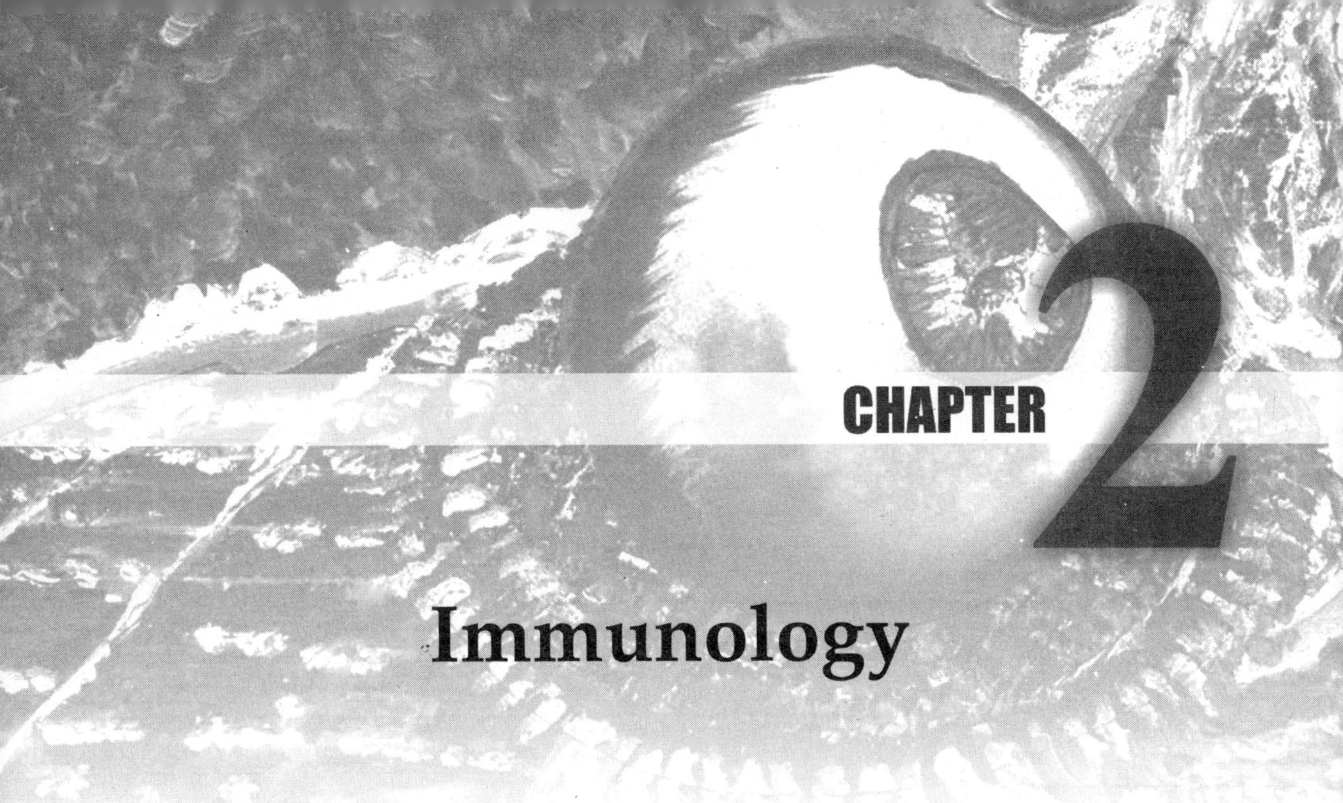

Immunology

IMMUNITY

Refers to resistance exhibited by host towards to injury caused by microorganism or its products.

Type: Innate Immunity and Acquired/Adaptive Immunity

Innate immunity	Acquired/Adaptive immunity
➢ Resistance to infection that an individual possess from birth by its genetic or constitutional makeup. ➢ Which can be: – Species specific – Racial specific – Individual specific	➢ Resistance to infection that an individual acquires during his life. ➢ Which can be: – Active or passive – Artificial or natural
➢ Occurs in minute	➢ Occurs in days
➢ Diversity limited	➢ Active against wide range of infection
➢ Non-specific	➢ Specific
➢ No memory	➢ Memory present
Components of Innate Immunity ➢ Phagocyte (monocyte, macrophage, neutrophils) ➢ Dendritic cell ➢ Natural killer cell ➢ Alternate complement pathway	**Components of Acquired Immunity** ➢ T cell ➢ B cell ➢ Classical complement pathway ➢ Antigen presenting cell

Innace Immunity	Acquired/Adaptive Immunity
➢ Acute phase protein (CRP, MBP, serum amyloid protein) ➢ Normal resident flora antagonism ➢ Inflammation, fever ➢ Skin and mucosal barrier	

Active Immunity	Passive Immunity
Produced actively by host immune system	Received passively
Induced by infection or immunogen	Induced by readymade antibody transferred
Long lasting	Short
Lag period present	No lag period
Memory present	No memory
Booster doses – useful	Subsequent doses – less affective
Negative phase may occur	No negative phase
In Immunodeficiency – not useful	Useful

Local Immunity

- ❖ Produced at mucosal surfaces – GIT or respiratory mucosa.
- ❖ Provided by IgA antibody.
- ❖ Induced by infection or by live vaccination.

Herd Immunity

- ❖ Overall immunity of a community to a pathogen.
- ❖ If Herd immunity is good – chance of epidemic is less.
- ❖ Eradication of a communicable disease – depends on good Herd immunity.
- ❖ Provided by mass vaccination by live vaccination to all individual at same time.

ANTIGEN

- ❖ ***Antigen*** **–** has two properties:
  - Immunogenicity – capacity to induce antibody.
  - Immunological reactivity (Antigenicity) – capacity to react with an antibody.
- ❖ ***Hapten***
  - Does not have immunogenicity but retain immunological reactivity, i.e., antigenic.
  - Hapten becomes immunogenic by combing with carrier molecule.
  - Simple hapten – Univalent, non-precipitating with its antibody, only blocks the site on antibody.
  - Complex hapten – Polyvalent, precipitating with its antibody.
- ❖ ***Epitope*** – Antigenic determinant that combines with antibody

IMMUNOLOGY

Antigenicity depends on:

- Size – Larger size, more antigenic.
- Chemical – decreasing order of Antigenicity – Protein > carbohydrate > lipid and nucleic acid.
- Susceptibility to tissue enzyme.
- Foreignness – More the foreignness of the antigen, more is the antigenicity.
- Route of entry.
- Genetic constituent.
- Specificity.

Heterophile specificity – Antigens of different species cross react with each other.

- ***Paul Bunnel*** – EBV with sheep RBC.
- ***Weil Felix*** – Proteus OX2, OX19, OX K with Rickettsia alkali stable polysaccharide.
- ***Cold Agglutination test*** – Mycoplasma with human O +ve RBC at 4°c.
- ***Streptococcus MG*** with Mycoplasma.
- ***Forssman antigen*** – Lipid – CHO complex, present all except rabbit. So anti-Forssman antibody can be prepared in rabbit.
- ***Non-treponemal test*** for syphilis like VDRL, RPR (Flocculation test).
  - Treponemal antibody detected by using Cardiolipin antigen prepared from beef heart.
- ***Autoimmune*** consequences:
  - Acute rheumatic fever and glomerulonephritis (Streptococcal antigens and human tissue).

Antibody

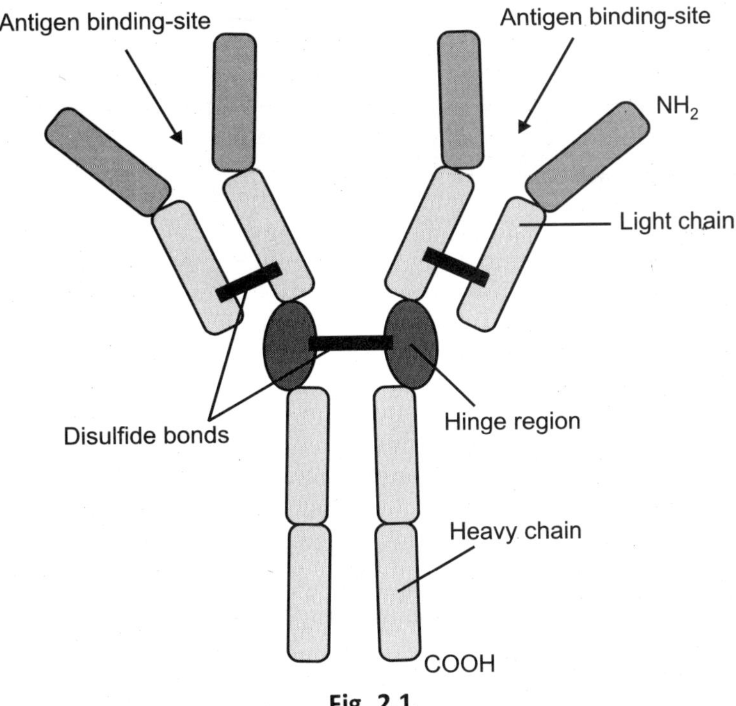

Fig. 2.1.

- Immunoglobulin is Y shaped, consisting of 2 heavy and 2 light chain.

- Papain digestion of Immunoglobulin produces:
  - 2 Fab portion – antigen binding site.
  - 1 Fc portion – perform biological function like complement attachment site, adherence to monocyte.
- Heavy chain:
  - Five types: α, γ, α, E, δ.
  - One of these five chains present in an immunoglobulin (Isospecificity).
- Light chain:
  - Two types – kappa and lambda.
  - One of these two chains present in an immunoglobulin.
- Hinge region – rich in cysteine, praline.

IgG Antibody

- *Possess highest* ***DHS***
  - **D**aily production
  - **H**alf life (23d)
  - **S**erum concentration (decreasing order – *GAMDE*), i.e., highest is IgG and lowest is IgE.
- *Types:* IgG1 > 2 > 3> 4 (Decreasing order of the serum concentration)
- Responsible for:
  - Precipitation
  - Neutralization
  - NK cell (ADCC)
  - Classical complement pathway ***(IgG3 highest).***
- Appear late, indicates past/chronic infection.
- IgG avidity increases with time. So, detection of less avidity IgG indicates relatively recent infection.
- Secreted in placenta, breast milk ***(Except IgG2).***

IgE Antibody

- Heat labile
- Lowest *DHS*
- Responsible for: Type I Hypersensitivity reaction
- Homocytotropic
- Reagin antibody.

IgA Antibody

- Second most abundant.
- *Types:*
  - IgA2 – Surface/mucosal IgA – Dimer joined by J chain and secretory piece (from epithelium)
  - IgA1 – Serum IgA – monomer, minor.
- Responsible for:
  - Alternate compliment binding
  - Mucosal/local immunity.

IgD Antibody

- Surface Immunoglobulin.
- Possess highest carbohydrate content.

IgM Antibody

- *Possess highest **MIS**:*
  - **M**olecular weight (900,000)
  - **I**ntravascular distribution (blood antibody) (80%)
  - **S**edimentation coefficient (19).
- Pentameric with 10 valency.
- 1st to appear following infection, indicates recent infection.
- 1st to appear in intrauterine life also (20 wk).
- *Responsible for* (or Mediates):
  - Agglutination
  - Haemolysis
  - Opsonization
  - Classical complement pathway.
- *Example:*
  - O antibody in typhoid
  - Antibody of ABO, Rh system.

Abnormal Immunoglobulin

- Bence Jones Protein
  - Coagulate at 5°C, redissolve at 7°C
  - Elevated in multiple myeloma
  - Due to unchecked proliferation of single clone of plasma chain
  - Made up ***light chain*** of immunoglobulin, i.e., Kappa or lambda (but never both in same patient)

Notes:

- **Epitope:** Antigenic determinant that combines with antibody.
- **Paratope:** Part of antibody (present in variable region) that combines with epitope of antigen.
- **Idiotope:** Based on antigenic determinant present on paratope known as idiotopes.

ANTIGEN ANTIBODY REACTION

Precipitation

- **Definition:** (Soluble Antigen + Antibody) at suitable temperature and pH → leads to formation of insoluble precipitate/floccules.

IMMUNOLOGY

Example of Precipitation Reaction

Ring Test

- Ascoli thermo precipitation test (anthrax).
- Lancefield grouping (*Streptococcus*).

Slide flocculation test: VDRL, RPR.

Tube flocculation test: Kahn test, standardization of toxin.

Immuno-diffusion (in gel):

- Produces visible band, so interpretation is easy.
- Can be preserved.
- Differentiate between antigens.

Example:

- Elek gel precipitation (*C diphtheriae* toxigenicity testing),
- Eiken test.

CIEP – αFetoProtein, Antigen of Cryptococcus and Meningococcus.

Agglutination

- **Definition:** (Insoluble or particulate Antigen + Antibody) – at suitable temperature and pH leads to clumps formation.

Example

Example of Agglutination Reaction

- Widal test – Enteric fever.
- Standard agglutination test – Brucella.
- Microscopic agglutination test – Leptospira.
- Cold agglutination test – Mycoplasma.
- Weil felix – Rickettsia.
- Paul Bunuel – EBV.
- Coomb test for incomplete (IgG) Antibody.
- Passive agglutination test (PHA):
    - Soluble antigen is coated on carrier particle like RBC, latex.
    - So that a precipitation reaction can be converted to an agglutination reaction and hence better visualized.

      Example: TPHA (syphilis), Rose Waaler test (Rheumatoid arthritis).
- *RPHA* (Reverse Passive Hemagglutination test):
    - Antibody is coated on a surface of carrier particle like RBC to detect antigens.

      Example: HBsAg.

Complement Fixation Test (CFT):

- Syphilis – Wasserman test
- CFT for viral diseases

- **Other complement dependent reaction**
  - Sabin Feldman test – Toxoplasma
  - T. pallidum immobilization test (TPI) – for Syphilis.

STRUCTURE AND FUNCTION OF IMMUNE SYSTEM

Lymphoid System – Lymphoid Organ + Lymphoid Cells

Lymphoid Organ:

- *Central/Primary:*
  - Thymus
  - Bursa of Fibricus (birds)/Bone Marrow (human).
- *Peripheral/Secondary:*
  - Spleen
  - Lymph node
  - MALT (GIT and Respiratory mucosa).

Lymphoid Cells:

- T Cell
- B Cells
- NK Cell.

Thymus:

- Developed from 3rd/4th pharyngeal pouch.
- *Divided to:*
  - Cortex – contains T lymphocytes, nurse cell.
  - Medulla – contains epithelial cells, lymphocytes, Hassal's corpuscle.
- Progenitor T cells passed through thymus during embryonic life.
- 1% of them released out, rest destroyed (self reacting T cells).
- Released T cells are educated – Acquire Thymic Ag – becomes T dependent T cells.
- *Defect in thymus*
  - Leads to low CMI.
  - Runt disease – affecting nude mice.
  - DiGeorge syndrome.

Bursa of Fabricus and Bone Marrow

- Bursa of fabricus – Birds.
- Bone marrow – humans.
- All lymphocytes originates in BM.
- T cell goes to thymus.
- B cell proliferates in BM.

Lymphocytes:

- Short lived lymphocyte – life span 2 week, Effector cells.
- Long lived lymphocyte – life span 2-3 years, memory cells.

- *Markers:*
  - CD 10, 19, 22, 23 – B cell markers.
  - CD 1, 2, 3, 4, 7, 8 – T cell markers.

T Lymphocyte:

- ***T cell Blast transformation occurs by:***
  - Anti CD3
  - Phytohemagglutinin
  - Concanavalin A.
- ***T cell development:***
- Starts from Yolk sac → Fetal liver → Bone marrow → Thymus.

Development of T Cell in Thymus:

- CD7 +ve Pre T cell enter thymus.
- Pro T cell converts to Pre T cell (CD2 and CD3 +ve).
- Pre T cell converts to Immature T cell – (CD1, 4, 8 and T cell receptor +ve).
- Self-reacting T cells are deleted.
- Mature T cells – (loose CD1) – CD4 T cells and CD8 T cells.
- *T cell receptor:*
  - TCR – made up α β or γδ.
  - TCR α β – most common (95%).
  - TCR γδ – present on intra epithelial lymphocyte and intracellular organism like MTB.

CD4 T Helper Cells:

- Recognizes antigens presented with MHC II molecule.
- 60% of total lymphocytes
  - TH1 cell – secrete IL2 and IFN γ
    - IFN γ– Activate macrophage, class switch over of B cell (IgG2b)
    - IL2 – T cell growth factor, DTH T cell, NK cell → LAK cell
    - TGF β
  - TH2 cell – secrete IL4, 5, 6, 10.
    - IL4 – Inhibit TH1, Chemo attractant, class switch to IgE, IgG.
    - IL5 – class switch IgA, Chemo attractant to Eosinophils.

CD 8 Expressing Cells:

- Recognizes antigens presented with MHC I molecule.
- 30% of total lymphocytes:
  - T cytotoxic cells (Tc cells) – causes Cytotoxic lysis of target cells.
  - T supressor cells (Ts cells) – suppresses immune response.

B Lymphocytes:

- B cell Blast transformation occurs by:
  - Endotoxin

- Anti Ig
- EBV
- Super antigen

❖ B cell accounts for 10-20% of total lymphocyte

❖ B cell also act as APC – mediated by surface IgM receptors

❖ CD40 of B cell attach to CD40L of T cell – leads to B cell maturation

❖ B cell possess:
- Fc Receptor
- CD21 – EBV receptor.
- CD2 – measles receptor.
- Microvilli present on B cell surface.

Macrophages:

❖ Derived from the bone marrow.

❖ *Has role in:*
- Phagocytosis
- Secretion of cytokines
- Antigen presentation

❖ *Example:*
- Peripheral blood – *Monocytes*
- Liver – *Kupffer cells*
- Brain – *Microglia*
- Kidney – *Mesangial cells*
- Bone – *Osteoclasts*
- Lung – *Alveolar macrophage*
- Any solid tissue – *Histiocytes*
- Inflammation site – *Multinucleated cell and epitheloid cell*

❖ *Kill cell by:*
- Phagocytosis and phagolysozome fusion and lysosomal degranulation
- Also by generating oxygen free radical.

Dendritic Cell

❖ Act as APC during primary immune response

❖ Bone marrow derived (separate lineage)

❖ Transport the presented antigen to lymph node

❖ Possess MHC II>MHC I, also possess B7

❖ Non-phagocytic in nature

❖ *Types:*
- Interdigitating
- Interstitial
- Langerhans

- *Follicular:*
  - Special type of dendritic cell.
  - Does not possess any MHC II.
  - Act on memory B cell.

NK Cell

- Natural killer cell/null cell/large granular (LGL)/lymphokine activated cell.
- NK cell → to LAK (Lymphokine activated killer cell) transformation is induced by IL2.
- Constitutes 5-10% of total lymphocyte.
- Possess indented nuclei and several granules.
- NK cells are not MHC restricted.
- Possess CD16 and CD56 markers.
- Used in treatment of – renal cell Ca.
- Mediates **ADCC** – Antibody dependent cytotoxicity
  - CD16 (FcR like) recognized Fc portion of antibody bound to a target cell.
  - Then, NK cell release perforin and granazyme which lyses the target cells.
- Responsible for cytotoxicity to virus infected cell and malignant cells, parasitic infection.

HLA/MHC

- Transplantation antigen – determining histocompatibility.
- HLA I, II, III.
- Play a central role in antigen recognition.
- MHC – located in short arm of chromosome 6 in humans.
- ***Class I MHC genes*** – Glycoprotein – all nucleated cells
  - Present peptide antigen to Tc cells (CD8 T cells).
  - Processing of virus infected cells and tumour cells.
- ***Class II MHC genes*** – Glycoprotein on all antigen presenting cells
  - Present peptide antigen to Th cells (CD4 T cells)
  - Regulates immune response
  - Plays a central role in initiation of the immune response to transplantation antigens.
- ***Class III MHC genes*** **–** Genes coding C2,C4, properdin, factor B, C3 convertase, TNF, HSP
- **Class I MHC**
  - Present in all nucleated cells.
  - Present the Ag to the CD8 cytotoxic T cells.
  - *Function* – Graft rejection, Cell mediated cytolysis, Hormone receptor.
  - Heavy α chain – 3 globular domain.
  - α_1-α_2 Groove – Ag peptide binding groove.
  - α_3 – CD8 Binding groove.
  - β_2 microglobulin.

IMMUNOLOGY

- **Class II MHC**
  - Present in APC (macrophage).
  - Present the Ag to the CD4 T helper cells.
  - Heterodimer.
  - α chain – globular domain – α_1, α_2.
  - β chain – β_1, β_2.
  - α_1 – β_1 Groove: Ag peptide binding groove.
  - β_2 – CD4 Binding groove.

IMMUNE RESPONSE

CD4 T Cell Mediated CMI

Microbe → captured by APC → broken down to peptides → combined with MHC II → → Presented to T cell with CD4

↓

1st signal – Antigen-MHC complex on APC to CD4 (CD3 also help) on Th cell

2nd signal – B7 (on APC) to CD28 (on T cell) ……. (can be blocked by CTLA4)

↓

CD4 T cell activated – differentiated to TH1 or TH2

↓

TH1 – secrete IL2 and IFNg

- IFN γ – Activate macrophage, stimulate B cell and class switch to IgG2b
- IL2 – T cell growth factor, activate DTH T cell, convert NK cell → LAK cell

TH2 – secrete IL4, 5, 6, 10

- IL4 – Inhibit TH1, class switch to **IgE, IgG**
- IL5 – class switch to **IgA.**

CD8 T Cell Mediated CMI

- Provides immunity against viral and tumor cell antigen
- These antigens are processed by virus infected cell or tumor cells and presented to their surface along with MHCI

↓

Presented to CD8 Tc cell

CD8 Tc cell activated and secrete granazyme and perforin

Forms pores and lyses the target cells

B Cell Mediated Humoral Immunity

- B cell also can act as APC for the 2nd antigenic challenge
- Memory B cell possess IgM surface receptors
  - 1st signal – MHC II peptide to CD4 of T cell
  - 2nd signal – B7/CD28
  - 3rd signal – CD40 of B cell/CD40L of T cell
- Stimulation of T cell leads to cytokine productions.
- Then, class switch over occurs – various class of immunoglobulins produced.
- *Function:*
  - Mediates Phagocytosis (Fc part) by opsonization.
  - Mediates ADCC (antibody dependent cell mediated cytotoxicity).
  - Mediates Complement mediated cytolysis.

Adjuvant

- Enhance immunogenicity of antigen.
- *Example:*
  - Freund's incomplete antigen – antigen coated to water phase of water in oil emulsion– leads to slow release of antigen, hence enhances immunogenicity.
  - Freund's complete Ag – Adding MTB Muramyl dipeptide antigen.
  - Aluminium hydroxide or phosphate.
  - LPS of B. pertussis.
  - Corynebacterium granulosum.

IMMUNOLOGY

HYPERSENSITIVITY REACTION

- **Hypersensitivity is defined as injurious consequences in the sensitized host, following contact with specific antigen.**

Character	Immediate	Delayed
Type	I, II, III	IV
Time	Minutes to hours	Days
Mediator	Antibodies	T cells
Route	Any route	Intradermal
Passive transfer	With serum	With transfer factor
Desensitization	Easy, but short lived	Difficult but long lasting

Type I Hypersensitivity Reaction – Mechanism

Sensitization phase – Priming dose of antigen (allergen) → processed by APC → antigenic peptide presented to T cell → Th 2 → secretes IL4 → Acts on B cell → IgE produced → Mast cell coated with Ig E (Fc)

Effector phase – Shocking dose → IgE (Fab) binds to Antigen → Mast cell degranulation

Mediators of type I Hypersensitivity Reaction:

- ❖ ***Primary Mediator***
  - Histamine
  - Eosinophils
  - Serotonin
  - Neutrophil chemotactic factor.
- ❖ ***Secondary Mediators***
  - Prostaglandin
  - Cytokines.

Example of Type I Hypersensitivity Reaction:

- ❖ Atopy
  - Asthma
  - Food allergy
  - Allerigic rhinitis (Hay fever)
  - Atopic eczema.
- ❖ Anaphylaxis.
- ❖ Theobald Smith phenomena.
- ❖ Schultz Dale phenomena.
- ❖ Prausnitz Kustner reaction.
- ❖ Casoni test.
- ❖ Wheal and flare reaction.

Type II Hypersensitivity Reaction

- ❖ **Compliment dependent cytolysis:**
  - Transfusion reaction
  - Auto immune hemolytic anemia
  - Erythroblastosis fetalis
  - Pernicious anemia.
- ❖ **Compliment dependent inflammation (C3a, C5a):**
  - Good Pasteur syndrome
  - Bullous pemphigus
  - Vasculitis.
  - Pemphigus vulgaris
  - Rheumatic fever
- ❖ **Compliment dependent phagocytosis**
- ❖ **ADCC – (Type VI)**
  - By NK cell
  - Useful for parasite removal, graft rejection.
- ❖ **Antibody dependent cellular dysfunction – (Type V)**
  - Stimulation – Grave's disease (LATS).
  - Inhibition – Myasthenia gravis (Anti Acetyl choline receptor Antibody).

Type III Hypersensitivity Reaction

- ❖ Immune complex mediated HSN reaction.
- ❖ Immune complex gets deposited in tissue.
- ❖ Usually complement gets bound to complex – so serum level of complement falls.
- ❖ Neutrophils are attracted and release enzymes.

- Two forms
  - Arthus reaction – local reaction
  - Serum sickness – systemic.

Example of Type III Hypersensitivity Reaction

- Hypersensitivity Pneumonitis (farmer's lung)
- Post streptococcal glomerulonephritis
- Subacute bacterial endocarditis
- Microbial antigen
  - *Streptococcus pyogenes*
  - *M. leprae*
  - *Treponema*
  - *Plasmodium*
  - *Trypanosoma*
  - HBV, HCV, EBV, Dengue.
- Connective tissue disorder – SLE, Rheumatoid Arthritis, PAN.
- Hyperacute graft rejection.
- Lepra reaction type 2.
- Henoch Schonlein purpura.

Type IV Hypersensitivity Reaction

- Delayed type of HSN.
- Mediated by CD4 Th1 cell.
- Cytokines involved – IL2.
- **Example:**
  - Tuberculin test
  - Lepra reaction I
  - Contact dermatitis
  - Frie test – for LGV
  - Montenegro test – for Leishmania.

FMGE MCQ's

Immunity

1. **Components of innate immunity that are active against viral cells include:** [*March 2009*]
   (a) Cytotoxic T cells (b) B cell
   (c) NK cells (d) All of the above.
2. **Herd Immunity is a feature of all of the following diseases except:** [*September 2008*]
   (a) Diphtheria (b) Polio
   (c) Tetanus (d) Measles.

3. Immunoglobulin is used for all of the following diseases except: [*March 2008*]

(a) Measles (b) Rabies

(c) Typhoid (d) Chicken pox.

4. Injectable tetanus toxoid is an example of which immunity: [*September 2006*]

(a) Reactive immunity (b) Active immunity

(c) Passive immunity (d) Herd immunity.

Antigen, Antibody and Antigen Antibody Reaction

5. Half life of IgG: [*March 2010*]

(a) 5 days (b) 6 days

(c) 8 days (d) 23 days.

6. IgM have how many four-peptide subunits: [*March 2010*]

(a) 3 (b) 4

(c) 5 (d) 6.

7. True regarding agglutination reaction are all except: [*September 2007*]

(a) It is less sensitive than precipitation reaction for detecting antibodies

(b) Works on the same principle as that of precipitation reaction

(c) It is the method used for cross matching and blood grouping

(d) Agglutination occurs optimally when antigens and antibody react in equivalent proportions.

8. Which one of the following is a major component in activation of the complement via alternative pathway? [*September 2007*]

(a) CI (b) C2

(c) C3 (d) C4.

9. Intravascular hemolysis is mediated by: [*September 2007*]

(a) IgA (b) IgD

(c) IgM (d) IgG.

10. Which immunoglobulin is present in the breast milk? [*September 2005*]

(a) IgA (b) IgE

(c) IgD (d) IgM.

11. True about IgM is: [*September 2005*]

(a) Mediates Prausnitz-Kustner reaction (b) Primary response

(c) Transported across placenta (d) Secondary response.

12. Southern blot test is for detection of: [*September 2005*]

(a) Antibodies against viral proteins (b) DNA

(c) RNA (d) Carbohydrate epitopes.

13. Complement fixation test is: [*September 2005*]

(a) WIDAL (b) Coombs test

(c) Wasserman reaction (d) VDRL.

Immune Response

14. E-rosetting is a means of identifying: [*March 2011*]

(a) T-cells (b) B-cells

(c) NK cells (d) Null cells.

15. Defect seen in Di George syndrome: [*September 2009*]

(a) Humoral immunity (b) Cell mediated immunity

(c) Thymic hyperplasia (d) Autoimmune hemolytic anaemia.

16. Cells associated with humoral immunity: [*September 2005*]

(a) NK cells (b) B cells

(c) T cells (d) Null cells.

Hypersensitivity Reaction

17. Erythroblastosis foetalis is which type of hypersensitivity: [*September 2009, 2007*]

(a) Type I (b) Type II

(c) Type III (d) Type IV.

18. Which immunoglobulin is involved in anaphylaxis? [*March 2007*]

(a) IgA (b) IgE

(c) IgG (d) IgM.

19. All are type II hypersensitivity reaction except: [*September 2007*]

(a) Steven Johnson's syndrome (b) Drug induced hemolytic anemia

(c) Drug induced thrombocytopenia (d) Hemolytic disease of newborn.

20. Hyperacute rejection of renal transplant is which type of hypersensitivity reaction: [*March 2007*]

(a) Type I hypersensitivity reaction (b) Type II hypersensitivity reaction

(c) Type III hypersensitivity reaction (d) Type IV hypersensitivity reaction.

21. Hyperacute rejection occurs most commonly in which organ: [*March 2007*]

(a) Liver (b) Kidney

(c) Lung (d) Heart.

22. Which of the following is true about anaphylaxis? [*September 2007*]

(a) It is mediated by allergen specific IgE

(b) Type-I hypersensitivity reaction

(c) Cytokines like IL4, IL5 and IL6 along with histamine is released

(d) All of the above.

23. Which of the following is type III hypersensitivity reaction? [*September 2006*]

(a) Prausnitz-Kustner reaction (b) Contact dermatitis

(c) Arthus reaction (d) Rh incompatibility.

24. Wheal and flare reaction is: [*September 2005*]

(a) Type I hypersensitivity (b) Type II hypersensitivity

(c) Type III hypersensitivity (d) Type IV hypersensitivity.

ANSWERS TO FMGE MCQ's

Immunology

1. Ans. (c) NK cells

[*Ref.:* Ananthnaranan, 8th ed., page no. 86]

- ❖ **Components of innate immunity that are active against virus infected cells and tumor cells – *NK cell.***
- ❖ **Components of acquired immunity that are active against virus infected cells and tumor cells – *T cell.***

Innate immunity: Resistance to infection that an individual possess from birth by its genetic or constitutional makeup.

Components of Innate Immunity:

- Phagocyte (monocyte, macrophage, neutrophils).
- Dendritic cell.
- Natural killer cell.
- Alternate complement pathway.
- Acute phase protein (CRP, MBP, serum amyloid protein).
- Normal resident flora at GIT and respiratory tract.
- Inflammation, fever.
- Skin and mucosal barrier, e.g., sebum.

2. Ans. (c) Tetanus

[*Ref.:* Ananthnaranan, 8th ed., page no. 89; Park, 21st ed., page no. 97]

- ❖ Herd immunity refers to an overall level of immunity in a community.
- ❖ Eradication of an infectious disease depends on development of a high level of herd immunity against the pathogen.
- ❖ Epidemics of a disease is likely to occur when herd immunity against that disease is very low, indicating the presence of a large number of susceptible people in the community.
- ❖ ***Elements that contributes to herd immunity are:***
  - Occurrence of clinical and subclinical cases in herd.
  - Ongoing immunization programme.
  - Herd structure – includes population.
- ❖ ***Herd immunity occurs with the following vaccines:***
  - Diphtheria
  - Measles, Mumps, Rubella
  - Small pox.
  - Pertusis
  - OPV

3. Ans. (c) Typhoid

[*Ref.:* Ananthnarayan, 8th ed., page no. 88; Park, 21st ed., page no. 97-98]

- ❖ ***No immunoglobulin is available for typhoid and paratyphoidal fever.***
- ❖ Administartion of immunoglobulins provides artificial passive immunity to individual.
- ❖ Immunoglobulins are important for immunocompromised individuals and also for post exposure treatment.

Types of Immunoglobulins available:

- ***Human Immunoglobulins:***
  - Hepatits A
  - Hepatits B
  - Measles
  - Mumps
  - Varicella.
- ***Non-human Immunoglobulins (Antisera):***
  - Botulism
  - Gas gangrene.
- ***Both Human Immunoglobulins and Antisera are available for:***
  - Diphtheria
  - Tetanus
  - Rabies.

4. Ans. (b) Active immunity

[*Ref.:* Ananthnarayan, 8th ed., page no. 86; Park, 21st ed., page no. 97]

- ***Active immunity*** is the resistance developed by an individual after contact with microorganisms. Or their antigenic products.
- This contact may be:
- ***Natural Active Immunity*** – Following clinical or subclinical infection.
- ***Artificial Active Immunity*** – Following immunization with live or killed vaccine or microbial products such as toxins and toxoids

Live attenuated vaccines – Viral	Live attenuated vaccines – Bacterial
❖ Oral polio (sabin) ❖ Measles, mumps, rubella ❖ Varicella ❖ Yellow fever ❖ Influenza	❖ BCG ❖ Type 21a (Typhoid oral) ❖ Plague ❖ Epidemic typhus
Killed vaccines – Viral	**Killed vaccines – Bacterial**
❖ Poliomyletis (Salk) ❖ Influenza ❖ Hepatitis A ❖ Rabies ❖ Japanese encephalitis ❖ Kyasanur forest disease	❖ Pertusis ❖ Cholera ❖ Anthrax ❖ Typhoid ❖ Plague
Toxoids	**Subunit vaccines**
❖ Diptheria ❖ Tetanus	❖ *Proteins:* • Acellular pertusis • Subunit influenza • Hepatitis B ❖ *Carbohydrate:* • Haemophilus influenzae type B (Hib) • Typhoid Vi antigen • Meningococci • Pneumococci

IMMUNOLOGY

Antigen, Antibody and Antigen Antibody Reaction

5. Ans. (d) 23 days

[*Ref.:* Ananthnarayan, 8th ed., page no. 98]

- ***Immunoglobulin G (IgG) has a half life of 23 days, longest among all the immunoglobulins.***
- Immunoglobulin G (IgG) is the most abundant class of immunoglobulins in the serum comprising of about 80% of the total serum immunoglobulin.
- There are four IgG subclasses IgG1, IgG2, IgG3 and IgG4, so numbered according to their decreasing concentrations in serum.

IgG Antibody

- ***Possess highest DHS:***
  - Daily production
  - Half life (23d)
  - Serum concentration (decreasing order – *GAMDE*), i.e., highest is IgG and lowest is IgE.
- *Types* – IgG1 > 2 > 3 > 4 (Decreasing order of the serum concentration).
- ***Responsible for:***
  - Precipitation
  - Neutralization
  - NK cell (ADCC)
  - Classical complement pathway *(IgG3 highest).*
- Appear late, indicates past/chronic infection
- IgG avidity increases with time. So, detection of less avidity IgG indicates relatively recent infection.
- Secreted in placenta, breast *(**Except IgG2**)*

6. Ans. (c) 5

[*Ref.:* Ananthnarayan, 8th ed., page no. 99]

- *Immunoglobulin M (IgM) is basically a pentamer composed of five monomeric IgM immunoglobulin and joined by one molecule of J chain.*
- Each monomeric IgM is composed of two light chains and two heavy chains (ì).

7. Ans. (a) It is less sensitive than precipitation reaction for detecting antibodies

[*Ref.:* Ananthnarayan, 8th ed., page no. 107-108]

- Agglutination reaction is more sensitive than precipitation reaction for detecting antibodies.

  –Ananthnarayan
- Both agglutination and precipitation reaction work on the same principle (Marrack's hypothesis).
- Marrack's hypothesis says that:
  - Antigen antibody reaction occurs optimally when antigens and antibody react in equivalent proportions (Zone of equivalence.).
  - Antigen antibody reaction is weak when antibody is excess (known as the *prozone phenomenon*) or when antigen is excess (known as postzone *phenomenon*).
- Agglutination reaction is the method used for cross matching and blood grouping.

Other Examples of Agglutination Reaction:

- *Widal test* – done for Enteric fever
- *Standard agglutination* test – done for Brucella
- *Microscopic agglutination test* – done for Leptospira
- *Weil felix* – done for Rickettsia
- *Paul Bunuel* – done for EBV
- *Coomb test* for incomplete (IgG) Antibody
- ***Passive agglutination test:*** Soluble antigen is coated on carrier particle like RBC, latex
    - TPHA (syphilis)
    - Latex *agglutination test*
    - Rose Waaler test (Rheumatoid arthritis).
- ***RPHA (Reverse Passive Hemagglutination test:***
    - Antibody is coated on a surface of carrier particle like RBC to detect antigens

      Example: HBsAg.

8. Ans. (c) C3

[***Ref.:*** **Ananthnaranan, 8th ed., page no. 119-120]**

- ***Alternate complement pathway takes place by the activator like bacterial endotoxin which binds to C3b that activates Factor B to Ba and Bb.***
- ***Factor Bb binds to C3b to form C3bBb complex which acts as C3 covertase of alternate complement pathway.***
- ***C1,C4,C2 factors are involved in classical complement pathway where as C4,C2 are involved in lectin complement pathway.***

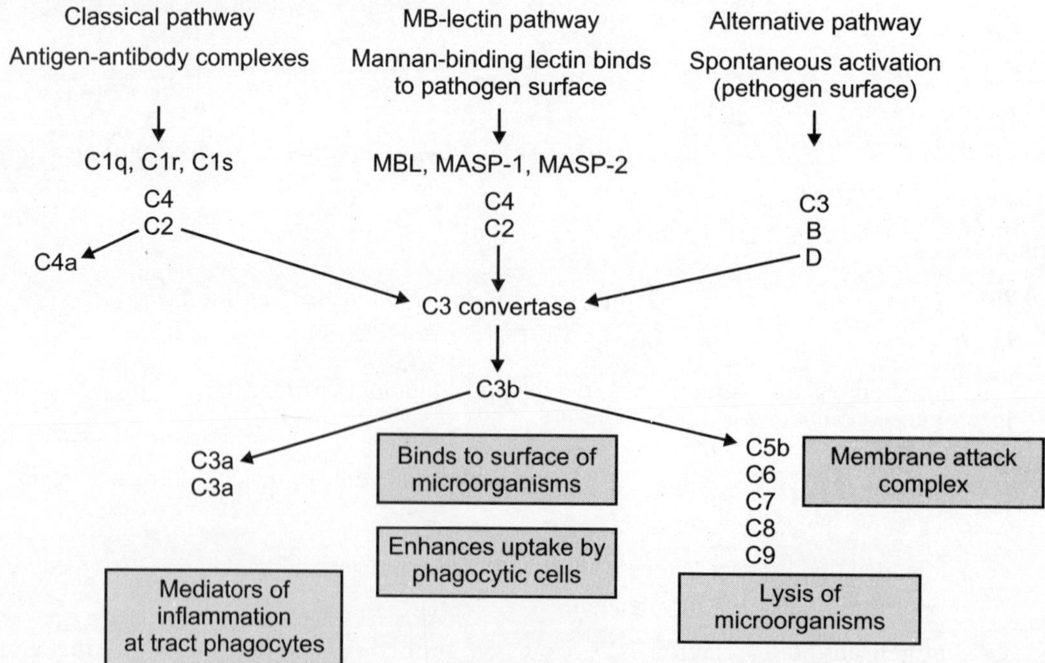

Fig. 2.2: ***Complement Pathways – Binds to the Surface***

IMMUNOLOGY

	Classical pathway	Alternate pathway	Lectin pathway
Activator	Antigen antibody complex	Zymosan, Endotoxin IgA, IgD, Cobra venom Nephritic factor	Carbohydrate residue of bacterial cell wall
1st complement activated	C1	C3b	C4
Sequence of complement activated	C1 → C4 →C2	C3b → B	C4 → C2
C3 convertase	***C14b2a***	***C3bBb***	***C4b2a***

9. Ans. (c) IgM

[*Ref.:* Ananthnaranan, 8th ed., page no. 99-100]

- **IgM has highest intravascular distribution (80%) and this responsible for immune hemolysis.**

10. Ans. (a) IgA

[*Ref.:* Ananthnaranan, 8th ed., page no. 99]

- **IgG and IgA antibody secretes in breast milk but only IgG antibody secretes in placenta.**

IgA Antibody

- 2nd most abundant antibody.
- Secretes in breast milk.
- *Types:*
  - Surface/mucosal IgA – Dimer joined by J chain and secretory piece (from epithelium).
  - Serum IgA – monomer, minor component.
- *IgA is responsible for:*
  - Alternate compliment.
  - Mucosal/local immunity.

11. Ans. (b) Primary response

[*Ref.:* Ananthnaranan, 8th ed., page no. 99]

- **IgM is the first immunoglobulin class produced in a primary response to an antigen. Where as IgG is produced in a secondary response.**
- IgM protects against invasion of blood by microbial pathogens.

IgM Antibody

- ***Possess highest MIS:***
  - Molecular weight (900,000)
  - Intravascular distribution (blood antibody) (80%)
  - Sedimentation coefficient (19)
- Pentameric with 10 valency
- 1st to appear following infection, indicates recent infection
- 1st to appear in intrauterine life (20 wk).

❖ ***Responsible for (or Mediates):***
- Agglutination
- Opsonization
- Haemolysis
- Classical complement pathway

❖ ***Examples:***
- O antibody in typhoid
- Antibody of ABO), Rh system.
- Reagin antibody (syphilis)

12. Ans. (b) DNA

[*Ref.:* Ananthnaranan, 8th ed., page no. 69, 115]

❖ Southern blot test is for detection of – DNA

❖ Northern blot test is for detection of – RNA

❖ Western blot test is for detection of – Protein (antibodies).

13. Ans. (c) Wasserman reaction

[*Ref.:* Ananthnaranan, 8th ed., page no. 110]

❖ The complement fixation reactions had been widely used for diagnosis of many infections, such as:
- **Wassermann test for syphilis.**
- Tests for antibodies to Mycoplasma pneumoniae, Bordetella pertussis, many different viruses, and to fungi such as Cryptococcus, Histoplasma, and Coccidioides.

Immune Response

14. Ans. (a) T-cells

[*Ref.:* Ananthnaranan, 8th ed., page no. 128]

❖ **E Rosette:** T cells have CD2 receptors on their surface that bind to sheep erythrocytes to form rosettes where as B cells do not.

❖ **EAC Rosette:** B cells can bind to sheep RBC coated with antibody and complement to form EAC Rosette due to presence of C3 receptor (CR2) on their surface.

Differences between T-cells and B-cells:

Property	T-cell	B-cell
Antigen recognition receptors	T cell receptors	Surface IgM/IgD receptor
Surface glycoprotein antigens	CD3	CD19
Receptor for Fc fragment of IgG	–	+
EAC rosette	–	+
SRBC rosette (E rosette)	+	–
Thymus specific antigens	+	–
Microvilli on surface	–	+
Blast transformation with:		
• Concovalin	+	–
• Phytohaemagglutinin	+	–
• Endotoxin	–	+

15. Ans. (b) Cell mediated immunity

[*Ref.:* Ananthnaranan, 8th ed., page no. 125, 157]

Di-George syndrome is a classic example of a pure T-cell deficiency characterized by congenital aplasia of thymus and parathyroids leading to deficiency of cell mediated immunity and tetany and hypocalcemia.

16. Ans. (b) B cells

[*Ref.:* Ananthnaranan, 8th ed., page no. 138]

- Humoral immunity is mediated by – B cells
- Cell mediated immunity is mediated by – T cells.

Hypersensitivity Reaction

17. Ans. (b) Type II

[*Ref.:* Ananthnaranan, 8th ed., page no. 166]

Example of Type II HSN

- **Compliment dependent cytolysis**
  - Transfusion reaction
  - *Erythroblastosis fetalis*
  - Auto immune hemolytic anemia
  - Pernicious anemia.
- **Compliment dependent inflammation (C3a, C5a)**
  - Good Pasteur syndrome
  - Pemphigus vulgaris
  - Bullous pemphigus
  - Rheumatic fever
  - Vasculitis.
- **Compliment dependent phagocytosis**
- **ADCC – (Type VI)**
  - By NK cell
  - Useful for parasite removal, graft rejection.
- **Antibody dependent cellular dysfunction – (Type V)**
  - Stimulation – Grave's disease
  - Inhibition – Myasthenia gravis.

18. Ans. (b) IgE

[Ref.: Ananthnaranan, 8th ed., page no. 163]

Example of Type I HSN

- Atopy
  - Asthma
  - Food allergy
  - Allerigic rhinitis (Hay fever)
  - Atopic eczema.

- Anaphylaxis
- Theobald Smith phenomena
- Schultz Dale phenomena
- Prausnitz Kustner reaction
- Casoni test.

19. Ans. (a) Steven Johnson's syndrome

[*Ref.:* Ananthnaranan, 8th ed., page no. 166]

- Steven Johnson's syndrome, e.g., of Type III HSN.

20. Ans. (b) Type II HSN

[*Ref.:* Internet source]

- **Hyperacute rejection** occurs usually within the first few hours post-transplantation and is mediated by preformed antibodies against ABO or MHC antigens of the graft (which are formed due to previous exposure to the graft from the same donor).
- Usually it occurs with:
  - **Kidney transplantation (most common)**
  - Skin transplantation
  - Blood transfusion.

21. Ans. (b) Kidney

[*Ref.:* Internet source]

- Refer Q. No. 20

22. Ans. (d) All of the above

[*Ref.:* Ananthnaranan, 8th ed., page no. 163]

Anaphylaxis: It is an acute life threatening reaction usually affecting multiple organs. Multiple organ systems are usually affected, including the skin (pruritus, flushing, urticaria, angioedema), respiratory tract (bronchospasm and laryngeal edema) and CVS (hypotension and cardiac arrhythmias).

- It is an, e.g., of Type-I hypersensitivity reaction.
- It is mediated by IgE antibody.
- Cytokines like IL4, IL5 and IL6 along with histamine is released.

Mechanism of Type I HSN

Priming dose of antigen (allergen) → processed by APC → antigenic peptide presented to Th cell → Th cell differentiates to Th2 → ***Th2 secretes IL4*** → Acts on B cell → IgE produced → mast cell coated with IgE (Fc)

Shocking dose → IgE (Fab) binds to antigen → Mast cell degranulation

- **Mast degranulation releases mediators**
- **Primary mediator**
  - Histamine
  - Eosinophils
  - Serotonin
  - Neutrophil chemotactic factor.
- **Secondary mediators**
  - Prostaglandin
  - Cytokines.

IMMUNOLOGY

23. Ans. (c) Arthus reaction

[*Ref.:* Ananthnaranan, 8th ed., page no. 162-169]

- Prausnitz-Kustner reaction, e.g., Type-I hypersensitivity reaction.
- Contact dermatitis, e.g., Type-IV hypersensitivity reaction.
- Arthus reaction, e.g., Type-III hypersensitivity reaction.
- Rh incompatibility, e.g., Type-II hypersensitivity reaction.

24. Ans. (a) Type I hypersensitivity

[*Ref.:* Ananthnaranan, 8th ed., page no. 166]

The 'wheal and flare' response is seen in cutaneous anaphylaxis which an, e.g., Type-I hypersensitivity reaction.

PRACTICE MCQ's

Immunity

1. The innate immunity shows all the following features except that:

(a) It is the first line of defense of immune system

(b) Phagocytic cells are components of innate immunity

(c) It is non-specific

(d) T cells are components of innate immunity.

2. Administration of Hepatitis vaccine induces:

(a) Natural active immunity
(b) Artificial passive immunity
(c) Artificial active immunity
(d) Natural passive immunity.

Antigen, Antibody and Antigen Antibody Reaction

3. Antibody transfer mother to fetus:

(a) IgG
(b) IgM
(c) IgD
(d) IgA.

4. First immunoglobulin to appear following infection:

(a) IgG
(b) IgM
(c) IgA
(d) IgE.

5. Mucosal secretion contains:

(a) IgA
(b) IgE
(c) IgM
(d) IgG.

6. Atopy is mediated by:

(a) IgE
(b) IgD
(c) IgM
(d) IgA.

Immune Response

7. Mononuclear phagocytes are produced by:

(a) Thymus
(b) Spleen
(c) Bone marrow
(d) Liver.

8. T-cell maturation takes place in:

(a) Peyer's patch
(b) Lymph node
(c) Thymus
(d) Bursa of fabricius.

9. NK cell provides immunity against:

(a) Virus
(b) Bacteria
(c) Fungus
(d) Chlamydia.

Hypersensitivity Reaction

10. Which is an example of type III hypersensitivity?

(a) Contact dermatitis
(b) Hemolytic anemia
(c) Serum sickness
(d) Good Pasture syndrome.

11. The example of type II hypersensitivity reaction is:

(a) Arthus reaction
(b) SLE
(c) Autoimmune hemolytic anemia
(d) Contact dermatitis.

12. Which of the following is an example of type IV hypersensitivity?

(a) Granulomatous reaction
(b) Shwartzman reaction
(c) Arthus reaction
(d) Serum sickness.

13. All of the following are immune complex disease except:

(a) Serum sickness
(b) Farmer's lung
(c) SLE
(d) Casoni test.

ANSWERS TO PRACTICE MCQ's

Immunity

1. Ans. (d) T cells are components of innate immunity

[*Ref.:* Ananthnaranan, 8th ed., page no. 86]

- ❖ T & B cells are components of acquired immunity.

2. Ans. (c) Artificial active immunity

[*Ref.:* Ananthnaranan, 8th ed., page no. 86]

- ❖ Hepatitis vaccine is composed of recombinant HBsAg and is an example of artificial active immunity.

Antigen, Antibody and Antigen Antibody Reaction

3. Ans. (a) IgG

[*Ref.:* Ananthnaranan, 8th ed., page no. 98]

IMMUNOLOGY

4. Ans. (b) IgM

[*Ref.:* Ananthnaranan, 8th ed., page no. 99]

5. Ans. (a) IgA

[*Ref.:* Ananthnaranan, 8th ed., page no. 98-99]

- Mucosal or local immunity is mediated by secretory IgA.

6. Ans. (a) IgE

[*Ref.:* Ananthnaranan, 8th ed., page no. 100]

Immune Response

7. Ans. (c) Bone marrow

[*Ref.:* Ananthnaranan, 8th ed., page no. 132]

- The mononuclear phagocytic system consists of monocytes circulating in the blood and macrophages in the tissues. They are synthesized from bone marrow.

8. Ans. (c) Thymus

[*Ref.:* Ananthnaranan, 8th ed., page no. 128]

- T cells and B cells are originated from bone marrow.
- The maturation of B cell occurs in bone marrow whereas the maturation of T cell occurs in thymus.

9. Ans. (a) Virus

[*Ref.:* Ananthnaranan, 8th ed., page no. 131]

- NK Cell and cytotoxic CD8 T cells provide immunity against virus infected cells and tumor cells.

Hypersensitivity Reaction

10. Ans. (c) Serum sickness

[*Ref.:* Ananthnaranan, 8th ed., page no. 167]

11. Ans. (c) Autoimmune hemolytic anemia

[*Ref.:* Ananthnaranan, 8th ed., page no. 166]

12. Ans. (a) Granulomatous reaction

[*Ref.:* Ananthnaranan, 8th ed., page no. 168]

13. Ans. (d) Casoni test

[*Ref.:* Ananthnaranan, 8th ed., page no. 163]

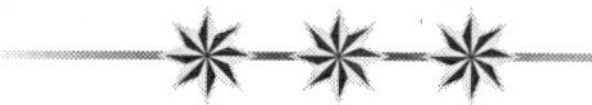

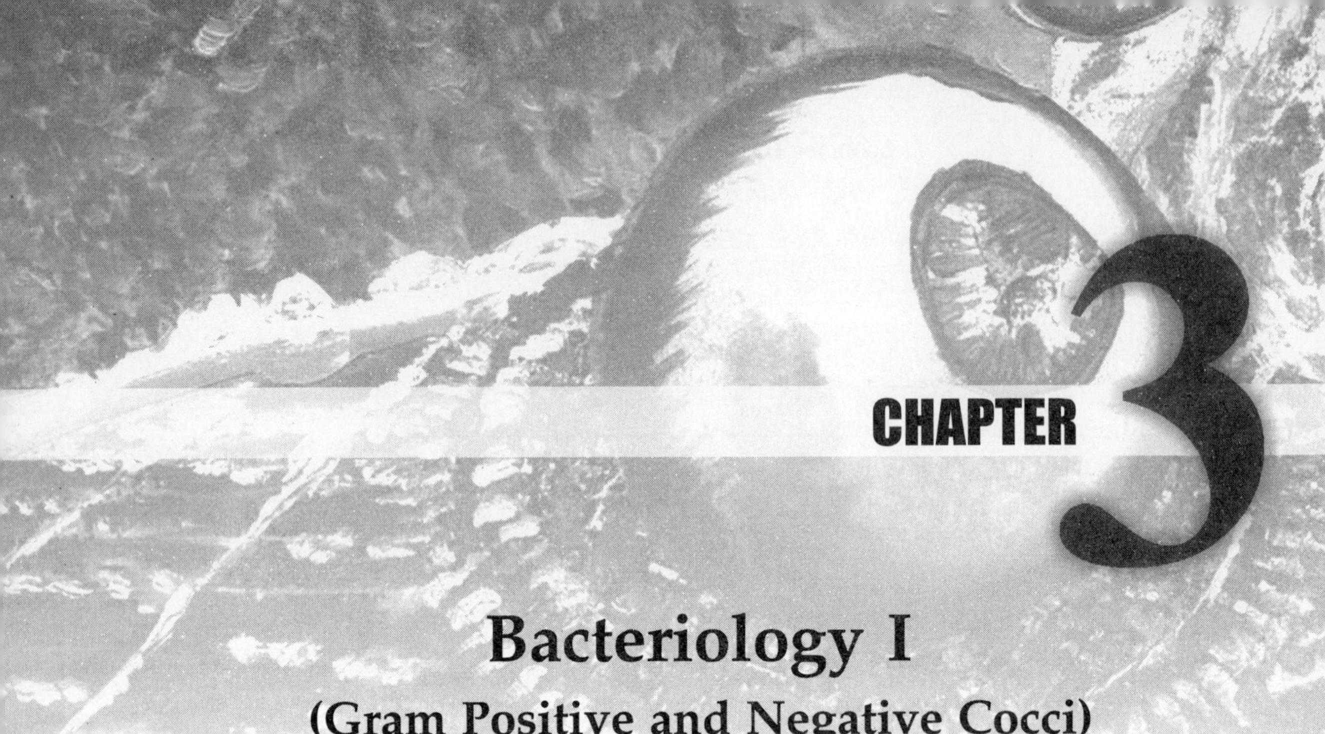

Bacteriology I
(Gram Positive and Negative Cocci)

COCCI (GRAM POSITIVE AND GRAM NEGATIVE)

Classification of Bacteria

- Clostridium
- Non-sporing anaerobes.

Classification	Definition	Examples
Obligate aerobes	Grows only in presence of oxygen	Bacillus Mycobacterium tuberculosis Pseudomonas Brucella Nocardia
Micro-aerophilic	Require 5% of oxygen	Campylobacter Helicobacter
Facultative anaerobes	Grows in presence or absence of oxygen	Most of the pathogenic bacteria like Staphylococcus, E. coli etc
Obligate anaerobes	Grows only in absence of oxygen Lack catalase enzyme	Clostridium Non sporing anaerobes

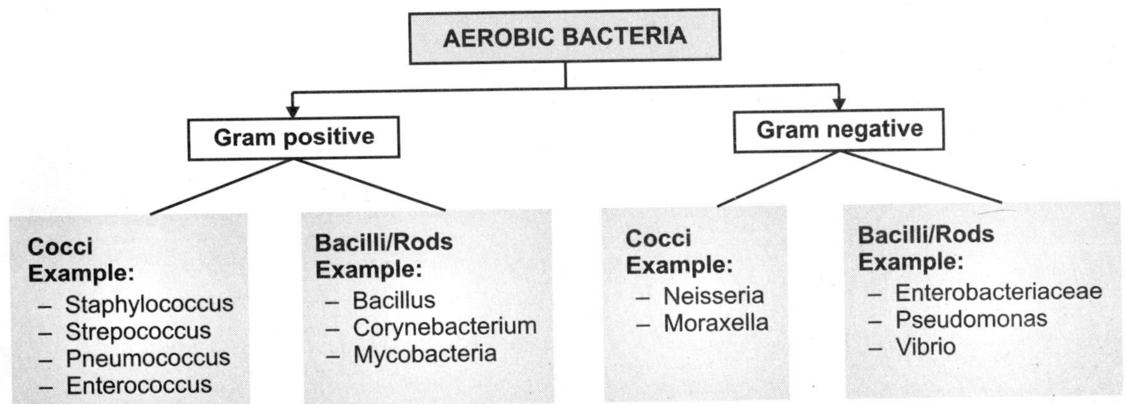

GRAM POSITIVE COCCI

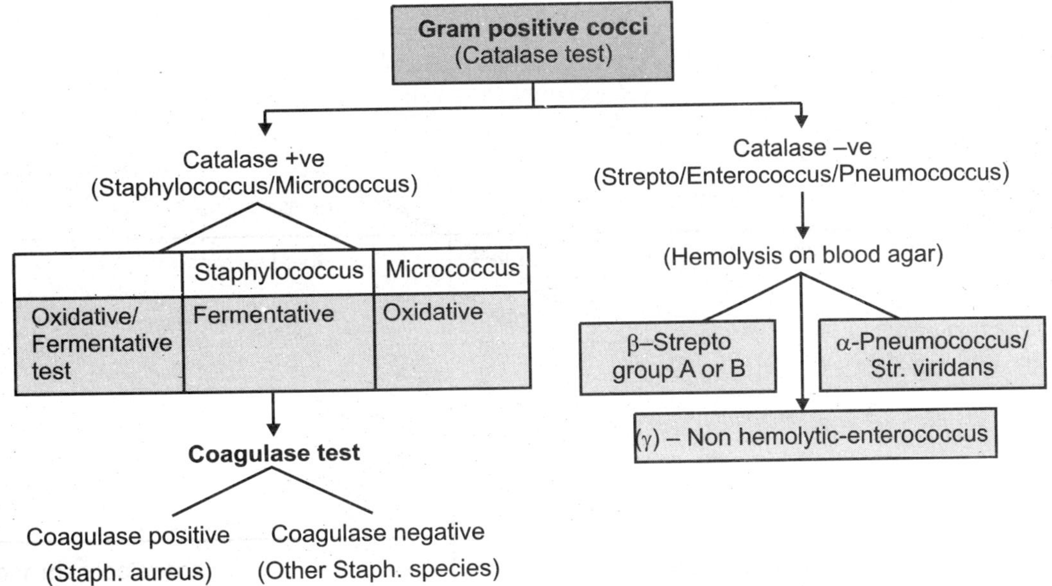

STAPHYLOCOCCUS

- Catalase +ve, Gram positive cocci arranged in cluster.
- 'Staphylo' means grape like cluster:
  - They are arranged in cluster because the cell divides in multiple plane.
  - In contrast Streptococcal cell divides in one plane, hence they arrange in chain.

Media for Staphylococcus:

- Nutrient agar – S. aureus produces ***Golden yellow pigmentation*** is due to β carotene.
- Blood agar – S. aureus shows *pin head shaped colony with narrow zone of β haemolysis.*
- MacConkey agar – S. aureus shows minute pink lactose fermenting colonies.
- *Selective medium:*
  - Salt milk agar (8-10% NaCl).
  - Mannitol salt agar-with 7.5% NaCl.
  - Ludlam's medium.

Antigenic Structure and Virulence Factors

Hemolysin	Activity
α Hemolysin	❖ Gets inactivated at 70°C but reactivated **paradoxically** at 100°C (due to denaturation of a heat labile inactivator at 100°C).
β Hemolysin	❖ *Mechanism* – Sphingomyelinase in nature. ❖ ***Lyses sheep RBC,*** but not human or rabbit RBC. ❖ Exhibits **hot-cold** phenomenon.
γ Hemolysin	❖ Has two components.
δ Hemolysin	❖ Detergent like action.
Leucocidins/***Panton valentine*** toxin	❖ Has two components.
Synergohymenotropic toxin: Examples inculde bicomponent toxins like γ and leucocidins.	

Extracellular enzymes	Activity
Coagulase enzyme	❖ Enzyme is secreted into the surrounding medium. ❖ Requires coagulase reacting factor (CRF) present in plasma. ❖ It is responsible for tube coagulase test.
Other enzymes: • Staphylokinase (fibrinolysin) • Hyaluronidase	

Cell wall associated structures	Activity
Clumping factor/Bound coagulase	❖ It is responsible for slide coagulase reaction.
Protein A	❖ It Binds to Fc region of IgG leaving Fab free to bind to Antigen – ***Basis of Co-agglutination reaction.***
Other factors: Capsular polysaccharide, Peptidoglycan, Teichoic acid.	

Toxins	Activity
Epidermolytic toxin (Exfoliative toxin)	❖ Causes Scalded skin syndrome (SSS). ❖ Severe forms like – **Ritter** disease (newborn), **TEN** (adult). ❖ Milder – Pemphigus neonatorum, bullous impetigo.
Enterotoxin	❖ Cause food poisoning ❖ It is a ***preformed toxin,*** i.e., already secreted into the contaminated food, so that it starts acting as soon as ingested. ❖ Incubation period of staphylococcal food poisoning : **1-6 hr.**

	❖ Produces vomiting due to vagus nerve and vomiting centre stimulation. ❖ It is a Heat stable toxin (not destroyed after heating food) ❖ MC Enterotoxin to cause food poisoning is type-A
Toxic shock syndrome toxin (TSST)	❖ Also known as Enterotoxins F/Pyrogenic exotoxin C. ❖ *Risk factor* – with females using vaginal tampon during menstruation. ❖ *Clinical feature* – Rash, desquamation and multi-organ failure. ❖ *Treatment* – Clindamycin.

Coagulase Test:

- **Tube Coagulase Test:**
  - Due to Coagulase Enzyme.
  - Coagulase Enzyme is secreted into the surrounding medium.
  - Requires coagulase reacting factor (CRF) present in plasma for action.
- **Slide Coagulase Test:**
  - Due to clumping factor present in the cell wall.
  - No need of CRF.

MRSA (Methicillin resistant *Staphylococcus aureus*):

- *Mechanism of Resistance* – MRSA is due to chromosomally mediated **Mec *A gene*** which codes for altered PBP 2a (Penicillin Binding protein 2a) present in cell wall which has less affinity for β lactam drugs.
- Hence MRSA strains are resistant to all β lactam drugs.
- Vancomycin is DOC.
- Others drugs that can be given: Teichoplanin, Linezolid, streptogramin.

***S. aureus* is the most common agent of:**

- Skin and soft tissue infection
- Osteomyelitis
- Surgical wound infection
- Botryomycosis
- Pneumatocele
- Native valve Endocarditis.

Endocarditis

Most common cause of

- Native valve endocarditis – *S. aureus.*
- Early prosthetic valve endocarditis (<12 months) – *Staphylococcus epidermidis.*
- Late prosthetic valve endocarditis (>12 months) – *Streptococcus viridans.*
- Endocarditis in IV drug users – *Staphylococcus aureus.*
- Subacute endocarditis – *Streptococcus viridians.*

Points to remember

- Most common site of colonization of Staphylococcus aureus – Skin.
- Most common way to of hospital spread – Hospital staff to Patients.
- Most common way to prevent the hospital spread – Hand washing.
- Most common method for typing of Staphylococcus aureus – Phage typing (pattern method).

BACTERIOLOGY I

- Plasmid mediated beta lactamase resistance in Staphylococcus aureus transferred by – Transduction (MC).

Coagulase Negative Staph. (CONS) – Normal flora of skin.

S. epidermidis

- Most common CONS – Accounts for 60-70% of CONS infection.
- Causes – Early onset prosthetic valve Endocarditis.

S. saprophyticus

- *Causes* – UTI in young sexually active female.
- Novobiocin Resistant.

STREPTOCOCCUS

- Catalase –ve, gram positive cocci arranged in chains.
- **Selective media:** Crystal violet – Blood agar.
- **Transport media:** Pike's media.

Classification:

On the basis of Hemolysis, Streptococci are divided into three groups:

- *∝ haemolytic* – Viridans group, common in throat.
- *β haemolytic* – Most of the pathogenic Streptococci fall into this group.
- *γ haemolytic* – No hemolysis seen, include Enterococcus.

Lancefield's grouping (To classify β haemolytic Streptococci):

- On the basis of group specific **carbohydrate antigen** in cell wall β haemolytic Streptococci are further divided in to 20 serological types A to V except **I and J.**

Griffith Typing (To classify Group A β haemolytic Streptococci):

- Strep. Group A is subdivided based on proteins M protein (>80 M types are present).

Species	Lancefield Group	Typical Hemolysis	Important Lab Characteristics
S. pyogenes	A	Beta	❖ Bacitracin – sensitive ❖ Hippurate hydrolysis negative ❖ CAMP test negative
S. agalactiae	B	Beta	❖ Bacitracin – resistant ❖ Hippurate hydrolysis positive ❖ CAMP test positive

Strep. pyogenes (Group A)

Virulence factor	Activity
Streptococcal pyrogenic exotoxin – SPE	❖ Subtyped to three types (SPE A, B and C). ❖ Type **A and C** are bacteriophage coded, **B** toxin is chromosomal coded. ❖ Causes scarlet fever and toxic shock syndrome.

BACTERIOLOGY I

Streptolysin O	❖ It is produced by group A, C and G Streptococci. ❖ **It is Oxygen labile.** ❖ Chemically it is similar to Pneumolysin, tetanolysin, perfringolysin. ❖ It is strongly antigenic and rise of antistreptolysin O antibody (ASO) >200u, indicates recent streptococcal infection except skin infections (pyoderma) and acute glomerulonephritis (AGN).
Streptolysin S	❖ It is oxygen stable, serum soluble. ❖ It produces hemolysis on the surface of an aerobic blood agar plate. ❖ Not antigenic.
Streptokinase	❖ It is fibrinolysin (activate plasminogen) in nature. ❖ Causes rapid spread of infection by preventing the formation of fibrin barrier. ❖ This property is used therapeutically in treatment of coronary thrombosis.
Deoxyribonuclease	❖ Also known as Streptodornase (four types – A, B, C, D). ❖ Anti-DNAase B antibody is useful for the retrospective diagnosis of skin infections (pyoderma) and AGN where ASO is usually low.

Pathogenicity:

❖ **Group A Streptococcus is most common cause of:**
- Pharyngitis/sore throat.
- Scarlet fever.
- Impetigo – Seen in young individual.
- Erysipelas.
- Cellulitis.
- Puerperal sepsis.
- Toxic shock syndrome (S. aureus is most common cause, next is Streptococcus).

❖ **It can also cause non-suppurative sequelae like:**
- ARF (Acute rheumatic fever).
- Acute glomerulonephritis – can occur either after skin or throat infection.

Property	Acute rheumatic fever (ARF)	Acute glomerulonephritis (AGN)
Site	Throat	Skin > Throat
Prior sensitization	Essential	Not
Serotype	Any	Restricted serotype causes AGN
Immune response	Marked	Moderate
Complement level	Unaltered	Low
Genetic susceptibility	Present	No
Repeated attack	Common	Not so

BACTERIOLOGY I

Penicillin prophylaxis	Indicated	Not so
Course	Progressive	Spontaneous resolution
Prognosis	Variable	Good

Group B Streptococci

- *S. agalactiae* is the most common cause of ***neonatal meningitis.***
- It colonizes the maternal genital tract, thus can be transmitted to baby during delivery.
- Presumptive identification of *S. agalactiae done by:*
    - CAMP +ve.
    - Hippurate hydrolysis test +ve.
    - Bacitracin resistant.

Enterococcus

- γ haemolytic (No haemolysis).
- Can grow in presence of **6.5% NaCl, 40% bile, at pH 9.6 and at 45°C, PYR +ve.**
- Most strains are **resistant to penicillin**, amino glycoside and sulfonamides.
- **Penicillin resistant** can be overcome by combination therapy with aminoglycoside (Synergistic).
- Disease produced – UTI, endocarditis, intra abdominal infection, meningitis.

Streptococcus viridans

- α hemolytic, mostly they are mouth commensals.
- *S. mutans* – causes dental caries.
- *S. sanguis* – causes subacute endocarditis.

Streptococcus pneumoniae

- α hemolytic.
- Gram positive cocci in pair.
- Lanceolate (flame) shaped.

Character	S. pneumoniae	S. viridians
Morphology	Lanceolate, pair	Round/oval, long chain
Capsule	Present	Absent
Blood agar at 48 hr	Draughtsman	Convex
Liquid medium	Uniform turbidity	Granular turbidity
Bile solubility	Soluble	Insoluble
Inulin fermentation	Fermenter	Non-fermenter
Optochin	Sensitive	Resistant
Animal pathogenicity	Pathogenic	Non-pathogenic

Antigenic Structure

- Capsular polysaccharide antigen – detected by ***Quellung reaction*** (capsular swelling when mixed with respective antisera and methylene blue).

BACTERIOLOGY I

- C-Carbohydrate Antigen –

  C reactive protein (CRP) is so named as it precipitates with C-Carbohydrate antigen.
- Pneumolysin.
- Autolysin.

Pathogenicity

- Can be commensal in nasopharynx and throat.
- PC60 – Most common cause of lobar pneumonia – ***most virulent and is type-3*** (this type 3 strain produces mucoid colonies).
- Most common cause of pyogenic meningitis.

Vaccine

- ***Polysaccharide vaccine:***
  - 23 valent, covers 90% of strains.
  - Not useful for < 2 yr as it is poorly immunogenic to children.
  - Contraindicated – lymphoreticular malignancy, pregnancy.
  - Indication:
    - After splenectomy.
    - Sickle cell anemia patient.
    - Patients with diabetes mellitus, chronic heart/lung/renal/liver disease.
- ***Conjugated vaccine*:**
  - 7 valent – covers 60% of strains, can be given <2 yr.

GRAM NEGATIVE COCCI

Example: Neisseria, Moraxella and Veillonella.

Neisseria

- Catalase and oxidase +ve.
- Diplococci.

N. meningitidis	N. gonorrhoeae
Capsulated	Non-capsulated.
Lens shaped/Half moon shaped (Diplococci with adjacent sides flattened).	Kidney shaped.
Ferment Glucose and Maltose ***(M for only M).***	Only ferments glucose.
Rarely have plasmids.	Usually possess plasmid coding drug resistance genes.
Exists in both intra and extracelular forms.	Predominantly intracellular form.

N. meningitides (Meningococcus)

Virulence Factors

- *Capsular polysaccharide*
  - Inhibits phagocytosis

- Serotyped to 13 serogroups
- Most common serogroup causing disease → A B, C, Y, 29E, W 135

❖ *Endotoxin and LOS (Lipooligosaccharide)*

➢ It differs from LPS of enterobacteriaceae by lacking the repetitive O side chain.

➢ Produce Water house – *Friderichsen Syndrome.*

Pathogenicity

❖ ***Most common group associated:***

➢ Group A – epidemics

➢ Group C – sporadic

➢ Group B – both.

❖ Humans – only reservoir.

❖ ***Most common source – human carriers*** (Nasopharyngeal carrier).

❖ Mode of transmission – Droplet infection.

❖ Most common Route – ***hematogenous*** (most common) followed by olfactory nerve and conjunctiva.

❖ Deficiency of ***terminal complement components*** (C5- C9)→ increase risk of *Neisseria* infection.

❖ High prevalence area– ***sub-Saharan belt of Africa.***

❖ Seasonal variation – most common in ***winter spring.***

❖ Case fatality ratio is **80%.**

Clinical Feature:

❖ *Fulminant meningococcemia:*

➢ Water house – Friderichsen Syndrome.

➢ Characterized by DIC, shock, B/L adrenal hemorrhage.

➢ Occurs due to endotoxin/LOS (not capsule).

❖ *Meningitis* – Common in 3-5 year age.

Diagnosis

❖ *Sample* – CSF, blood (early stage) and nasopharyngeal swab (for carriers).

❖ *Culture media* – Chocolate agar, Muller Hilton agar, Thayer Martin media.

❖ *Transport media* – Stuart's medium.

Treatment

❖ Cefotaxime and ceftriaxone – DOC for treatment.

❖ Rifampicin (DOC), ciprofloxacin – For carriers and prophylaxis.

Polyvalent vaccine

❖ Contains group A, C, Y, W-135 capsular antigens.

❖ *No vaccine available for Group B* (because Group B capsule is poorly immunogenic).

❖ Polyvalent vaccine is not useful – below 3 year (capsule is poorly immunogenic <3 year).

❖ C/I – Pregnancy.

N. gonorrhea (Gonococcus)

- Typed based on Pili divided to four types ($T_1 - T_4$).
- Intra species typing – done by ***Auxotyping.***
- Incubation period of gonorrhoea – 2-8 days.

Antigenic Structure

- Pili – important role in attachment, are antiphagocytic
- Outer membrane protein
- IgA 1 protease
- Lipo-oligosaccharide
- Transferrin.

Clinical Feature

- Babies born to infected mother – Causes Ophthalmia neonatorum
    - Gonococcal Ophthalmia neonatorum (occurs in first 2 days, purulent discharge)
    - Chlamydial Ophthalmia neonatorum (occurs after 1st week, mucous discharge).
- Male: Most common manifestation is ***urethritis*** *does not involve testes*
- Female: ***Cervicitis*** *(adult vagina is resistant to Gonococcus, so less severe in female).*
- *Complication:*
    - ***DGI (Deep Gonococcal Infection)*** **–** Mainly arthritis (rarely endocarditis).
    - Water can perineum.
    - Fitz Hugh Curtis syndrome (perihepatitis).

Sample

- Urethral discharge.
- Endocervical swab (high vaginal swab not recommended).
- Rectal swab.

Transport media – Charcoal impregnated swabs/medium (Stuart/Amies media).

Selective Media

- Modified Thayer Martin.
- Modified New York city medium.

Treatment (DOC) – Cefotaxime and ceftriaxone.

Mostly resistant to Penicillin due to Penicillinase production.

FMGE MCQ's

Staphylococcus

1. **Which of the following organism is responsible for vesicular eruptions and 'honey-coloured' crusts over face:** [*March 2011*]

   (a) TB bacilli
   (b) Staphylococcus aureus
   (c) Hansen's bacilli
   (d) Herpes zoster.

BACTERIOLOGY I

2. **Which of the following is gram positive:** [*March 2010, 05*]
   (a) Veillonella
   (b) Bacteroides
   (c) Fusobacterium
   (d) Actinomyces.
3. **Gram positive cocci are:** [*March 2009*]
   (a) Staphylococci
   (b) Streptococcus
   (c) Pneumococcus
   (d) All of the above.
4. **Staphylococcus aureus is a normal inhabitant of:** [*March 2005*]
   (a) Throat
   (b) Nose
   (c) Perianal skin
   (d) GIT.
5. **Toxic shock syndrome is most commonly caused by:** [*March 2005*]
   (a) Sterptococcus pneumoniae
   (b) Staphylococcus aureus
   (c) Vibrio cholerae
   (d) Clostridium tetani.
6. **Pneumatocoele is most commonly caused by:** [*September 2005, 2010*]
   (a) Streptococcus pneumoniae
   (b) Klebsiella
   (c) Hemophilus influenzae
   (d) Staphylococcus aureus.
7. **Bacteria most commonly involved in prosthetic valvular heart disease within two months of surgery is:** [*March 2007*]
   (a) Staphylococcus epidermidis
   (b) Enterococci
   (c) Streptococcus viridans
   (d) Hemophilus.
8. **Which of the following is commonly responsible for toxic shock syndrome in female patient:** [*September 2008*]
   (a) Streptococcus-group B
   (b) Pseudomonas
   (c) H. influenzae
   (d) Staphylococcus aureus.
9. **Most common cause of acute bacterial endocarditis is:** [*September 2009*]
   (a) Staphylococcus aureus
   (b) Streptococcus viridans
   (c) Streptococcus intermedius
   (d) Candida albicans.
10. **Which of the following is true for Staphylococcus aureus food poisoning:** [*September 2008*]
    (a) Incubation period of over 20 hours
    (b) Immediate antibiotic therapy is required
    (c) Heat labile enterotoxin is responsible
    (d) Common with dairy products.
11. **Panton-valentine leucocidin is seen in infection with:** [*September 2009*]
    (a) Streptococci
    (b) Staphylococci
    (c) Gonococci
    (d) Pneumococci.
12. **A person has episodes of vomiting 3 hrs after consuming milk. Organism responsible for this may:** [*March 2009*]
    (a) Clostridium perfringenes
    (b) Bacillus cereus
    (c) Salmonella typhi
    (d) Staphylococcus.

Streptococcus

13. **Which of the following is prophylactic treatment of rheumatic heart disease?** [*March 2011*]
    (a) Ampicillin
    (b) Penicillin G
    (c) Benzathaine penicillin
    (d) Phenoxy-methyl penicillin.

14. Causative agent of sore throat is: [*September 2005*]

(a) Staphylococcus aureus
(b) Streptococcus pyogenes
(c) H. influenzae
(d) Corynebacterium diphtheriae.

15. Streptococcus is classified based on: [*September 2007*]

(a) Catalase
(b) Cultural characteristics
(c) Cell wall carbohydrate
(d) Bile solubility.

16. Pikes medium is used for transport of: [*March 2005*]

(a) Staphylococci
(b) Streptococci
(c) Shigella
(d) E. coli.

17. Which is not a major criteria for diagnosis of acute rheumatic fever: [*March 2009*]

(a) Carditis
(b) Polyarthritis
(c) ASO raised
(d) Subcutaneous nodule.

18. An infant with neonatal meningitis has a positive CAMP test, the causative agent is: [*September 2007*]

(a) Staphylococci
(b) E. coli
(c) Strept. agalactiae
(d) Klebsiella.

19. Dental caries is due to: [*March 2004*]

(a) Streptococcus sanguis
(b) Streptococcus mitis
(c) Streptococcus mutans
(d) Streptococcus salivarius

20. Draughtman concentric rings on culture are produced by: [*September 2010*]

(a) Yersina pestis
(b) H. ducreyi
(c) B. pertusis
(d) Pneumococi.

21. Quellung reaction is seen with: [*March 2004*]

(a) Pneumococcus
(b) Gonococcus
(c) Streptococcus
(d) Staphylococcus.

22. Culture of Streptococcus Viridans resemble: [*September 2008*]

(a) Staphylococcus
(b) Strept. pyogenes
(c) Pneumococcus
(d) Enterococcus fecalis.

23. Which of the following microorganism is the most common cause of lobar pneumonia: [*March 2005*]

(a) Klebsiella pneumoniae
(b) Streptococci
(c) Pneumococci
(d) Staphylococci.

24. Anti streptolysin O test is diagnostic in: [*March 2004*]

(a) Acute rhematic fever
(b) SLE
(c) Rhematoid arthritis
(d) Acute glomeruloneohritis.

Neisseria

25. Which organism can penetrate intact cornea: [*September 2009*]

(a) Pneumococcus
(b) Gonococci
(c) Pseudomonas
(d) Staphylococci.

ANSWERS TO FMGE MCQ's

Staphylococcus

1. Ans. (b) Staphylococcus aureus

[*Ref.:* Internet source (http://emedicine.medscape.com/article/965254-overview]

Vesicular eruptions and 'honey-colored' crusts over face is characterized of staphylococcus aureus impetigo.

- ❖ Impetigo is an acute, highly contagious gram-positive bacterial infection of the superficial layers of the epidermis.
- ❖ Impetigo occurs most commonly in children and hot, humid climates.
- ❖ Impetigo occurs in two forms: bullous and nonbullous.
- ❖ Nonbullous impetigo is the more common form, constituting approximately 70% of impetigo cases.
- ❖ Nonbullous impetigo is caused by ***Staphylococcus aureus*** followed by group A beta hemolytic streptococci.

2. Ans. (d) Actinomyces

[*Ref.:* Ananthnarayan, 8th ed., page no. 15, 391]

Example of gram positive cocci	Example of gram negaitive cocci
❖ Staphylococcus ❖ Streptococcus ❖ Pneumococcus ❖ Enterococcus	❖ Neisseria ❖ Moraxella ❖ Veillonella
Example of gram positive bacilli	**Example of gram negaitive bacilli**
❖ *Corynebacterium* ❖ *Bacillus* ❖ *Clostridium* ❖ *Listeria* ❖ *Actinomycetes* ❖ *Mycobacterium* ❖ *Erysepelothrix* ❖ Non-sporing Anaerobes–like Propionibacterium	❖ Enterobacteriaceae ❖ Vibrionaceae ❖ Pseudomonads ❖ Haemophilus, Brucella, Bordetella ❖ Spirochete, Rickettsia, Chlamydia and Mycoplasma ❖ Helicobacter, Campylobacter and Legionella ❖ Non-sporing Anaerobes – like Bacteroides, . Fusobacterium

3. Ans. (d) All of the above

[*Ref.:* Ananthnarayan, 8th ed., page no. 15]

- ❖ See above explanation

4. Ans. (b) Nose

[*Ref.:* Ananthnarayan, 8th ed., page no. 200]

- Most common source of Staph infection – carriers.
- Most common site of colonization is ***anterior nare*** followed by perianal skin, vagina, groin, axilla.
- Most common species in human skin – *S. epidermidis.*

5. Ans. (b) Staphylococcus aureus

[*Ref.:* Ananthnarayan, 8th ed., page no. 199]

- *Staphylococcus aureus* is the most common agent to cause Toxic Shock Syndrome followed by Strept. pyogenes.
- This syndrome is caused by Toxic Shock Syndrome toxin (TSST) of *S. aureus* and Streptococcal pyrogenic exotoxin (SPE) of Strept. pyogenes.
- These toxins are **super antigens,** which stimulate the release of large amount of interleukins IL1 and IL2 in the body.
- TSS is an acute and potentially life threatening condition similar to gram-negative sepsis and septic shock, a multisystem disease characterized by fever, hypotension, myalgia, vomiting, diarrhoea, mucosal hyperaemia and an erythematous rash followed by desquamation of the skin, particularly on palms and soles.
- This condition is more often documented among **menstruating ladies** using highly absorbent **vaginal tampons**, the vaginal swab from these ladies shows a heavy growth of Staph. aureus. However, it is also seen in men with infection of skin and mucosa in extra-genital sites.

6. Ans. (d) Staphylococcus aureus

[*Ref.:* Harrison, 18th ed., 1164, 17th ed., 895]

Pulmonary Pneumatocele:

- Shaggy thin-walled, air-filled, cyst like emphysematous lesion.
- Most often, they occur as a sequela to acute pneumonia, commonly caused by Staphylococcus aureus.
- However, pneumatocele formation also occurs with other agents, including – Streptococcus pneumoniae, Haemophilus influenzae, Escherichia coli, group A Streptococci, Serratia marcescens, Klebsiella pneumoniae, adenovirus, and tuberculosis.

7. Ans. (a) Staphylococcus epidermidis

[*Ref.:* Harrison 18th ed., 1053, 17th ed., 790]

- Most common cause of Early prosthetic valve endocarditis (<12 month) – Staph. epidermidis.
- Most common cause of Late prosthetic valve endocarditis (>12 months) – Streptococcus viridans.
- Overall most common cause of prosthetic valve endocarditis- S. epidermidis.
- ***Most common Agents of Endocarditis:***
  - Most common cause of Native valve endocarditis – *S.aureus.*
  - Most common cause of Subacute endocarditis – *Str. viridans.*

8. Ans. (d) Staphylococcus aureus

[*Ref.:* Ananthnarayan, 8th ed., page no. 199]

- See previous explanation.

9. Ans. (a) Staphylococcus aureus

[*Ref.:* Harrison 18th ed., page no. 1053; 17th ed., page no. 790]

- See previous explanation.

10. Ans. (d) Common with dairy products

[*Ref.:* Ananthnarayan, 8th ed., page no. 198]

- "Common source of food that contaminates with Staphylococcal enterotoxin are milk and milk products (dairy products), meat and fish." *–Ananthnarayan*
- Staphylococcal enterotoxin is heat stable. So cooking the contaminated food and leaving at room temperature for some time leads to toxin accumulation.
- Incubation period of of S. aureus food poisoning is 1-6 hour due to preformed toxin.
- Fluid replacement is the 1st line of treatment, immediate antibiotic therapy is not required.

11. Ans. (b) Staphylococcus

[*Ref.:* Ananthnarayan, 8th ed., page no. 198]

- *Leucocidins* or *Panto-valentine (PV)* toxin is one of the most important hemolysin produced by *S. aureus* which causes marked necrosis of the skin.
- Panto-valentine (PV) toxin and gamma hemolysin of *S. aureus* have two components. Hence known as synergohymenotropic toxin.

12. Ans. (d) Staphylococcus

[Ref.: Ananthnarayan, 8th ed., page no. 198]

- ***Episodes of vomiting 3 hrs of food indicates preformed toxin mediated food poisoning:***
  - *S. aureus* – most common source is dietary food (milk and milk products).
  - *Bacillus cereus* (emetic type) – most common source is Chinese fried rice.

Streptococcus

13. Ans. (c) Benzathaine penicillin

[*Ref.:* Jawetz, 24th ed., page no. 240]

- Antistreptococcal chemoprophylaxis is very useful in persons who have suffered an attack of rheumatic fever.
- This involves giving one injection of benzathine penicillin intramuscularly, every 3–4 weeks, or daily oral penicillin or oral sulfonamide.
- The first attack of rheumatic fever infrequently causes major heart damage; however, such persons are particularly susceptible to reinfections with Streptococci that precipitate relapses of rheumatic activity and give rise to cardiac damage.
- Chemoprophylaxis in such individuals, especially children, must be continued for long time.

14. Ans. (b) Streptococcus pyogenes

[*Ref.:* Ananthnarayan, 8th ed., page no. 209]

- ***S. pyogenes is the most common bacteria causing pharyngitis or sore throat.***
- Pharyngitis is characterised by inflammation of pharyngeal mucosa with exudate formation, tender enlarged cervical lymph nodes, fever and leucocytosis.

- ❖ The condition is commonly seen in children and spreads by droplet nuclei.
- ❖ The complications of streptococcal pharyngitis may lead to cervical lymphadenitis, sinusitis, otitis media, peritonsillar abscess, retropharyngeal abscess, meningitis endocarditis and pneumonia.

15. Ans. (c) Cell wall carbohydrate

[*Ref.:* Ananthnarayan, 8th ed., page no. 205]

- ❖ Streptococci are classified based on hemolysis on blood agar to $\propto$, β, γ haemolytic Streptococci.
- ❖ β hemolytic Streptococcus is classified to group A-V based on C carbohydrate antigen ***(Lancefield classification).***
- ❖ M protein is used to further classify group A Streptococcus ***(Griffith types).***

16. Ans. (b) Streptococcus

[*Ref.:* Ananthnarayan, 8th ed., page no. 211]

- ❖ *Pikes transport medium containing crystal violet and sodium azide is a frequently used transport medium for transporting throat swab for culture of S. pyogenes.*

17. Ans. (c) ASO raised

[Ref.: Harrison, 18th ed., page no. 1171-79; 17th ed., page no. 889]

WHO Criteria for Diagnosis of Rheumatic Fever	Revised Jones Criteria (1992)
Major manifestations	❖ Carditis ❖ Polyarthritis ❖ Chorea ❖ Erythema marginatum ❖ Subcutaneous nodules
Minor manifestations	❖ Clinical: fever, polyarthralgia ❖ Laboratory: elevated ESR or leukocyte count ❖ Electrocardiogram: prolonged P-R interval
Supporting evidence of a preceding streptococcal infection within the last 45 days	❖ Elevated or rising ASLO or other streptococcal antibody ❖ A positive throat culture ❖ Rapid antigen test for group A streptococcus ❖ Recent scarlet fever

18. Ans. (c) Strept. agalactiae

[*Ref.:* Ananthnarayan, 8th ed., page no. 214-15]

- ❖ ***Infant with neonatal meningitis has a positive CAMP test is suggestive of S. agalactiae (Group B Streptococci) infection.***

***S. agalactiae* (Group B Streptococci)**

- ❖ The most common cause of *neonatal meningitis.*
- ❖ It colonizes the maternal genital tract, thus can be transmitted to baby during delivery.

BACTERIOLOGY I

❖ Presumptive identification of S. *agalactiae done by:*
- CAMP test +ve
- Hippurate hydrolysis test +ve
- Bacitracin resistant.

19. Ans. (c) Streptococcus mutans

[*Ref.:* Ananthnarayan, 8th ed., page no. 216]

❖ S. mutans is an important causative agent of dental caries. It splits dietary sucrose producing acid and a dextran. The acid damages the dentine. The dextran binds together exfoliative epithelial cells, mucus, food debris and bacteria to form dental plaques.

20. Ans. (d) Pneumococci

[*Ref.:* Ananthnarayan, 8th ed., page no. 219]

❖ *Pneumococcus produces* ***draughtman shaped or carom coin shaped*** *colony on blood agar on prolonged incubation for 48 hrs.*

21. Ans. (a) Pneumococci

[*Ref.:* Ananthnarayan, 8th ed., page no. 219]

Capsular swelling reaction:

❖ This is also known as 'Quellung reaction' due to swelling (Latin *quellung* means swelling) of the capsule suspension observed in the test.

❖ This reaction was first described by Neufeld in the year 1902. In this test a drop of type specific antiserum is added to a drop of suspension of pneumococci on a glass slide along with a drop of methylene blue solution.

❖ The capsule, in the presence of the specific homologous antiserum, becomes apparently swollen, clearly delineated and refractile.

22. Ans. (c) Pneumococci

[*Ref.:* Ananthnarayan, 8th ed., page no. 216]

❖ **Streptococcus Viridans and Pneumococci both produces alfa Haemolytic colony on blood agar.**

23. Ans. (c) Pneumococci

[Ref.: Ananthnarayan, 8th ed., page no. 221]

❖ **S. pneumoniae is the leading cause of lobar pneumonia.**

24. Ans. (a) Acute rhematic fever

[*Ref.:* Ananthnarayan, 8th ed., page no. 212]

❖ Rise of Antistreptolysin O antibody (ASO) >200u, indicates recent streptococcal infection except skin infections (pyoderma) and acute glomerulonephritis (AGN).

❖ Anti DNAse B antibody is used as indicator of recent streptococcal skin infections (pyoderma) and acute glomerulonephritis (AGN)

25. Ans. (b) Gonococcus

[Ref.: Internet source, Handbook of Ocular Disease and Management]

- ❖ N. gonorrhoeae's ability to penetrate an intact corneal epithelium makes the risk of corneal infection and ulceration high.
- ❖ Organisms can penetrate an intact cornea.
  - Neisseria gonorrhoeae
  - Corynebacterium spp (diptheroides)
  - Haemophilus aegypticus.

PRACTICE MCQ's

Staphylococcus

1. Hot cold phenomenon is seen due to which toxin:

(a) Alpha lysin (b) Beta lysin
(c) Gamma lysin (d) Theta lysin.

2. Toxic shock syndrome was first discovered in:

(a) Tampoon users (b) Diabetic septicemia
(c) Drug addicts (d) None.

3. The most common mechanism of drug resistance in Staphylococci:

(a) Conjugation (b) Plasmids
(c) Transduction (d) Translation.

4. Novobiocin resistant Staph is:

(a) Staph aureus (b) Staph epidermidis
(c) Staph hemolyticus (d) Staph saprophyticus.

Streptococcus

5. Quellung reaction is associated with:

(a) Capsular delineation (b) Capsular degeneration
(c) Capsular absence (d) Carbohydrate antigen.

6. Most common cause of community acquired pneumonia:

(a) Strep pneumoniae (b) Kleb pneumoniae
(c) Vibrio cholera (d) H. influenzae.

7. Streptococcus pneumoniae true is:

(a) Bile insoluble and optochin sensitive
(b) Vaccine is made from capsular polysaccharide
(c) Vaccine is indicated in pregnancy (d) Catalase and oxidase positive.

8. Which of the following is lanceolate:

(a) Cl. tetani (b) S. aureus
(c) Pneumococci (d) Meningococci.

9. Neonatal meningitis acquired during passage through birth canal is due to:

(a) Streptococcus agalactiae (b) S. equisimilus

(c) S. pyogenes (d) Pnemococci.

10. True statement about Enterococcus faecalis except:

(a) Grows in 6.5% NaCl solution (b) PYR +ve

(c) Easily destroyed at 60°C for 30 minutes (d) Possess teichoic acid in cell wall.

ANSWERS TO PRACTICE MCQ's

Staphylococcus

1. Ans. (b) Beta lysin

[*Ref.:* Ananthnarayan, 8th ed., page no. 198

- Beta lysin exhibits hot cold phenomena, i.e., hemolysis due to beta hemolysin starts at 37°C, but gets exaggerated at 4°C.

2. Ans. (a) Tampoon users

[*Ref.:* Ananthnarayan, 8th ed., page no. 199]

3. Ans. (c) Transduction

[*Ref.:* Ananthnarayan, 8th ed., page no. 197]

4. Ans. (d) Staph saprophyticus

[*Ref.:* Ananthnarayan, 8th ed., page no. 202]

Streptococcus

5. Ans. (a) Capsular delineation

[*Ref.:* Ananthnarayan, 8th ed., page no. 220]

6. Ans. (a) Strep pneumoniae

[*Ref.:* Ananthnarayan, 8th ed., page no. 221]

7. Ans. (b) Vaccine is made from capsular polysaccharide

[*Ref.:* Ananthnarayan, 8th ed., page no. 221-23]

8. Ans. (c) Pneumococci

[*Ref.:* Ananthnarayan, 8th ed., page no. 219]

9. Ans. (a) Streptococcus agalactiae

[*Ref.:* Ananthnarayan, 8th ed., page no. 214-15]

10. Ans. (c) Easily destroyed at 60°C for 30 minutes

[*Ref.:* Ananthnarayan, 8th ed., page no. 215-16]

- Enterococcus is heat stable, i.e., it can tolerate 60°C for 30 minutes.

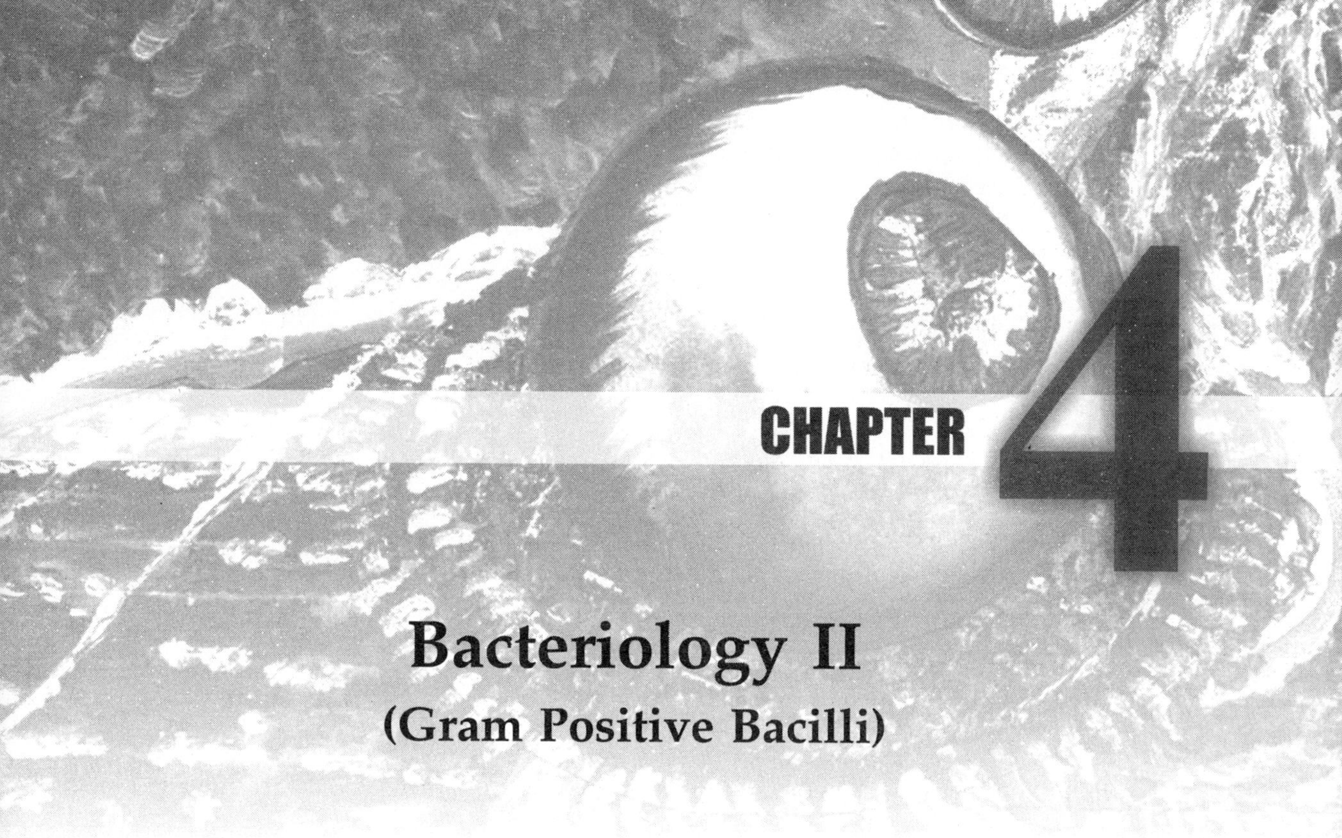

Bacteriology II
(Gram Positive Bacilli)

Example of Gram Positive Bacilli include:

- *Corynebacterium*
- *Clostridium*
- *Listeria*
- *Bacillus*
- *Mycobacterium*
- *Actinomycetes.*

CORYNEBACTERIUM

- *Corynebacterium. diphtheriae* is also known as ***Kleb Loeffler bacillus.***
- ***Arrangement:*** Club shaped, Chinese letter and cuneiform arrangement.
- ***Metachromatic granules (volutin granule):*** They possess metachromatic granules on both the ends made up inorganic polyphosphates which is also known as ***Babes Ernst or Polar body.***
- ***Special stain*** to demonstrate metachromatic granules – Albert, Ponder, Neisser stain.

Table: On the basis of morphology on Tellurite medium

McLeod classification	Gravis	Intermedius	Mitis
Colonies on PTA	***Daisy head***	***Frogs eggs colony***	***Poached egg***
Fermentation of starch	+ve	–ve	–ve
Toxigenic strains	100%	95-99%	80-85%
Occurrence	Epidemic	Epidemic	Endemic
Hemolysis	Variable	Non-hemolytic	Hemolytic

Diphtheria Toxin:

- ***Mechanism of action:*** Possess two fragments – A and B
  - Fragment A – ADP ribosylation of elongation factor 2→ Inhibit EF 2→ inhibits protein synthesis.
  - Fragment B – For transportation of fragment A inside cell.
- Toxin production depends on optimum ***iron concentration*** (0.1 mg per litre optimum).
- DT is coded by b **phage (tox phage).**
- Park William 8 strain of *C. diphtheriae* is used as a source of toxin for diphtheria toxoid (DPT vaccine).
- Diphtheria Bacilli is non invasive but **DT** is released locally and absorbed in circulation and produce systemic manifestation. So ***diphtheria is toxemia but not bacteremia.***
- ***Skin/local lesions*** – Produced by non-toxigenic strains, so vaccination has no role in preventing cutaneous diphtheria.
- ***Exotoxin A of Pseudomonas*** *resembles DT in its mechanism.*

Clinical Diphtheria

- Clinical diphtheria can be produced by three species of *Corynebacterium* because all of them possess diphtheria toxin.
  - *C. diphtheriae.*
  - *C. ulcerans.*
  - *C. pseudotuberculosis.*

Pathogenicity

- Diphtheria is a natural infection affecting ***only to man.***
- Clinically it is characterized by – Pseudo membrane formation on tonsil, posterior pharyngeal wall.
- ***Main source of infection – Nasal carriers.***
- ***Faucial diphtheria – Most common, but laryngeal diphtheria – dangerous***, requires tracheostomy.
- 1st muscle involved – ***palatopharynges.***

Lab Diagnosis

Diagnosis:

- Diphtheria is an emergency, treatment is required immediately.
- Diagnosis is usually clinical, not to wait for lab confirmation.
- Gram staining of throat swab is done and culture followed by toxigenicity testing.
- Laboratory methods include direct smear and isolation by culture followed by detection of toxin.

Direct Smear

- **Gram stain:** Showing gram positive bacilli with Chinese letter arrangement.
- **Albert stain:** To demonstrate metachromatic granules.

Culture

- ***Loffler's serum slope (Enriched medium)***
  - Growth occurs early (6-8 hours)
  - Granules are best developed in this medium.

- ***Potassium tellurite agar –0.04% (Selective medium)***
  - Black colonies are formed in two days due to tellurite reduction.
  - It is the best medium for detection of carriers, convalascent and cases.

Toxigenicity or Virulence test of C. diphtheria:

- ***In vivo tests:*** Guinea pig or rabbit used.
- ***In vitro tests:*** Elek gel precipitation test.

Shick test:

- It is a susceptibility test before starting immunization (now not in use).
- Toxin given intradermally on forearm.
- If erythema and indurations occur on test arm, ↑ size by 7th day, it indicates the test is positive and the person is susceptible to diphtheria and needs immunization.

	Vaccine	Antibiotic
Carrier	Not affective	Affective
Treatment of diphtheria	Affective	Not affective (Except early stage)
Treatment of cutaneous Diphtheria	Not affective	Affective

Treatment:

- Diphtheria is due to toxin not due to organism. (Except Cutaneous diphtheria which can be produced by non-toxigenic strains also.)
- Antibiotics do not neutralize circulating toxin, so antibiotics have no role after the toxin is formed (6 hour) in preventing the disease.
- However, antibiotics can prevent cutaneous diphtheria.
- Penicillin is given for treatment of cases.
- Erythromycin is active for treatment of carriers.

Prevention:

- Vaccine is directed against Diphtheria toxin, so it can prevent all type of Diphtheria except Cutaneous diphtheria and also it ***can not prevent carrier stage.***

DPT- Diphtheria Toxoid, Tetanus Toxoid and Pertussis (whole cell or acellular component)

- *Two types of DPT available – Adsorbed toxoid and fluid toxoid:*
  - *Adsorbed toxoid* is more immunogenic than fluid toxoid.
  - *Aluminum phosphate* is used in adsorbed toxoid – which is more immunogenic than hydroxide adsorbed toxoid.
  - ***Thiomersal*** used as preservative.
- Both whole cell killed B. pertussis and acellular pertussis component increases potency of DT and TT (acts as adjuvant).
- Whole cell killed B. pertussis is ***encephalogenic*** and ***short lasting*** immunity while acelluar pertussis component (DTaP) is devoid of neurological complication.
- Acelluar pertussis component consists of pertussis toxoid, agglutinogen, fimbrial antigen.
- *Dose* – 0.5 ml given IM.
- *Schedule:* 5 dose-3 dose at 6/10/14 week followed by DPT booster at 16-24 week and 5 year.

> *Quadruple vaccine* – (DPT + Haemophilus influenze b (Hib). In this vaccine, DT and TT increases immunogenicity of Hib.
> *Absolute contraindication to DPT* – Hypersensitivity and progressive neurological disorder.

Non-diphtheria Corynebacterium

- ***C. pseudotuberculosis*** *(Preisz Nocard bacilli)* – affect sheep and horse
- ***C. minutissimum (causes erythrasma)***
- ***C. jeikeium (multidrug resistant)***
- ***C. parvum, e.g., of immunomodulator.***

BACILLUS

- Bacillus spp are strict aerobic gram positive spore forming bacilli.
- Two species are pathogenic – *B. anthracis and B. cereus.*
- All bacillus are motile except – *B. anthracis.*
- All bacillus are non-capsulated except – *B. anthracis.*

B. anthracis

- Highly pathogenic.
- Non-motile.
- Capsulated.
- Produces zoonotic disease especially involving herbivorous animals.

Cultural Characteristics

- ***Bacillus anthracis can be differentiated from other Bacillus species by various ways:***
  - *Mc Fadyean reaction:* polypeptide capsule can be seen when stained with polychrome methylene blue.
  - Gram staining: ***bamboo sticks*** appearance, chain of bacilli.
  - On nutrient agar plate: ***medusa head appearance*** colony (under low power microscope).
  - Gelatin stab: ***inverted fir tree*** appearance.
  - Solid media with penicillin: ***String of pearl*** appearance.
  - Blood agar: ***non-hemolytic colony.***
- Selective medium: ***PLET media***.
- *Spores found in soil or in culture but never in animal body.*

Virulence Factor

Anthrax toxin: It has three fraction:

- *Edema factor* – acts by ↑cAMP.
- *Protective factor* – helps in binding (antibody to it is protective).
- *Lethal factor.*
- Alum precipitated toxoid vaccine – prepared by including protective antigen.

Capsule

- Made up polyglutamate.
- Inhibits phagocytosis.

BACTERIOLOGY II

- Live attenuated spore vaccine (Sterne, Mazucchi) prepared by deleting the capsule genes.

Pathogenesis of Anthrax: It is a zoonotic disease (cattle and sheep)

Man acquires infection through:

- *Cutaneous type:* by small cuts or skin abrasion, use of shaving razors used for animal, insect bite.
- *Pulmonary type:* by spore inhalation.
- *Intestinal type:* occurs following eating meat of animal dying of anthrax.
- Rarely by insect bite.
- All three form can lead to – hemorrhagic meningitis and septicemia (less in Cutaneous type).

	Cutaneous anthrax	Pulmonary anthrax
Also known as	Hide Porter's disease	Wool Sorter's disease
Mode of transmission	Cutaneous exposure to animal	Inhalation of spores
Main clinical feature	Malignant pustule (black eschar surrounded by non pitting edema)	Hemorrhagic mediastinitis
Occupational exposure	Dock worker, butcher, abattoir, farmer	Wool factory
Frequency	Most common (95%)	Rare
Prognosis	Self-limiting	Fatal

- Anthrax can be agent of bioterrorism – recently used by Afghanistan (spores enclosed in paper were mailed).
- Ascoli thermo precipitin test – to demonstrate anthrax antigen.

Bacillus Cereus

- Motile, lacks capsule, causes food poisoning.
- Selective media- **MYPA** (mannitol, egg yolk, phenol red polymyxin agar).
- Produces two types of entrotoxin – Diarrheal type and Emetic type.

B. cereus	Diarrheal type	Emetic type
Incubation period	8-16 hour	1-5 hour (preformed toxin)
Food	Cooked meat/vegetable	Rice (Chinese fried rice)
Toxin	Heat labile	Heat stable
Clinical feature	Diarrhea, fever, rarely nausea	Vomiting, abdominal cramps
Serotype	2, 6, 8, 9, 10, 12	1, 3, 5

CLOSTRIDIUM

- *Clostridia* are gram positive, spore forming, anaerobes.
- All *Clostridia* are motile and exhibit stately motility except: *Cl. tetani VI* and *Cl. perfringens.*

- *Arrangement of spore* – Most of them possess subterminal spores except.
  - *Cl. tetani* – Spherical and terminal drum stick appearance.
  - *Cl. tertium* – Oval and terminal and tennis racket shaped.
  - *Cl.bifermentans* – Central.
- All are non-capsulated (except *Cl. perfringens, Cl. butyricum).*
- Most of the *Clostridia* are found normally in feces.

Clostridium Perfringens

- Non-motile, capsulated.
- Spores are oval, subterminal.
- They are toxigenic and invasive.
- Possess four major (lethal) toxins – α, β, ε, i.
- α toxin (lecithinase or phospholipase C) – principle virulence factor.
- Blood Agar – Produces ***Target*** Haemolysis.
- ***Shows Naegler reaction*** – due α toxin – opalescence on egg yolk media (inhibited) by antisera.

Infections:

1. Gas Gangrene

- Gas gangrene is a rapidly spreading oedematosus myonecrosis condition occurring in association with severe wounds of extensive muscle which has been contaminated with *Cl. perfringens* or other pathogenic clostridia like *Cl. novyi and Cl. septicum.*
- The condition occurs following:
  - Road accidents, wars or any other injury involving crushing of large muscle mass and contamination with pathogenic *Clostridia.*
  - Rarely, the condition may occur following surgical operations.
- *Established causes:*
  - *Cl. perfringens* type-A (most common cause of gas gangrene)
  - *Cl. novyi*
  - *Cl. septicum.*
- Gas gangrene is usually polymicrobial.
- Incubation period – Varies from hours to 6 weeks [shortest for *Cl. perfringens* (48 hour)].
- Pain and crepitus – characteristic.
- Gas gangrene strains of *Cl. perfringens* do not produce spore in tissue nor in culture media.
- *Gram staining:*
  - Gram positive bacilli without spore – *Cl. perfringens.*
  - Citron body and boat shaped gram positive bacilli – *Cl. septicum.*
  - Gram positive bacilli with oval subterminal spore – *Cl. novyi.*
- **Treatment**
  - ***Surgery*** (mainstay of treatment)
  - ***Other treatment modalities include:***
    - DOC – Penicillin + Clindamycin,

BACTERIOLOGY II

- Hyperbaric O_2
- Anti gas gangrene serum.

2. Food Poison

- Caused by Type A strains of *Cl. perfringens*
- Produces enterotoxin
- Heat resistant spores can be found contaminated with food.

3. Necrotizing Enteritis (Pigbel):

- Due to b toxin of type C strains of *Cl. perfringens.*

Clostridium Tetani

- All are motile (except type VI).
- Shows swarming on blood agar.
- Possess terminal and spherical spore (drum stick appearance).

Two Toxins

- Tetanospasmin – Blocks release of inhibitory transmitters glycine and GABA → leads to spastic paralysis.
- Telanolysin – No role in pathogenesis.

Tetanus:

- More common in warm climate and rural area with fertile soil.
- 1st symptom – masseter tone (trismus/lock jaw) then descending tetanus.
- Hands feet are spared.
- Mentation is unimpaired.
- Incubation period – 6-10 days.
- Shorter incubation period – graver the prognosis.
- Noninfectious – *no person to person spread.*
- Diagnosis is *always clinical, microscopy is unreliable.*

Treatment: All type of wounds need surgical toilet followed by:

Immunity Category	Wound < 6hr, clean, non-penetrating, no/negligible tissue damage	Other complicated wounds
Category A	Nothing required	Nothing required
Category B	Toxoid 1 dose	Toxoid 1 dose
Category C	Toxoid 1 dose	Toxoid 1 dose + HTIG
Category D	Toxoid complete dose	Toxoid complete dose+ HTIG

A: Taken complete course of TT/booster with in past 5 year.

B: Taken complete course of TT/booster with in past > 5 year – <10 year.

C: Taken complete course of TT/booster with in past >10 year.

D: Not Taken complete course of TT/booster or immunity status not known.

Antibiotic

- Can kill the organism but cannot neutralize the toxin once it is formed.
- Used only to eradicate the source of toxin.
- Has no role in treatment if toxin is already produced (after 6 hr).
- Drugs – Penicillin/metronidazole/clindamycin/erythromycin

Prevention

- Tetanus toxoid (TT) – three doses at 1-2 months interval followed by two boosters after one year and five year followed by two doses of TT at 10 yr & 16 yr.
- Others – DPT, human tetanus immunoglobulin (HTIG), combined immunization

Clostridium Botulinum

Botulinum toxin

- Most toxic known to man.
- **Mechanism of action –** *Blocks release of acetylcholine – leads to flaccid paralysis.*
- Botulinum toxin is subtyped to eight types (A-G).
- Type A, B and E – commonly causes Human disease.
- All types except C2 are-neurotoxin, ***C2-enterotoxin.***
- Type *C, D – bacteriophage coded.*
- ***Toxin used therapeutically*** – For the treatment for strabismus, blepharospasm.

Types

- ***Food borne botulism***
  - Due to *preformed toxin* contaminated with canned food
  - *Symptoms:* ***(5Ds):***
    - Diplopia
    - Dysphasia
    - Dysarthria
    - Descending (symmetric) paralysis
    - ↓ Deep tendon reflexes
    - Constipation (not diarrhea).
- ***Wound botulism*** – Due to contamination of spores to the wound surface.
- ***Infant botulism***
  - Due to spore ingestion.
  - Also known as Floppy Child syndrome.
  - *Source* – ***Honey.***
  - Affect usually <6 months age.

Clostridium Difficile

- Causes ***pseudo membranous colitis*** after prolong intake of broad spectrum antibiotics like Clindamycin, Ampicillin.
- DOC – Metronidazole followed by Vancomycin.

BACTERIOLOGY II

- Mechanism is due to liberation two types of Toxins: *Enterotoxin and Cytotoxin.*
- Toxin can be demonstrated – effect on Hep2 or ELISA.
- Since it can be found as a part of normal flora. So, *culture though is highly sensitive but not specific.*
- *Demonstration of toxin* – specific for the diagnosis.

LISTERIA MONOCYTOGENES

- Gram +ve coccobacilli, catalase +ve.
- Shows ***Tumbling*** type of motility.
- *Listeria* is motile at 25°C but nonmotile at 37°C ***(differential motility).***
- Growth improves if cultured in thioglycollate broth at **4°C (known as cold enrichment).**
- It can grow in refrigerated food and can tolerate preserving agents.
- **Lab diagnosis**
  - Media – Blood agar, chocolate agar, **PALCAM** agar.
  - ***Anton test*** – instillation to rabbit eye causes conjuntivitis.
- **Treatment**
  - DOC – Ampicillin (also penicillin).
  - Cephalosporin – not affective.

ACTINOMYCETES

- Gram +ve branching filamentous bacteria.
- Actinomyces is non acid fast and anaerobic.
- *Nocardia* – Aerobe and acid fast (1% sulfuric acid).

Actinomyces

- Causes lumpy jaw in cattle.
- Most common agent – *A. israelii.*
- They are commensal of the mouth therefore causes endogenous infection.
- Microscopy – **Sulphur granules** which are composed of organisms, i.e., gram positive bacilli.
- **Types** – Most common Cevicofacial (lower jaw), others – thoracic, abdominal, pelvic (in IUCD users).
- *A. israelii* produces
  - **Spidery molar teeth** colony in solid media.
  - **Fluffy ball** at bottom of liquid medium.

Nocardia

- Strictly aerobic.
- Partially acid fast to 5% sulfuric acid.
- Urease +ve.

- Causes exogenous infection.
- *Nocardia* – Grow on ***Sabouraud's dextrose agar.***
- Produces dry wrinkle red pigmented colony.
- For isolation of *Nocardia*, **paraffin bait technique** used.
- *Nocardia* causes:
  - Mycetoma.
  - Pulmonary infection.
  - CNS infection.

FMGE MCQ's

Corynebacterium

1. Chinese letter arrangement is seen in: [*September 2011*]

(a) Mycobacterium tuberculosis
(b) Mycobacterium leprae
(c) Corynebacterium diphtheriae
(d) Yersinia pestis.

2. Best culture media used for corynebacterium diphtheriae is: [*March 2007, Sept 2007*]

(a) LJ media
(b) Potassium tellurite media
(c) Loeffler's serum slope
(d) McConkey.

3. Chinese letter arrangement is seen in: [*March 2009*]

(a) M. tuberculosis
(b) Corynebacterium diphtheria
(c) Chlamydia trachomatis
(d) M. leprae.

4. Diphtheria toxin's mechanism of action is: [*September 2009*]

(a) Inhibiting glucose synthesis
(b) Inhibiting protein synthesis
(c) Promoting acetylcholine release
(d) Altering cyclic GMP levels.

5. Vaccine associated with encephalitis? [*September 2008*]

(a) DPT vaccine
(b) BCG vaccine
(c) Measles vaccine
(d) OPV.

6. Elek's gel precipitation test is for: [*September 2008*]

(a) Gonococcus
(b) Corynebacterium diphtheriae
(c) H. influenzae
(d) Anthrax.

7. Which of the following is known as Preiz Nocard bacillus: [*March 2006*]

(a) Corynebacterium diphtheriae
(b) Corynebacterium pseudotuberculosis
(c) H. influenzae
(d) Salmonella.

Bacillus

8. Inverted fir tree appearance is characteristic: [*March 2009*]

(a) Bacillus anthracis
(b) Hemophilus influenzae
(c) Yersinia pestis
(d) Brucella.

BACTERIOLOGY II

9. Woolsorter's disease is: [*September 2005*]

(a) Pneumonic form of anthrax
(b) Pneumonic plague
(c) Hydatid disease of the lung
(d) Caused by psittacosis.

10. Medusa head colonies on nutrient agar is seen in: [*September 2004*]

(a) Pneumococcus
(b) Legionella
(c) Brucella
(d) Bacillus anthracis.

Clostridium

11. Most common cause of gas gangrene is: [*September 2009*]

(a) Clostridium histolyticum
(b) Clostridium bifermentans
(c) Clostridium fallax
(d) Clostridium perfringens.

12. Which of the following is not manifested on day 1 after birth: [*March 2009*]

(a) Jaundice
(b) Neonatal tetanus
(c) Sepsis
(d) Meconium aspiration syndrome.

13. Swarming growth is shown by which gram positive bacilli: [*September 2009*]

(a) Clostridium tetani
(b) Clostridium welchii
(c) Proteus
(d) All of the above.

14. Elemination of tetanus in villages, true is: [*September 2006*]

(a) Rate more than 1/1000 live births
(b) Attended deliveries less than 50%
(c) Attended deliveries more than 50%
(d) Rate less than 0.1/1000 live births.

15. Pseudomembranous colitis is caused by: [*September 2005, 2010]*

(a) Pneumocystis carinii
(b) Clostridium difficile
(c) Escherichia coli
(d) Streptococcus pneumoniae.

16. Which of the following statement is true about *bacteroides*: [*September 2004*]

(a) It is gram positive bacilli
(b) It is strictly aerobic
(c) It possesses endotoxin
(d) Presence in stool culture indicates need for treatment.

ANSWERS TO FMGE MCQ's

Corynebacterium

1. Ans. (c) Corynebacterium diphtheriae

[*Ref.:* Ananthnarayan, 8th ed., page no. 232]

- Grams staining of corynebacterium show bacteria in short chains or clumps and angling each other like V or L shaped arrangements resembling characteristic Chinese letters.
- "Coryne" means irregular club-shaped.

2. Ans. (b) Potassium tellurite media

[*Ref.:* Ananthnarayan, 8th ed., page no. 233]

BACTERIOLOGY II

Potassium tellurite agar is a selective medium, so can suppress the normal flora of throat hence is the best medium for detection of carriers, convalescent and cases of diphtheria.

Culture media for C. diphtheriae →

- ❖ ***Loffler's serum slope (Enriched medium)→***
  - Growth occurs early (6-8 hours).
  - Granules are best developed in this medium.
- ❖ ***Potassium tellurite agar – (Selective medium) →***
  - ➢ 0.04% tellurite is used as selective agent.
  - ➢ Black colonies are formed in 2 days of incubation due to tellurite reduction.
  - ➢ It is the best medium for detection of carriers, convalascent and cases.

3. Ans. (b) Corynebacterium diphtheriae

[*Ref.:* Ananthnarayan, 8th ed., page no. 232]

- ❖ Refer previous (Q. 1) explanation.

4. Ans. (b) Inhibiting protein synthesis

[*Ref.:* Ananthnarayan, 8th ed., page no. 233-34]

- ❖ **Fragment A of diphtheria toxin catalyses ADP ribosylation of diphtheamiole, a novel amino acid present on elongation factor 2 (EF2). This leads to the inhibition of protein synthesis.**

Mechanism of Action of Diphtheria Toxin

- ❖ Possess two fragments – A and B.
- ❖ Fragment A – ADP ribosylation of elongation factor 2 – Inhibit on elongation factor 2 (EF 2) – inhibits protein synthesis.
- ❖ Fragment B – for transportation of fragment A inside cell.
- ❖ Toxin production depends on optimum *iron concentration* (0.1 mg per litre optimum).
- ❖ DT is coded by *bacteriophage.*
- ❖ Park William 8 strain of *C. diphtheriae* is used as a source of toxin for diphtheria toxoid.
- ❖ Pseudomonas exotoxin A has similar mechanism like Diphtheria toxin.

5. Ans. (a) DPT Vaccine

[*Ref.:* Park, 21st ed., page no. 152; 20th ed., page no. 142]

- ❖ **The most severe complication following DPT is neurological complication like encephalitis, encephalopathy, prolonged convulsion and Reye's syndrome mainly due to Pertussis component with estimated risk of 1:170,000 doses administrated.**

DPT – Diphtheria Toxoid, Tetanus Toxoid and Pertussis (whole cell or acellular component)

- ➢ *Two types of DPT available – Adsorbed toxoid and fluid toxoid*
  - *Adsorbed toxoid* is more immunogenic than fluid toxoid.
  - *Aluminum phosphate* is used in adsorbed toxoid – which is more immunogenic than hydroxide adsorbed toxoid.
  - ***Thiomersal*** used as preservative.

BACTERIOLOGY II

6. Ans. (b) Corynebacterium diphtheriae

[*Ref.:* Ananthnarayan, 8th ed., page no. 237]

- **Elek's gel precipitation test is an in vitro toxigenicity test used for corynebacterium diphtheria.**

Elek's Gel Precipitation Test:

- An immunoprecipitation test, developed in 1949.
- It is a neutralization reaction between toxin and antitoxin *in vitro.*
- The test is performed on a petri dish containing horse serum agar.
- A rectangular strip of filter paper impregnated with of diphtheria anti-toxin (1000 units/ml) is placed across the medium before the medium is solidified.
- The strain of *C. diphtheriae* to be tested for toxicity is streaked on the medium at right angle to the filter paper strip. A known toxigenic strain of *C. diphtheriae* (positive controls) and non-toxigenic strain of *C. diphtheriae* (negative control) are also inoculated along with the test strain at right angles of the strip.
- The plate is incubated at 37°C for 24-48 hours.
- After incubation the toxin produced by growth of the test strain diffuse into the agar and meets the antitoxin at optimal concentration and line of precipitation can be seen. In strains which are negative, no precipitin lines are seen.

7. Ans. (b) Corynebacterium pseudotuberculosis

[*Ref.:* Ananthnarayan, 8th ed., page no. 239]

- ***Corynebacterium pseudotuberculosis is known as Preiz Nocard bacillus.***
- **It is pathogen for animals especially livestock causes *pseudotuberculosis in sheep and suppurative lymphadenitis in horses.***
- Also know, Kleb-Loeffler's bacilli – Corynebacterium diphtheriae.

Bacillus

8. Ans. (a) Bacillus anthracis

[*Ref.:* Ananthnarayan, 8th ed., page no. 243]

In a gelatin stab, bacillus anthracis produces a growth down the stab line with lateral spikes, longer near the surface, giving an inverted fir tree appearance.

Bacillus anthracis can be differentiated from other bacillus species by various ways

- *Mc Fadyean reaction* – polypeptide capsule can be seen when stained with polychrome methylene blue.
- Gram staining: ***bamboo sticks*** appearance, chain of bacilli.
- On nutrient agar plate – ***medusa head appearance*** colony (under low power microscope).
- Gelatin stab: ***inverted fir tree*** appearance.
- Solid media with penicillin – ***string of pearl*** appearance.
- Blood agar: ***non-hemolytic colony.***

9. Ans. (a) Pneumonic form of anthrax

[*Ref.:* Ananthnarayan, 8th ed., page no. 245]

- ***Inhalational (Pneumonic) anthrax is also known as Wool Sorters' disease. The condition occurs after inhaling spores into the lungs.***
- The spores are present in the dust or in filaments of wool from infected animals, particularly in wool factories.
- Spores are ingested by alveolar macrophages and are carried to the mediastinal lymph nodes.
- Anthrax in the lungs does not cause pneumonia, but it does cause hemorrhagic mediastinitis and pulmonary edema.

	Cutaneous anthrax	Pulmonary anthrax
Also known as	Hide Porter's disease	Wool Sorter's disease
Mode of transmission	Cutaneous exposure to animal	Inhalation of spores
Main clinical feature	Malignant pustule (black eschar surrounded by non pitting edema)	hemorrhagic mediastinitis
Occupational exposure	Dock worker, butcher, abattoir, farmer	Wool factory
Frequency	Most common (95%)	Rare
Prognosis	Self-limiting	Fatal

10. Ans. (d) Bacillus anthracis

[*Ref.:* Ananthnarayan, 8th ed., page no. 243]

- On nutrient agar after 24 hr of incubation, B. anthracis produces grayish and granular colonies measuring 2-3 mm in diameter. Under low power of the microscope, the edge of the colony appear as long, interlacing chains of bacilli, resembling locks of matted hair, which gives them a **'medusa head' appearance** with an uneven surface and wavy margin.

Clostridium

11. Ans. (d) Clostridium perfringens

[*Ref.:* Ananthnarayan, 8th ed., page no. 254]

- *Cl. perfringens is the most common causes of gas gangrene.*
- Gas gangrene is a rapidly spreading edematous myonecrosis condition occurring in association with severe wounds of extensive muscle which has been contaminated with *Cl. perfringens* or other pathogenic clostridia like *Clostridium novyi and Clostridium septicum.*
- The condition occurs following road accidents or any other injury involving crushing of large muscle mass, and contamination with pathogenic clostridia. Rarely, the condition may occur following surgical operations. Extensive wounds with heavy contamination of clostridia bacteria contributed to a high number of cases seen during wars.
- Gas gangrene is rarely caused by a single Clostridium species. The aetiology of gas gangrene is usually due to multiple *Clostridium* species, and is commonly associated with anaerobic streptococci and facultative anaerobes such as *Staphylococci*, *Escherichia coli* and *Proteus.*
- ***But among all, Cl. perfringens is the most common species causing gas gangrene.***

12. Ans. (b) Neonatal tetanus

[*Ref.:* Park, 21th ed., page no. 284]

- **Neonatal tetanus manifests at 8th day following delivery, hence is also known as *"8th Day disease"*.**

13. Ans. (a) Clostridium tetani

[*Ref.:* Ananthnarayan, 8th ed., page no. 257]

- Clostridium tetani is gram +ve bacilli and can swarm on blood agar.
- Proteus is *gram –ve bacilli* and can swarm on blood agar.
- Clostridium welchii is gram +ve bacilli but does not swarm on blood agar.

Bacteria that produces Swarming on blood agar:

- Clostridium tetani
- Proteus
- Vibrio parahemolyticus
- Vibrio alginolyticus
- Serratia.

14. Ans. (d) Rate less than 0.1/1000 live births

[*Ref.:* Park, 21th ed., page no. 284]

Neonatal tetanus elimination is based on:

- Rate less than 0.1/1000 live births.
- TT coverage – >90%.
- Attended deliveries – > 75%.

15. Ans. (b) Clostridium difficile

[*Ref.:* Ananthnarayan, 8th ed., page no. 263]

- **Cl. difficile that is responsible for the development of antibiotic-associated diarrhea and colitis known as *pseudomembranous colitis* following broad spectrum antibiotics like clindamycin.**

> - ***Pseudomembranous colitis***
> - Mechanism is due to liberation two types of toxins by clostridium difficile : *Enterotoxin and Cytotoxin.*
> - Since clostridium difficile can be found as a part of normal flora.
> - So, *culture though is highly sensitive but not specific.*
> - *Demonstration of toxin* – specific for the diagnosis.
> - DOC – Metronidazole followed by Vancomycin.

16. Ans. (c) It possesses endotoxin

[*Ref.:* Ananthnarayan, 8th ed., page no. 267]

Bacteroides are:

- *Gram negative bacilli.*

- *Non-sporing strict anaerobe.*
- Since they are *gram negative,* possess endotoxin in cell wall.
- They are the *most common commensal present in GIT.*
- So, they can always be present in stool culture and it does not indicate need for treatment.

Bacteroides

- Most common anaerobes isolated in clinical specimen.
- Virulence factor – capsular polysaccharide and LPS.
- Classified to:
  - Porphyromonas (Asaccharolytic).
  - Prevotella (moderately Saccharolytic).
  - Bacteroides proper (Saccharolytic) – B. fragilis.

Also know, the anaerobic/aerobic Ratio in human GIT flora:

- 1:1 (stomach, ileum, jejunum, saliva).
- 10^3 : 1 (terminal ileum and colon and gingival crevices).
- 10:1 (female genital tract).

PRACTICE MCQ's

1. Culture media for corynebacterium diphtheriae:

(a) Loeffler's serum slope
(b) TCBS media
(c) Wilson blair media
(d) Lowenstein Jensen medium.

2. Malignant pustule is seen in infection with:

(a) Clostridum tetani
(b) Bacillus anthracis
(c) Bacillus cereus
(d) Yersinia pestis

3. Erythrasma is caused by:

(a) Corynebacterium minutissimum
(b) Corynebacterium xerosis
(c) Corynebacterium ulcerans
(d) Corynebacterium diphtheriae.

4. Drum stick appearance of spore (terminal and spherical) seen in:

(a) Cl. tetani
(b) Cl. tertium
(c) Cl. perfringens
(d) Cl. histolyticum.

5. Diptheria toxin acts by

(a) Increasing levels of cAMP
(b) Inhibiting protein synthesis
(c) Inhibitng acetylcholine release
(d) Inhibiting glucose transport.

ANSWERS TO PRACTICE MCQ's

1. Ans. (a) Loeffler's serum slope

[*Ref.:* Ananthnarayan, 8th ed., page no. 233]

2. Ans. (b) Bacillus anthracis

[*Ref.:* Ananthnarayan, 8th ed., page no. 245]

Cutaneous lesions of B. anthracis is painless characteristic black eschar surrounded by non-pitting, gelatinous edema called 'malignant pustule'.

Malignant pustule:

- The disease begins as a painless; pruritic papule which becomes a 1-2 cm vesicle within 2 days.
- The vesicle is filled with clear or serosanguineous fluid containing very rare leucocytes and numerous large, gram positive bacilli.
- A characteristic ***non pitting, gelatinous*** edema surrounds the lesion. The vesicle enlarges and satellite vesicles may develop.
- Subsequently, the vesicle ruptures, undergoes necrosis and enlarges, forming an ulcer covered by a characteristic black eschar.
- The skin in surrounding areas may become edematous and necrotic but not purulent.
- The name anthrax, meaning coal, comes from the eschar which is black coloured.
- The lesion is called malignant pustule after their characteristic appearance, although the lesions are neither malignant nor pustular.
- ***Lesions are painless*** but on occasion are slightly pruritic.
- Occasionally, multiple bullae develop along with marked toxic effects, and the lesions especially on the face or neck becomes massively oedematous.

3. Ans. (a) Corynebacterium minutissimum

[*Ref.:* Ananthnarayan, 8th ed., page no. 239]

- *Erythrasma is a localized infection of stratum corneum usually affecting axilla and groin caused by corynebacterium minutissimum.*

4. Ans. (a) Cl. tetani

[*Ref.:* Ananthnarayan, 8th ed., page no. 249]

- **Arrangement of Spore:** Most of the Clostridia possess subterminal spores except:
  - *Cl. tetani* – Spherical and terminal drum stick Appearance.
  - *Cl. tertium* – Oval and terminal – tennis racket shaped.
  - *Cl. bifermentans* – Central.

5. Ans. (b) Inhibiting protein synthesis

[*Ref.:* Ananthnarayan, 8th ed., page no. 234]

- Refer text.

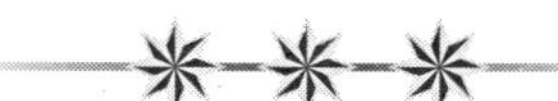

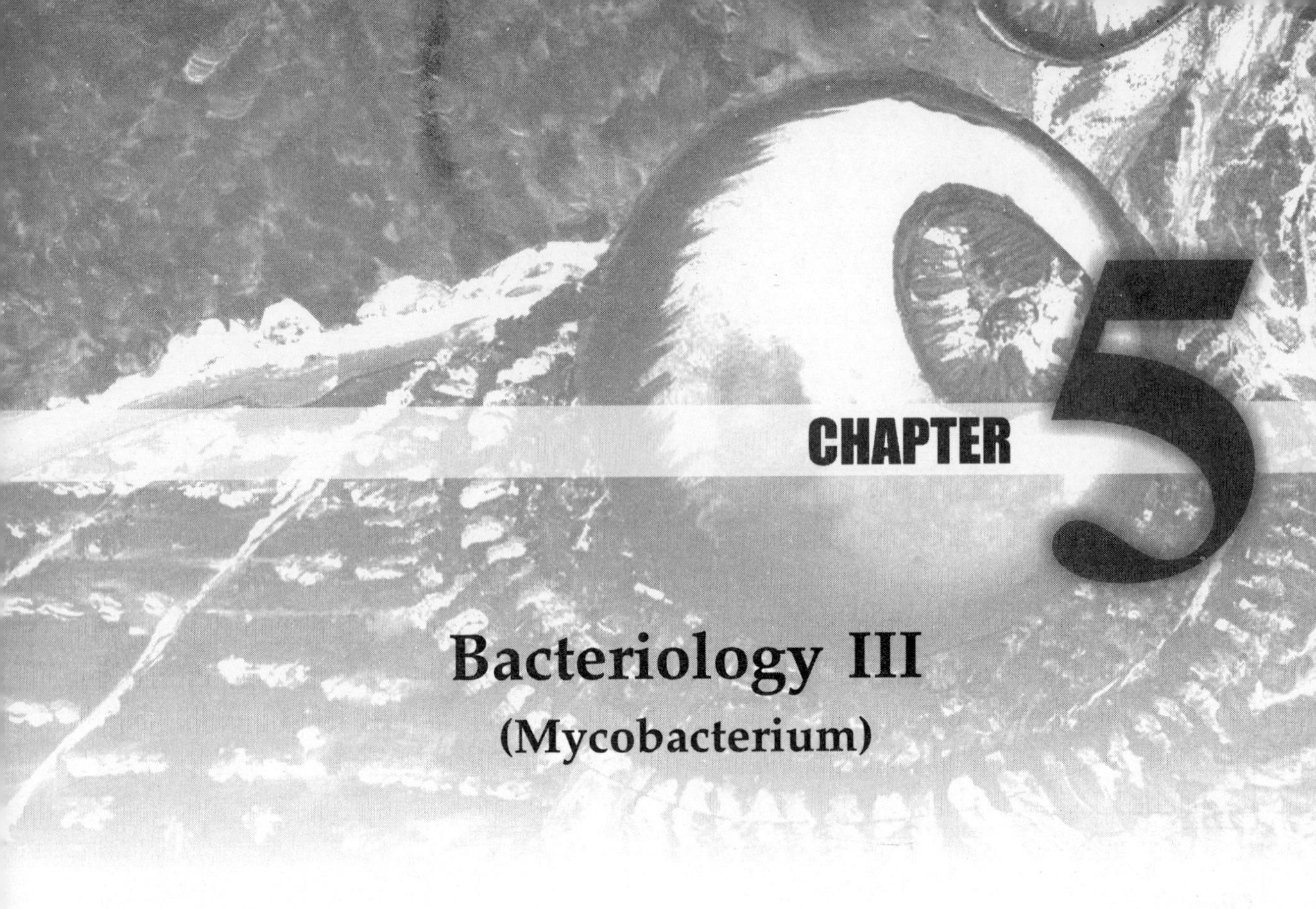

Bacteriology III
(Mycobacterium)

- ❖ **Mycobacterium:** Name was derived from their branching filamentous form and mould like pellicle in liquid media.

Acid Fast Organism

Acid fastness is due to mycolic acid and integrity of cell wall.

Examples-

- ❖ *Mycobacteria:*
  - *M. tuberculosis*
  - *M. leprae*
  - *Non-tuberculous Mycobacteria*
- ❖ *Nocardia*
- ❖ *Rhodococcus*
- ❖ *Spore*
- ❖ *Sperm head*
- ❖ *Parasite:*
  - *Cryptosporidium*
  - *Cyclospora*
  - *Isospora*
  - *Tinea scolex.*

MYCOBACTERIUM TUBERCULOSIS

- ❖ Generation time – 14-15 hours.
- ❖ Incubation period – 6-8 week.

***M tuberculosis* complex** – include genetically related species:

- ❖ *M. tuberculosis*
- ❖ *M. bovis* (bovine tubercle bacillus).
- ❖ *M. africanum* (intermediate between M. tuberculosis and M. bovis).
- ❖ *M. microti* (vole tubercle bacillus).

M. tuberculosis	M. bovis
Shape – Curved, long, beaded, less uniformly stained	Straight, short, stout, uniformly stained
Rough, tough, buff colony	White, smooth, moist colony
Eugonic growth	Dysgonic growth
Niacin test +ve Nitrate test +ve	Niacin –ve Nitrate –ve
Not pathogenic to rabbit	Pathogenic to rabbit
Obligate aerobe	Microaerophilic
Both are equally pathogenic to human	

Clinical Feature

Pulmonary Tuberculosis

Primary Pulmonary tuberculosis:

- ❖ Affect children.
- ❖ Subpleural focus in lower lobe of lungs (Ghon) + hilar LN↑ = **called as primary complex.**
- ❖ Ghon focus + Fibrosis and calcification – Ranke complex.

Post primary pulmonary tuberculosis:

- ❖ Affect adult.
- ❖ Upper lobe focus (Simons focus).
- ❖ LN spread rare, hematogenous spread seen.
- ❖ Necrosis, cavitations seen.
- ❖ Infra clavicular lesion – Assman focus.

Extrapulmonary TB

- ❖ Most common site LN (cervical) followed by pleural TB.
- ❖ Skeletal TB – Most common site is spine.
- ❖ TB meningitis.
- ❖ GI TB – Most common site caecum, ileum.
- ❖ TB pericarditis – Most common cause of chronic constrictive pericarditis.
- ❖ Scrofuloderma – Skin lesion d/t breakdown of underlying TB foci (usually lymph node).
- ❖ ***Lupus vulgaris:***
  - ➢ Most common TB skin lesion
  - ➢ Female

BACTERIOLOGY III

- ➢ Face and neck
- ➢ Apple jelly nodule
- ➢ ↑ Risk for malignant (Sq cell Ca).

Laboratory Diagnosis

- ➢ ***Two sputum samples*** are collected – early morning and spot.
- ➢ **Digestion and decontamination procedures for sputum:**
  - Petroff's method (4% Na OH).
  - Others – N acetyl cysteine, Oxalic acid.

AFB smear: Ziehl Neelsen staining – detection limit 10^4 bacilli/ml of sputum.

- ➢ RNTCP (Revised National Tuberculosis Control Programme) recommended method.
- ➢ *Used for:*
  - Monitoring the treatment.
  - Assessing the severity of the disease.
  - Determining the infectiousness of the patient.

Fluorescent staining – Auramine/rhodamine. Used for rapid screening.

Culture: Detection limit ***10 to 100*** viable organism

- More specific and sensitive than smear.
- But takes 6-8 weeks time to grow.

Solid media

- ➢ Egg based – ***Lowenstein Jensen***, Dorset egg media.
- ➢ Blood Based Media, e.g., Tarshis.

Automated culture method – Detects growth faster

- ➢ BATEC.
- ➢ BacT/ALERT.
- ➢ Polymerase Chain Reaction (PCR) – More sensitive and quick.
- ➢ Serology – Not much useful.

Diagnosis of Latent TBL:

Tuberculin Test:

- ➢ **Mantoux test:** The test is performed by intradermal injection of 0.1 ml or 5 TU purified protein derivative (PPD) to forearm. Induration and erythema is produced after 72 hr.
- ➢ Test is read after 72 hr and only induration is measured (not erythema)
- ➢ ***Induration:***
  - >10 mm – **Positive**
  - 6-9 mm – (**equivocal/doubtful**) due to BCG/NTM
  - <5 mm – **Negative.**

- ***Other Tuberculin Test:***
  - Heaf test (multiple puncture)
  - Tine test – Disposable prong with dried PPD.
- ***Positive Tuberculin Test Indicates:***
  - Past exposure in adult.
  - Active infection in infants.
  - Prevalence of infection in a community.
- ***False –ve Tuberculin Test:***
  - Early/advanced TB
  - Miliary TB
  - Post measles
  - ↓ immunity.
- ***False + Tuberculin Test:***
  - After BCG vaccination.
  - Atypical mycobacterial infection.
- Repeated test at different site – false –ve/equivocal reaction may turn +ve.

BCG Vaccination

- Name derived from – Bacilli Calmette Guerin.
- Efficacy varies from 0-80%.
- Immunity last for 15-20 yr.
- ***BCG strain*** (***Danish 1331 strain***) – Derived from live attenuated ***M. bovis*** grown in glycerol bile potato medium.
- ***Dose: 0.1 mg/0.1 ml strength (0.05 ml for <4 week).***
- ***Mode of administration – Intradermally to arm just above the insertion of deltoid. Normal saline is recommended*** as diluents for BCG vaccine
- The site for injection should be cleaned thoroughly with soap ***but disinfectant or antiseptic should not be used***.
- Tuberculin test is positive after ***8 weeks of BCG vaccination*** but in some it might require 14 weeks.
- ***Indication of BCG Vaccination***
  - Newborn soon after birth
  - No need after two year as natural immunity develops following exposure to environmental TB bacilli.
- ***Contraindication of BCG Vaccination***
  - Patient with active HIV
  - ↓Immunity
  - AFB +ve mother
  - Generalized eczema.

Sensitivity Testing:

- Resistance ratio method.
- Absolute concentration method.

- Proportion method – RNTCP recommended.
- Radio metric method.
- Molecular methods.

Drug Resistance in Tuberculosis

- ***Main mechanism of Drug Resistance in Tuberculosis is – Mutation in M. tuberculosis genome.***

MDRTB (Multi drug resistance **Tuberculosis**) – Resistant to INH and Rifampicin +/Resistant to other 1st line drug like Ethambutol, Streptomycin and Pyrazinamide.

XDRTB (Extended drug resistance **Tuberculosis**) – MDRTB + Resistant to quinolone + Resistant to aminoglycoside (amikacin/capreomycin/kanamycin).

Neonatal Tuberculosis

- Before delivery:
  - If mother chest X-ray and sputum AFB +ve then, mother is given ATT.
- After delivery:
  - If mother chest X-ray and sputum AFB +ve then, mother to be given ATT + baby for 9-12 months) + screening of household contacts.
  - Separation from mother or with hold of breast feeding is not recommended.

NTM/MOTT/ATYPICAL MYCOBACTERIA

Atypical (Environmental) Mycobacteria

Runyon group		Species
I. Photo chromogen	Pigmentation only in light	M. marinum, M. asciaticum, M. simiae, M. kansasii (MASK)
II. Scoto chromogen	Pigmentations in light and dark	M. scrofulaceum, M. szulgai, S.gordonae (SSG)
III. Non-chromogen	No pigmentation	MAC, M. xenopi M. ulcerans
IV. Rapid growers	Grows within a week	M. chelonei, M. fortuitum

Diseases Caused by Atypical Mycobacterium:

- ***Post trauma/injection abscess*** – *M. chelonei, M. fortuitum.*
- ***Swimming pool granuloma*** – *M. marinum.*
- ***Buruli ulcer*** – *M. ulcerans.*
- Mycobacteria causing Johnes disease – *M. paratuberculosis.*
- Lymphadenopathy – *M. avium intracellulare, M. scrofulaceum.*
- Pulmonary disease – *M. avium intracellulare, M. kansasii.*
- Disseminated disease – *M. avium intracellulare.*

MYCOBACTERIUM LEPRAE

- Non-cultivable on artificial medium.
- Generation time – 20 days.

- Grows well in cooler part of body (skin, testes, peripheral nerve, anterior eye).
- Acid fast to 5% H_2SO_4.
- Arrangement of the lepra bacilli:
  - Intracellularly as parallel **cigar** like bundles of bacilli bound with lipid like glia **(globi)** which is present inside foamy macrophage (known as **Virchow's leprae cell).**
- Bacteriological index (BI) – Total number of leprae bacilli.
- Morphological index (MI) – The percent of solid uniformly stained live bacilli in tissues.
- morphological index is more meaningful for assessing the progress of patients on chemotherapy.

Epidemiology

- *Transmission* – nasal secretion.
- *Incubation Period* – 2-5 year.
- Not highly communicable, intimate and prolong contact necessary.
- *Most affected area* – Southeast Asia and Brazil. In India (Most common: Bihar > Orissa > UP).

Animal Model

- Foot pad of mouse (Shepard model).
- Nine banded armadillo is highly susceptible to leprosy, due to low body temperature.

Classification

- Ridley Jopling classification – TT, BT, BB, BL, LL.
- Madrid classification – LL, TT, borderline/dimorphous, indeterminate (early unstable type).
- Indian classification – Madrid + pure neuritic type.

Lepromatous	Tuberculoid
AFB +++ Multibacillary	AFB +/–, Paucibacillary
Skin lesion many, poorly marginated, Leonine facies seen	Few, sharply demarcated and symmetric
Nerve lesion – late	Early anesthetic skin lesion
Lepromin test: –ve	Lepromin test +ve
Humoral – Auto Antibodies +ve	Humoral – Auto Antibodies –ve
CMI – low	CMI – normal
Biological false +ve VDRL test in syphilis	Biological false +ve VDRL test –ve
Involve any organ – *except CNS and lungs,* also warm area of skin (axilla, groin, scalp)	*MC nerve involved* – Ulnar > post auricular medial popliteal N – never involved.

Lepromin Test

- 0.1 ml lepromin given i/d.
- Early/Fernandez Reaction – 2-3 days – Induration like tuberculin (DTH) – indicates past infection (not useful).
- Late/Mitsuda Reaction 3-4 weeks – nodule, necrosis, ulcer.
- It measure of CMI induced by injected lepromin (does not say about the past exposure).

- Uses of lepromin test:
  - Classify lesions of leprosy
  - Assess prognosis
  - Assess resistance to leprosy in individuals.

Type I: Lepra Reaction:

- Type of hypersensitivity reaction IV.
- Seen with borderline leprosy.
- If occurs before t/t – ***down grading reaction*** occurs towards LL.
- If occurs after t/t – ***upgrading reaction*** occurs towards TT.
- Most common feature- edema.
- $\uparrow$ T cell ($\gamma\delta$ TCT).
- Most common nerve – Ulnar Nerve.
- Treatment DOC – glucocorticoid.

Type II: Reaction:

- Type of hypersensitivity reaction III.
- Seen with Lepromatous variety (BL, LL).
- Usually follows sulfonamide therapy, but may precede treatment.
- Most common feature – crop of painful erythematous papule and nodule [Erythematous nodosum leprosum (ENL)].
- Central cytokine involves – TNFα.
- Treatment: DOC – thalidomide, glucocorticoid, clofazemine and antipyretics.

Lab diagnosis:

- Sample: Total six sample:
  - Minimum four skin (slit skin smear)
  - Ear lobule
  - Nasal mucosa.
- Acid fast staining with 5% sulfuric acid as decolorizer.
- Grading of smear is done based on MI.
- Mouse food pad inoculation.
- Antibody to PGL1(Phenolic Glycolipid).

Treatment:

Paucibacillary	(I, TT, BT)	Rifampicin (monthly) + dapsone daily – for 6months
Multibacillary	(BB,BL, LL)	Rifampicin (monthly) + dapsone daily + clofazemine daily – till two years or smear –ve
Single lesion	ROM therapy (Rifampicin + Ofloxacin + Minocycline) – single dose	

FMGE MCQ's

1. **Apple jelly nodule is a feature of:** [*March 2011*]
   (a) Aspergillosis (b) Rhinoscleroma
   (c) Erysipelas (d) Lupus vulgaris.
2. **Cavitation of the lungs is not a feature of:** [*March 2011*]
   (a) Bronchiectasis (b) Primary pulmonary tuberculosis
   (c) Secondary pulmonary tuberculosis (d) Bronchogenic carcinoma.
3. **Mantoux test is an example of:** [*March 2008*]
   (a) Hypersensitivity reaction type I (b) Hypersensitivity reaction type II
   (c) Hypersensitivity reaction type III (d) Hypersensitivity reaction type IV.
4. **Culture medium for cultivation of Mycobacterium tuberculosis is:** [*September 2005*]
   (a) Ludlam's medium (b) Loeffler's serum
   (c) Thayer-Martin medium (d) LJ medium.
5. **Confirmatory test for tuberculosis is:** [*September 2006*]
   (a) Gram's staining (b) AFB
   (c) Guinea-pig inoculation (d) Tuberculin testing.
6. **M. avium intracellularae is an example of:** [*September 2009*]
   (a) Non-chromogens (b) Scotochromogens
   (c) Photochromogens (d) Rapid growers.
7. **Swimming pool granuloma is caused by:** [*March 2010, 2009*]
   (a) Mycobacterium chelonae (b) Mycobacterium kansasii
   (c) Mycobacterium marinum (d) Mycobacterium ulcerans.
8. **Ghon's focus reflects:** [*September 2005*]
   (a) Miliary tuberculosis (b) Primary complex
   (c) Tuberculous lymphadenitis (d) Post primary tuberculosis.
9. **Mycobacterium leprae can be cultured in:** [*September 2006*]
   (a) Testes of guinea pig (b) LJ medium
   (c) Footpad of mice (d) Testes of albino rats.
10. **BCG should be given:** [*September 2005*]
    (a) Immediately after birth (b) At the age of 1 month
    (c) At the age of 6 months (d) At the age of 1 year.
11. **BCG vaccine is diluted with:** [*September 2005*]
    (a) Normal saline (b) Distilled water
    (c) Dextrose (d) Colloids.
12. **The animal model frequently used for M. Leprae is:** [*March 2010*]
    (a) Mice (b) Guinea pig
    (c) Rabbits (d) Golden hamsters.
13. **Drug resistance in tuberculosis is due to:** [*September 2005*]
    (a) Transformation (b) Transduction
    (c) Conjugation (d) Mutation.

14. Buruli ulcer is caused by: [*September 2002*]

(a) Streptococcus
(b) Spirillium minus
(c) M. ulcerans
(d) Brucella.

15. Which does not cause skin involvement: [*September 2007*]

(a) M. tuberculosis
(b) M. ulcerans
(c) M. marinum
(d) M. kansasii.

16. Which of the following is scotochromogen: [*March 2010*]

(a) M. scrofulaceum
(b) M. ulcerans
(c) M. kansasii
(d) M. fortuitum.

17. The mycobacteria which grows in culture within 1 weeks are: [*September 2010*]

(a) M. kansasii
(b) M. leprae
(c) M. chelonei
(d) M. avium intracellulare.

ANSWERS TO FMGE MCQ's

1. Ans. (d) Lupus vulgaris

[*Ref.:* Wikipedia]

Apple jelly nodules are minute, yellowish or reddish brown, translucent nodules, seen on diascopic examination of the lesions of lupus vulgaris.

Lupus vulgaris:

- Most common type of cutaneous tuberculosis.
- Presents as painful cutaneous tuberculosis skin lesions with nodular appearance, most often on the face around nose, eyelids, lips, cheeks and ears.
- Small sharply defined reddish-brown lesions (called as apple-jelly nodules).
- Lesions persist for years, leading to disfigurement and sometimes skin cancer.

2. Ans. (b) Primary pulmonary tuberculosis

[*Ref.:* Ananthnarayan, 8th ed., page no. 351]

"Cavitaion is a feature of post primary (secondary) Pulmonary tuberculosis, it is never seen in primary tuberculosis."

Primary pulmonary tuberculosis	Post primary pulmonary tuberculosis
Occurs due to 1st time exposure to Tb bacilli	Due to endogenous reactivation or exogenous reinfection
Affect children	Affect adult
Lower lobe of lungs (*Ghon focus*)	Upper lobe focus (Simons focus)
Ghon focus + Hilar lymphadenopathy = k/a Primary complex	LN spread rare
Necrosis, cavitations never seen	Necrosis, cavitations seen
Ghon focus + associated fibrosis and calcification– k/a Ranke complex	Infra clavicular lesion– k/a *Assman focus*

3. Ans. (d) Hypersensitivity reaction type IV

[*Ref.:* Ananthnarayan, 8th ed., page no. 356]

- ❖ A positive mantoux (tuberculin test) indicates hypersensitivity type IV of the individual to tubercle protein.

Tuberculin Test

- ➢ *Mantoux test:* The test is performed by intradermal injection of 0.1 ml or 5 TU purified protein derivative (PPD) to forearm. Induration and erythema is produced after 72 hr.
- ➢ Test is read after 72 hr and only induration is measured (not erythema).
- ➢ *Induration:*
  - >10 mm – Positive.
  - 6-9 mm – (equivocal/doubtful) due to BCG/NTM)
  - <5 mm – Negative.
- ➢ *Other Tuberculin test:*
  - Heaf test (multiple puncture).
  - Tine test – disposable prong with dried PPD.

4. Ans. (d) LJ medium

[*Ref.:* Ananthnarayan, 8th ed., page no. 348]

- ❖ ***Lowenstein Jensen (LJ) medium is the RNTCP recommended culture medium for tuberculosis.***
- ❖ LJ medium without starch is most widely used and is also the medium recommended by the international union against tuberculosis (IUAT).
- ❖ The LJ medium consists of coagulated whole egg, asparagines, malachite green, mineral salt and glycerol or sodium pyruvate. Malachite green inhibits growth of bacteria other than my.cobacterium.

Other options:

- ❖ *Ludlam's medium:* Selective medium for Staphylococcus aureus.
- ❖ *Loeffler's serum:* Enriched medium for Corynebacterium diphtheriae.
- ❖ *Thayer-Martin medium:* Selective medium for Neisseria.

5. Ans. (c) Guinea-pig inoculation

[*Ref.:* Ananthnarayan, 8th ed., page no. 355]

- ❖ Ideal methods for confirmatory test for tuberculosis:
  - Culture followed by Biochemical test like niacin test
  - Molecular test detecting the specific M. tuberculosis specific genes.
- ❖ *Acid fast stain* – Though the typical beaded long slender filamentous form is more suggestive of M.tuberculosis but since it is just a staining method, it cannot be considered as a confirmatory test.
- ❖ *Animal inoculation* – Pathogenicity testing by inoculation in guinea pigs was earlier widely used for confirmation of diagnosis of tuberculosis. But guinea pig inoculation is now regarded as obsolete because it is cumbersome, costly and less sensitive than culture.
- ❖ Tuberculin test is indicates of past exposure and it cannot be used for diagnosis (except in children).

6. Ans. (a) Non-chromogens

[*Ref.:* Ananthnarayan, 8th ed., page no. 359]

- ❖ Non-photochromogens are the mycobacteria which donot produce pigment in dark, or on exposure to light. These include ***Mycobacterium avium* complexes (MAC), *M. xenopi* and *M. ulcerans*.**

Classification of Atypical (Environmental) Mycobacterium:

Runyon group		Species
I. Photo chromogen	Pigmentation only in light	*M. marinum,* *M. asciaticum,* *M. simiae,* *M. kansasii* ***(MASK)***
II. Scoto chromogen	Pigmentations in light and dark	*M. scrofulaceum,* *M. szulgai,* *S. gordonae* ***(SSG)***
III. Non-chromogen	No pigmentation	*MAC,* *M. xenopi,* *M. ulcerans*
IV. Rapid growers	Grows within a week	*M. chelonei,* *M. fortuitum,* *M. smegmatis*

7. Ans. (c) Mycobacterium marinum

[*Ref.:* Ananthnarayan, 8th ed., page no. 359]

- ❖ *M. marinum is the causative agent of swimming pool or fish tank granuloma. This condition is associated with development of superficial granulomatous lesions in the skin.*
- ❖ Also know, ***swimming pool conjunctivitis*** – caused by Chlamydia trachomatis and Adenovirus.

8. Ans. (b) Primary complex

[*Ref.:* Ananthnarayan, 8th ed., page no. 351]

- ❖ Primary tuberculosis is commonly found in the lower lobe or in the lower part of the upper lobe of the lungs. This subpleural focus is known as Ghon's focus.
- ❖ This focus is also associated with enlargement of the hilar lymphnodes.
- ❖ Both Ghon's focus and enlarged lymph nodes constitute the ***primary complex*** which usually develops in 3-8 weeks after infection by tubercle bacilli.

9. Ans. (c) Footpad of mice

[*Ref.:* Ananthnarayan, 8th ed., page no. 364]

- ❖ The mouse foot pad inoculation method is now being used as a standard procedure for cultivation and maintenance of *M. leprae.*
- ❖ Intradermal inoculation of lepra bacillus into foot pad of mice results in development of granuloma at the site of inoculation in 1 month to 6 months.
- ❖ The mouse foot pad model has been used to test the maximum required concentration of anti leprosy drugs and sensitivity of the bacilli to new anti leprosy drugs.

- ❖ Also remember:
  - M. leprae cannot be cultivable in artificial culture media or cell lines.
  - It does not follow Koch's postulate.
- Only way of maintenance of M. lepare is animal models – like food pad of mice and nine banded Armadillo.

10. Ans. (a) Immediately after birth

[*Ref.:* Ananthnarayan, 8th ed., page no. 357; Park, 21st ed., page no. 177, 20th ed., page no. 171]

- ❖ BCG vaccine is recommended to infants ***usually soon after birth*** or as early as possible before 12 months age and there is no need to give BCG after 2 years of time. *–Ananthnarayan*

11. Ans. (a) Normal saline

[*Ref.:* Ananthnarayan, 8th ed., page no. 357; Park's, 21st ed., page no. 176-77; 20th ed., page no. 171]

- ❖ **Normal saline is recommended as diluents for BCG vaccine as distilled water is irritant.**
- ❖ The site for injection should be cleaned thoroughly with soap **but disinfectant or antiseptic should not be used.** If alcohol is used then it should be evaporated before the vaccination is given.

BCG Vaccination

- ❖ Name derived from – Bacilli Calmette Guerin.
- ❖ Efficacy varies from 0-80%.
- ❖ Immunity last for 15-20 year.
- ❖ **BCG strain (Danish 1331 strain):** Derived from live attenuated *M bovis* grown in glycerol bile potato medium.
- ❖ **Dose:** 0.1 mg/0.1 ml strength (0.05 ml for <4 week).
- ❖ **Mode of administration:** Intradermally to arm just above the insertion of deltoid.
- ❖ ***Normal saline is recommended*** **as diluents for BCG vaccine.**
- ❖ The site for injection should be cleaned thoroughly with soap *but disinfectant or antiseptic should not be used.*
- ❖ If alcohol is used to clean skin, it should be allowed to dry up.
- ❖ Tuberculin test is positive after *8 weeks of BCG vaccination* but in some it might require 14 weeks.
- ❖ ***Indication of BCG Vaccination*:**
  - Newborn soon after birth.
  - No need after two year as natural immunity develops following exposure to environmental TB bacilli.
- ❖ ***Contraindication of BCG Vaccination:***
  - Patient with active HIV.
  - AFB +ve mother.
  - ↓Immunity.
  - Generalized eczema.

12. Ans. (a) Mice

[*Ref.:* Ananthnarayan, 8th ed., page no. 364]

- *The mouse foot pad inoculation method is now being used as a standard procedure for cultivation and maintenance of M. leprae.*

13. Ans. (d) Mutation

[*Ref.:* Ananthnarayan, 8th ed., page no. 357]

- Emergence of natural drug resistance in M. tuberculosis is a major problem in chemotherapy of tuberculosis. This occurs by mutation with a frequency of once appropriately 10^8 cell division. This can be affectively checked by multidrug therapy. *–Ananthnarayan*

Drug	Mutation occurs in gene
INH (Isoniazid)	Kat G gene, Inh A gene, ahp C
R (Rifampicin)	rpo B gene (RNA polymerase B)
Z (Pyrazinamide)	Pnc A (Pyrazinamidase)
E (Ethambutol)	emb A, B, C (Arabinosyl transferase)
S (Streptomycin)	Ribosomal protein subunit 12 (rpSL)

14. Ans. (c) M. ulcerans

[*Ref.:* Ananthnarayan, 8th ed., page no. 361]

- *M. ulcerans* is a skin pathogen which was originally isolated from human ulcerative skin lesions in Australia (1958). Subsequently this species causing similar cutaneous lesions have been documented from Uganda (known as ***Buruli Ulcer***) and other places like Nigeria, Congo, Malaysia, New Guinea and Mexico *–Ananthnarayan*
- *M. ulcerans* grows slowly on LJ medium in 4-8 weeks when incubated at 31-34°C.
- It is the only known mycobacterial species to produce exotoxins.
- ***Buruli's ulcer:*** Ulcers of the skin are typically seen on the legs or on the arms. After an incubation period of few weeks, initially the infection begins by minor injuries on the skin through which mycobacteria gain access. The infection begins with the appearance of an indurated nodule at the site of inoculation which breaks down forming indolent ulcer. Diagnosis of the condition is made by the microscopy of the smears, collected from the edge of the ulcer. Large numbers of acid-fast and alcohol-fast bacilli are seen in the stained smear by microscopy. Finally, the ulcer heals with the formation of scars.

15. Ans. (d) M. kansasii

[*Ref.:* Ananthnarayan, 8th ed., page no. 359]

- **M. kansasii causes disease identical to pulmonary tuberculosis. It does not affect the skin.**

Mycobacteria that affects skin:

- M. ulcerans – Buruli's ulcer.
- M. marinum – Swimming pool conjunctivitis.
- M. tuberculosis – Lupus vulgaris.
- M. leprae – Leprosy.

M. kansasii

- ❖ Causes disease identical to pulmonary tuberculosis.
- ❖ This condition is associated with formation of cavity and scarring, usually in the upper lobe of the lungs.
- ❖ This species is the second most common NTM next to *Mycobacterium avium* complex as causative agent of lung diseases.
- ❖ These strains have been frequently isolated from ***tap water*** and the infected tap water is believed to be the major source of infection.

Human infections caused by NTM	Diseases
M. kansasii	Pulmonary disease
M. marinum	Swimming pool granuloma
M. simiae	Pulmonary disease (rare)
M. scrofulaceum	Lymphadenopathy
M. gordoni	Puimonary disease (rare)
M. szulgai	Pulmonary disease and bursitis (occasional)
M. xenopi	Chronic pulmonary disease
M. avium complex	Pulmonary disease, lymphadenopathy, disseminated disease
M. ulcerans	Buruli ulcer
M. fortuitum & M. chelonae	Post-trauma chronic abscesses

16. Ans. (a) M. scrofulaceum

[*Ref.:* Ananthnarayan, 8th ed., page no. 359]

- ❖ Scotochromogens are characterized by their ability to produce yellow, orange or red pigmented colonies on the LJ medium even when incubated in the dark.
- ❖ These species are widely distributed in the environment. M. scrofulaceum, M. gordonae and M. szlugai are the important species.

17. Ans. (c) M. chelonei

[*Ref.:* Ananthnarayan, 8th ed., page no. 360]

- ❖ Rapid growers is a heterogenous group of mycobacteria which produce visible growth on LJ medium rapidly within 1 week of incubation at 37°C.
- ❖ These species are **M. fortuitum, M. chelonei, M. abscesses, M. smegmatis and M. phlei.**

PRACTICE MCQ's

1. Dorset egg medium is used for cultivation of:

(a) Staphylococcus
(b) Streptococcus
(c) Gonococcus
(d) M. TB.

2. True about M. tuberculosis is:

(a) Strict aerobes
(b) Gram negative
(c) Thin cell wall
(d) Endotoxin present.

3. Acid fastness of tubercle bacilli is attributed to:

(a) Presence of mycolic acid
(b) Integrity of cell wall
(c) Both of the above
(d) None of the above.

4. Reactivation of TB is almost exclusively a disease of:

(a) Bone
(b) Lymph nodes
(c) Lung
(d) Brain.

5. The commonest focus of Scrofuloderma is:

(a) Lung
(b) Lymph node
(c) Larynx
(d) Skin.

6. Collection of urine sample of a patient of TB/kidney:

(a) 24 hrs urine
(b) 12 hrs urine
(c) In early morning
(d) Any time.

7. Rapid examination of tubercle bacilli is possible with:

(a) Ziehl-Neelsen stain
(b) Kin young stain
(c) Auramine-Rhodamine stain
(d) Giemsa stain.

8. Tuberculin test positive is depended on:

(a) Erythema
(b) Nodule formation
(c) Induration
(d) Ulcerative change.

9. The following test is not used for diagnosis of leprosy:

(a) Lepromin test
(b) Slit skin smear
(c) Fine needle aspiration cytology
(d) Skin biopsy.

10. Mitsuda reaction is read after:

(a) 3 days
(b) 3 hours
(c) 3 weeks
(d) 3 months.

11. Johne's bacillus is:

(a) Corynebacterium pseudotuberculosis
(b) M. paratuberculosis
(c) H. aegypticus
(d) K. pneumoniae.

12. Lepra cells found in lepromatous leprosy are:

(a) Neutrophils
(b) Lymphocytes
(c) Macrophages
(d) Plasma cells.

ANSWERS TO PRACTICE MCQ's

1. Ans. (d) M. TB

[*Ref.:* Ananthnarayan, 8th ed., page no. 348]

The examples of solid medium for M. tuberculosis are:

- Egg containing media [Lowenstein Jensen (LJ) medium, Petragnini and ***Dorset egg medium***]

BACTERIOLOGY III

- ❖ Blood containing media (Tarshis medium)
- ❖ Serum containing media (Loeffler's)
- ❖ Potato based media (Powlowsky medium).

2. Ans. (a) Strict aerobes

[*Ref.:* Ananthnarayan, 8th ed., page no. 347-48]

- ❖ **M. tuberculosis is:**
  - Strict aerobes (M. bovis is microaerophilic).
  - Gram positive (hence no endotoxin).
  - Thick cell wall (due to mycolic acid).

3. Ans. (c) Both of the above

[*Ref.:* Ananthnarayan, 8th ed., page no. 348]

- ❖ *Acid fastness of tubercle bacilli is attributed to lipid rich unsaponified waxy cell wall made up mycolic acid and also due to integrity of cell wall.*

4. Ans. (c) Lung

[*Ref.:* Ananthnarayan, 8th ed., page no. 351]

- ❖ Reactivation of TB is almost exclusively occurs in Lung (Post primary Pulmonary tuberculosis) which may be due to endogenous reactivation or exogenous reinfection.

5. Ans. (b) Lymph node

[*Ref.:* Ananthnarayan, 8th ed., page no. 352]

- ❖ Scrofuloderma is a TB skin lesion occurs d/t breakdown of underlying TB foci (usually lymph node).

6. Ans. (c) In early morning

[*Ref.:* Ananthnarayan, 8th ed., page no. 355]

- ❖ Urine is the specimen of choice for diagnosis of genito-urinary tuberculosis.
- ❖ This is collected either as three consecutive early morning samples or a single sample of completely voided urine in 24 hours and centrifuged & the sediment is used for culture.

7. Ans. (c) Auramine – Rhodamine stain

[*Ref.:* Journal-Lancet Inf. Dis. 2006, Iss. 9]

- ❖ *Auramine* – Rhodamine stain is a more rapid method of screening than Ziehl-Neelsen stain because it is screened at high power (40x).
- ❖ So that more fields can be seen in the same time hence it is used when the number of samples are more.
- ❖ However, RNTCP recommends Ziehl-Neelsen stain.

8. Ans. (c) Induration

[*Ref.:* Ananthnarayan, 8th ed., page no. 336]

- ❖ **Tuberculin test** is read after 72 hr and only induration is measured (not the erythema)

- *Induration :*
  - >10 mm – **Positive.**
  - 6-9 mm – **(equivocal/doubtful)** due to BCG/NTM.
  - <5 mm – **Negative.**

9. Ans. (a) Lepromin test

[*Ref.:* Ananthnarayan, 8th ed., page no. 368]

- **Lepromin Test** is a measure of CMI induced by injected lepromin.
- It does not say about the past exposure neither is used for diagnosis.
- *Uses of Lepromin test:*
  - Classify lesions of leprosy
  - Assess prognosis
  - Assess resistance to leprosy in individuals.

10. Ans. (c) 3 weeks

[*Ref.:* Ananthnarayan, 8th ed., page no. 368]

- **Lepromin test** is done by injecting 0.1 ml lepromin antigen given intadermally.
- Reading is taken at two times:
  - Early/Fernandez Reaction: 2-3 days induration like tuberculin (DTH)
  - Late/Mitsuda Reaction: 3-4 weeks – nodule, necrosis, ulcer.

11. Ans. (b) M. paratuberculosis

[*Ref.:* Ananthnarayan, 8th ed., page no. 359]

- M. paratuberculosis is also called as Johne's bacillus.

12. Ans. (c) Macrophages

[*Ref.:* Ananthnarayan, 8th ed., page no. 364]

- The Lepra bacilli are seen singly and in groups intracellularly as well as extracellularly lying free outside the cell.
- The bacilli inside the cell are usually present in parallel bundles of 50 or more.
- Acid fast bacteria bound together by a lipid like substance known as glia. These masses of bacteria are known as ***globi.***
- The parallel rows of bacilli in the globi present a ***cigar like bundle appearance.***
- These are present inside large undifferentiated histiocytes which have a foamy appearance. These are known as ***Virchow's lepra cells.***

BACTERIOLOGY III

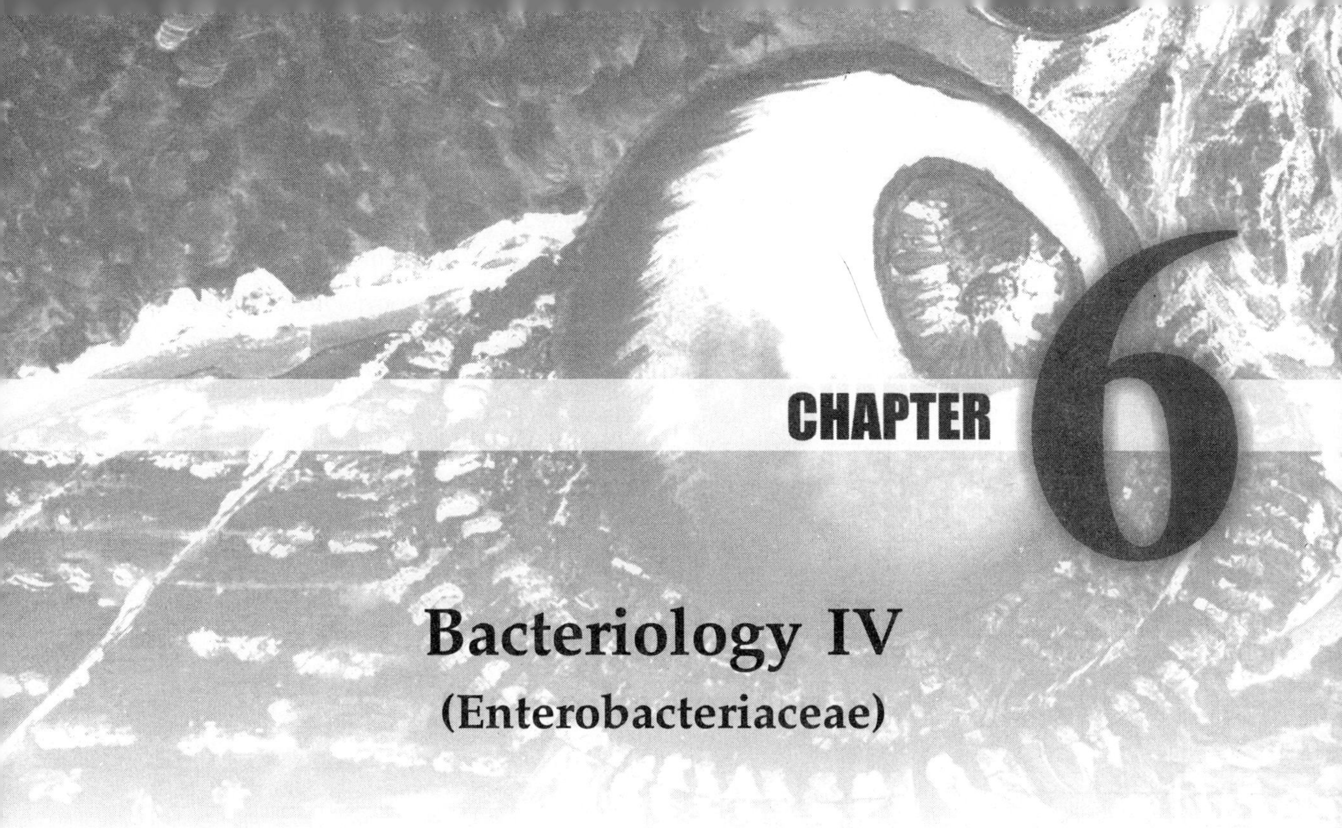

Bacteriology IV
(Enterobacteriaceae)

Members of Family Enterobacteriaceae includes:

- Escherichia
- Klebsiella
- Shigella
- Salmonella
- Proteus
- Yesinia.

Family Character:

All the members of family Enterobacteriaceae possess the following characters:

- Gram –ve bacilli
- Aerobic and facultative anaerobe
- Non-fastidious
- Glucose fermenting
- Catalase +ve (exception is Shigella dysenteriae Type 1)
- Oxidase negative
- Reduce nitrate to nitrite
- Motile (exception *Shigella, Klebsiella).*

Classification

Based on lactose fermentation (pink colony on MacConkey)

- Lactose fermenter – Escherichia, Klebsiella.
- Non-lactose fermenter – Shigella, Salmonella, Proteus, Yesinia.
- Late-lactose fermenter – Shigella sonnei.

ESCHERICHIA COLI

- Antigenic structure – E.coloi possesses the following antigens
  - Somatic Ag **O** – Heat stable, LPS, typed to 170 serotypes
  - Flagellar antigen **H** – heat labile, typed to 75 types
  - Capsular Ag **K** – attachment, typed to 103 types
  - Fimbrial Ag **F.**
- Normal colon commensal strains: bélongs to early O groups (1, 2, 3, 4 etc.)
- Enteropathogenic strains – belong s to later O groups (26, 55, 86, 111 etc.)
- Biochemical reactions: ***IMViC: ++–***
  - Indole +ve
  - MR +ve
  - VP –ve
  - citrate –ve.

Virulence Factors of E. coli:

- Uropathogenic E. coli:
  - K antigen; protects from phagocytosis
  - Hemolysin
  - ***Mannose resistant*** Fimbriae
  - ***P Fimbriae***.
- Diarrheagenic E. coli:
  - CFA (colonizing factor antigens) in ETEC
  - Enterotoxins – LT, ST, VT (explained below).

LT (heat labile toxin)	ST (heat stable toxin)	VT (Verocytotoxin)
B subunit – binds GM1 ganglioside receptor on intestinal epithelium	↑ cGMP	Inhibit ribosome and inhibit protein synthesis
Plasmid coded	Plasmid coded	Phage coded

Clinical Infections

UTI (Uropathogenic E. coli):

- Most common cause of UTI- E.coli.
- Most common serotypes causing UTI – "Early" O groups 1, 2, 4, 6, 7, 18, 75.
- Cystitis and lower UTI – mostly due to ascending infection, lack K Ag.
- Pyelonephritis and upper UTI – mostly due to descending infection, possess K antigen.
- Virulence factor:
  - Hemolysin
  - P fimbriae
  - Mannose resistant fimbriae
  - Siderophore.
- **Kass' concept of "significant Bacteriuria – >10^5/ml of urine".**

BACTERIOLOGY IV

Diagnosis:

If there is delay – urine can be **refrigerated or stored with 1.8% boric acid.**

Screening:

- Griess nitrite test
- Catalase
- Triphenyl tetrazolium phenyl test
- Leucocytes esterase test
- Wet mount (↑leucocytes).

➢ **Quantitative culture** (Pour plate method).

➢ **Semi quantitative culture** (standardized loop technique).

➢ **UTI is diagnosed when Bacteriuria:**

- 10^5/ml of urine (In asymptomatic)
- 10^4/ml of urine (In symptomatic, MSU)
- 10^2/ml of urine (In catheterized patient).

➢ **Any count is significant:**

- For suprapubic aspiration
- Gram positive organism
- If antibiotic started.

Diarrheogenic E. Coli

1. **EPEC (Enteropathogenic E. coli)**
   - ➢ Causes **infantile diarrhea,** sporadic diarrhea in adults.
   - ➢ Non-toxigenic, non-invasive.
   - ➢ Adhere to intestinal mucosa and disrupt brush border – attaching effacing lesions **(A/E lesions).**
2. **ETEC (Entero toxigenic E. coli)**
   - ➢ Acute watery diarrhea in infants and adults.
   - ➢ Most common cause of **traveller's diarrhea**
   - ➢ ***Pathogenesis:***
     - Toxins – LT, ST (plasmid mediated),
     - Fimbrial proteins (colonization factor Ag)
     - Non-invasive.
   - ➢ Diagnosis – typing, demonstration of toxins.
3. **EIEC (Entero invasive E. coli)**
   - ➢ Dysentery like disease in all ages.
   - ➢ *Pathogenesis:* Epithelial cell invasion by **virulence marker Antigen** (VMA).
   - ➢ Called atypical E. coli (lactose non-fermenter), resembles Shigella flexneri.
   - ➢ *Diagnosis* – HeLa and Hep2 cell invasion assay, Sereny's test.
4. **EHEC (Entero hemorrhagic E. coli)**
   - ➢ Strain involved – O157:H7.

- Produces blood diarrhea in all ages.
- *Pathogenesis* – Due to VTI and or VT2 (inhibit protein sysnthesis)
- *Complications* – Capillary microangiopathy leading to
  - HUS (Haemorrhagic Uremic Syndrome)
  - HC (Hemorrhagic Colitis).

5. **EAEC (Entero aggregative E. coli)**
   - Produse persistent diarrhea especially in developing countries.
   - Most are "O" un-type able but "H" type able strain.
   - Aggregated in a "Stacked Brick" formation on Hep2 cell lines.
   - EAST 1 (enter aggregative heat stable enterotoxins).

Treatment:

- UTI – Fluoroquinolones.
- Diarrhea – Fluid and electrolyte balance, no antibiotics.

KLEBSIELLA

- Capsulated.
- Lactose fermenter.
- Non-motile.
- Produce mucoid colonies.
- *K. pneumoniae* – **Urease +ve** – causes pneumonia, UTI, abdominal, wound and surgical site infection.
- *K. ozaenae* – causes ozaenae (foul smelling nasal discharge).
- *K. rhinoscleromatis* – causes rhinoscleroma.

PROTEUS

- Motile, non-lactose fermenter.
- Proteeae tribe includes – Proteus, Providencia and Morganella
- ***Biochemical reaction:***
  - ***Tribe character – PPA +ve*** (phenyl alanine deaminase +ve).
  - Urease +ve.
  - H_2S +ve – P. mirabilis and P. vulgaris.
- It has a fishy/seminal smell.
- Proteus can swarm on blood agar.

Organism which swarm:

- Proteus.
- Clostridium tetani.
- V parahemolyticus, V alginolyticus.
- Serratia.

- Proteus forms **Forms struvite stone** in bladder in alkaline urine.

BACTERIOLOGY IV

- Some non motile strains of proteus are used as the basis of **Weil felix reaction:**
    - OX 19, OX2 strains of Pr vulgaris.
    - OX K strain of Pr mirabalis.

SHIGELLA

- Non-motile.
- Non-lactose fermenter.
- Four species – *Sh. dysenteriae, Sh. flexneri, Sh. boydii, Sh. sonnei.*

Biochemical reaction

- All are catalase +ve except – Sh. dysenteriae type 1.
- All are mannitol fermenting except – Sh. dysenteriae.
- All are anerogenic except – Sh. flexneri biotypes new castle, Manchester.
- All are lactose non-fermenter except – Sh. sonnei (late lactose fermenter).
- Most hardier – Sh. sonnei.
- All four species cause bacillary dysentery.
- Most common in world – Sh. sonnei.
- Most common in India – Sh. flexneri.
- All can be typed by serotyping – except *Sh. Sonnei.*
- Colicin typing done for – *Sh. sonnei.*

- **Shigella dysenteriae Type 1:**
    - Called as Shiga bacillus.
    - Catalase negative.
    - Produce shiga toxin.
    - Causes HUS.
- **Shigella dysenteriae:** Type 2 – (Sh schmitzi) – indole +ve.
- **Shigella dysenteriae:** Type 3-7 – Large and sachs group.

Pathogenicity

- Endotoxin – LPS – Diarrhea, ulcers.
- Shiga toxin – by Sh. dysenteriae type – 1.
- VMA (virulence marker antigen) – possessed by all species (responsible for invasiveness).
- Infective dose – Low, 10-100 organisms (Salmonella and Vibrio – 10_6 – 10_8).

Complications:

Reactive Arthritis, Toxic Neuritis, Intussusception, Hemolytic uremic syndrome.

Diagnosis:

- Specimen – mucus flakes of stool
- Transport media – Sach's ***buffered glycerol*** saline
- Selective media:
    - DCA (Deoxycholate citrate agar)
    - XLD (Xylose lactose dextrose agar)
    - SS (Salmonella Shigella Agar)

- Enrichment Broth:
  - Gram negative broth
  - Selenite F broth
  - Tetrathionate broth.

Treatment:

- Mild: No treatment required.
- Severe: Ampicillin, Cotrimoxazole, ceftriaxone.

SALMONELLA

- All Salmonelle are Motile (by means of Peritrichous flagella) – except *S. gallinarum pullorum.*
- *Enteric fever* – Caused by S. typhi, S. paratyphi A, B, C.

Antigenic Classification

- Called as Kaufmann White Scheme – Based on ***O antigen,*** typed to > 2399 serotypes.

Molecular Classification

- DNA hybridization study – *Salmonella* are divided into seven group (pathogenic *Salmonella* is group 1).

Antigens of S. Typhi

H antigen → Flagellar antigen

- Heat labile, alcohol labile.
- Formaldehyde stable.
- Stronger immunogenic.
- H antibody appears late, goes late.
- Reacts to H Antibody – forms large loosed fluffy clumps.
- Exist in two alternative phases – Most of them are biphasic except (monophasic – S. typhi, S. paratyphi A).

O Ag → Somatic polysaccharide

- Heat stable.
- Formaldehyde labile.
- Less immunogenic.
- O antibody appears early, goes early – indicates recent infection.
- Reacts to O antibody – forms granular chalky clumps.

Vi Ag – Surface polysaccharide covering O Ag

- Heat labile when present it renders the bacterium inagglutinable by O antiserum.
- Possessed by S. Typhi and S. paratyphi C, S. dublin, citrobacter.
- Poorly immunogenic, but protective.
- Absence of Vi antibody in a proven case of enteric fever – carries poor prognosis.
- Persistance in coalescent stage – carier state.
- Epidemiological typing of S. typhi by Vi specific bacteriophage.

Enteric Fever:

- Characterized by
  - Step ladder – fever
  - Rose spots
  - Coated tongue
  - Headache
  - Altered mental status.

Lab Diagnosis

Culture – Samples like blood, faeces, urine, bone marrow, rose spots etc.

- **Selective media →**
  - DCA (Deoxycholate citrate agar)
  - XLD (Xylose lactose dextrose agar)
  - SS (Salmonella Shigella Agar)
  - ***Wilson Blair medium*** *– S. Typhi produces jet black colonies.*
- **Enrichment Broth:**
  - Gram negative broth
  - Selenite F broth
  - Tetrathionate broth.
- Need tryptophan as growth factor.

Other methods:

- Demonstration of **circulating** Ag.
- Demonstration of antibodies in serum (Widal test).

Week wise diagnosis of choice:

- 1st week – Gold standard is blood culture
  - Blood culture sensitivity – 90% in 1st week, 75% in 2nd week, 60% in 3rd week.
  - Clot culture – higher sensitive than blood culture.
  - Bone marrow or duodenal aspirate culture is done if blood culture is negative.
- End of 1st week – Widal test.
- 2nd and 3rd week – Widal test.
- 3rd and 4th week – Stool and urine culture.
- Stool culture:
  - +ve in both case/carrier.
  - +ve even after start of antibiotics.

Detection of Antibodies (Widal):

- Antibodies – appear by end of 1st week, peaks 3rd week then falls.
- 4 fold rise – between 1st and 3rd week is highly significant than single high titer
- Significant titre:
  - Titer of 1:100 of O agglutinins → significant.
  - 1:200 of H agglutinins → significant.

- H agglutinins appears late, goes late.
- O agglutinins appears early, goes early, rise in O antibody indicates recent infection.
- Anamnestic reaction – false +ve in unrelated infection.
- Patients treated with chloramphenicol – results in false –ve Widal test.

Carriers:

- Chronic carrier– called as presence of organism for >1 year.
- Prevalence of chronic carrier – 3% in India.
- Carriers mainly reside in biliary tract, gall bladder and rarely urinary tract.
- Fecal carriers are most common, but Urine carriers are more dangerous.
- Carriers are detected by:
  - Vi agglutinins (1:10) or
  - Fecal/urine culture.

Treatment:

- Ciprofloxacin
- Ceftriaxone
- Azithromycin.

Non-typhoidal Salmonella:

- Salmonella septicemia – Typically caused by *S. cholerasuis.*
- **Salmonella gastroenteritis:**
  - Zoonosis.
  - Transmitted by Food like meat, egg, milk.
  - S. typhimurium, commonest species (30-40%).

Vaccine:

- **Parental**
  - Killed **WC** (whole cell).
  - **TAB** – contains S. typhi, Paratyphi A, B.
  - Purified **Vi.**
- **Oral** – Ty2 1a **(Gal E mutant) – 3 capsules on alternate day.**

YESINIA PESTIS

- **Characters:**
  - Safety pin appearance (**Bipolar** staining) with ***Wayson's/methylene blue*** stain.
  - ***Optimum temp. 27°C*** but capsule grows best at **37°C.**
  - In broth – ***stalactite growth.***
  - Production of ***pigmented colonies*** on medium containing haemin (blood agar).

Plague:

- Zoonotic in rodents
- Three types:
  - Bubonic Plague
  - Septicemic Plague
  - Pneumonic Plague.

- Vector – Rat flea.
- **Incubation Period:**
  - Bubonic and Septicemic (2-7 days)
  - Pneumonic (1-3 days).
- **Mode of Infection:**
  - Bubonic (flea bite > contact with rodent),
  - Pneumonic – (Man – Man by Inhalational)
- *Most common variety – Bubonic.*
- *Highly infectious and fatal – Pneumonic.*
- India – outbreak in 1994 in Beed – Latur district (Maharashtra), then in 2002 (Shimla).

Lab Diagnosis

- Smear from bubo – bipolar staining (methylene blue staining).
- Fluorescent antibody staining.
- Culture – blood and bubo aspirate.
- Antibody to F1 Ag >128 titer.

Treatment: Streptomycin (DOC).

Vaccine:

- Killed vaccine (Haffkine Institute, Mumbai) – immunity lasts for 6 months.
- Live attenuated vaccine.

FMGE MCQ's

1. **Significant number of bacteria in urine is:** [*March 2011*]
   (a) 1000/ml (b) 10000/ml
   (c) 100000/ml (d) 1000000/ml.
2. **Traveller's diarrhea is caused due to:** [*September 2009, 2010*]
   (a) EIEC (b) EPEC
   (c) ETEC (d) EHEC.
3. **Vero toxin is produced by:** [*September 2010*]
   (a) Shigella dysenteriae serotype 1 (b) S. dysenteriae serotype 2
   (c) S. dysenteriae serotype 3 (d) S. dysenteriae serotype 4.
4. **The selective medium used for isolation of *Salmonella* is:** [*September 2009*]
   (a) Wilson and Blair agar (b) Cary-Blair medium
   (c) Thiosulphate citrate bile salt agar
   (d) Thayer martin medium.
5. **All Shigella species ferment mannitol except:** [*March 2009*]
   (a) Shigella dysenteriae (b) Shigella boydi
   (c) Shigella flexneri (d) Shigella sonnei.
6. **The stalactite growth in a liquid broth is characteristic of** [*March 2008*]

(a) Yersinia pestis
(b) Bacillus anthracis
(c) Salmonella
(d) Haemophilus.

7. Bipolar staining is characteristic of: [*March 2007*]
(a) Yersinia pestis
(b) E. coli
(c) Pseudomonas
(d) Proteus mirabilis.

8. True about significant bacteriuria is: [*March 2007*]
(a) Usually gram positive bacteria in urine
(b) Bacterial culture is non-specific
(c) More than 1 lac colony forming units/ml of midstream urine
(d) Multiple bacterial species are taken into account

9. Typhoid in first week is diagnosed by: [*Sept. 2007*]
(a) Widal test
(b) Stool culture
(c) Urine culture
(d) Blood culture.

10. All the following enrichment media are used for isolation of Salmonella except: [*March 2006*]
(a) Alkaline peptone water
(b) Selenite F broth
(c) Gram negative broth
(d) Tetrathionate broth.

11. Diagnostic test for Enteric fever is: [*September 2005*]
(a) VDRL
(b) Widal test
(c) Urine culture
(d) Gram's staining.

12. Intestinal perforation in Enteric fever occurs in: [*September 2005*]
(a) 1st week
(b) 2nd week
(c) 3rd week
(d) 4th week.

13. Enteric fever is caused by: [*September 2005, 2006*]
(a) Salmonella typhi
(b) Salmonella paratyphi A
(c) Salmonella paratyphi B
(d) All of the above.

14. Organism responsible for catheter predisposed UTI is: [*September 2005*]
(a) Pseudomonas
(b) E. coli
(c) Proteus
(d) All of the above.

15. Plague is transmitted by: [*September 2005*]
(a) Flea
(b) Soft tick
(c) Mites
(d) Hard tick.

ANSWERS TO FMGE MCQ's

1. Ans. (c) 100000/ml

[*Ref.:* Ananthnarayan, 8th ed., page no. 275]

Colony count of bacteria exceeding 100,000 (10^5) bacterial per ml of urine denotes significant bacteriuria and is suggestive of active UTI.

BACTERIOLOGY IV

Kass' concept of "significant Bacteriuria – >10^5/ml of urine" is based on:

- ❖ Colony count of bacteria exceeding 100000 (10^5) bacterial per ml of urine denotes significant bacteriuria and is suggestive of active UTI.
- ❖ Counts of 10000 bacteria or less per ml are of no significance and is due to contamination of urine during voiding.
- ❖ Bacterial counts between 10000 (10^3) and 100000 (10^5) are infrequent when the sample is collected properly and processed promptly. Such results are considered equivocal and the culture is repeated.
- ❖ Significant bacteria is applicable only to *E. coli* and other fram-negative bacteria and for urine collected by mid stream urine.
- ❖ It is not applicable to the urine collected directly from urinary bladder or by cystoscopy and also for gram positive bacteria such as *S. aureus,* in which even low counts may be significant.

2. Ans. (c) ETEC

[*Ref.:* Ananthnarayan, 8th ed., page no. 277]

- ❖ Enterotoxigenic ETEC is responsible for causing 'traveler's diarrhea in which individuals from developed countries visiting endemic areas often suffer from ETEC diarrhea.
- ❖ The disease is caused by through consumption of contaminated food or water. Person to person spread does not occur.

3. Ans. (a) Shigella dysenteriae serotype 1

[*Ref.:* Ananthnarayan, 8th ed., page no. 284]

- ❖ *Shiga toxin (verocytotoxin) is an exotoxin produced by S. dysenteriae type 1.*
- ❖ It is a heat labile protein and acts as enterotoxin and neurotoxin.
- ❖ It is coded by a bacteriophage.
- ❖ It is similar to verocytotoxin produced by entero hemorrhagic E. coli, i.e., acts by inhibiting protein synthesis.
- ❖ Major complication – *HUS (hemorrhagic uremic syndrome) and HC (hemorrhagic colitis).*

4. Ans. (a) Wilson and Blair agar

[*Ref.:* Ananthnarayan, 8th ed., page no. 288]

- ❖ **Wilson and Blair's bismuth sulphite agar is the medium of choice for Salmonella especially S. typhi,** produces **jet black colonies** surrounded by a metallic sheen due to production of hydrogen sulphide.
- ❖ *S. paratyphi A and other species which do not produce H_2S, form green colonies.*

Culture for Salmonella

- ❖ Differential medium:
  - MacConkey agar (produces NLF colonies).
- ❖ Selective media:
  - DCA (Deoxycholate citrate agar)
  - XLD (Xylose lactose dextrose agar)
  - SS (Salmonella Shigella Agar)
  - ***Wilson Blair medium.***

BACTERIOLOGY IV

- Enrichment Broth:
  - Gram-negative broth
  - Selenite F broth
  - Tetrathionate broth.
- Need tryptophan as growth factor.
- Shigella also has same culture media (except *Wilson Blair medium*).

5. Ans. (a) Shigella dysenteriae

[*Ref.:* Ananthnarayan, 8th ed., page no. 284]

- *Shigella ferments mannitol forming acid but no gas except Shigella dysenteriae hence Mannitol fermentation test is used to classify shigellae.*

Biochemical reaction of Shigella

- All are catalase +ve except – Sh. dysenteriae type 1
- All are mannitol fermenting except – Sh. dysenteriae
- All are anerogenic except – Sh. flexneri biotypes New castle, Manchester
- All are lactose non-fermenter except – Sh. sonnei (late lactose fermenter).

6. Ans. (a) Yersinia pestis

[*Ref.:* Ananthnarayan, 8th ed., page no. 321]

- Y. pestis produces a characteristic growth when grown in a flask of broth with oil or ghee (clarified butter) floated on top (ghee broth). The growth in the medium appears to hang down into the broth from the surface, resembling stalactites **(stalactite growth).**

7. Ans. (a) Yersinia pestis

[*Ref.:* Ananthnarayan, 8th ed., page no. 325]

- The lymph node aspirate smears of suspected cases of plague are stained with **Wayson stain** for demonstration of the typical **bipolar (safety pin)** morphology of Y. pestis.
- ***Bipolar (safety pin) appearance is produced by:***
  - Vibrio parahemolyticus.
  - Burkholderia mallei and pseudomallei.
  - Calymmatobacter granulomatis.
  - Yersinia pestis.

8. Ans. (c) More than 1 lac colony forming units/ml of midstream urine

[*Ref.:* Ananthnarayan, 8th ed., page no. 275]

- Colony count of bacteria exceeding 1,00,000 (10^5) bacterial per ml of urine denotes significant bacteriuria and is suggestive of active UTI.
- Significant bacteria is applicable only to E. coli and other gram-negative bacteria and for urine collected by mid stream urine.
- It is not applicable to the urine collected directly from urinary bladder or by cystoscopy, and also for gram-positive bacteria such as S. aureus, in which even low counts may be significant. Usually gram positive bacteria in urine.
- Bacterial culture is always recommended to find out the specific causative agent of UTI.

- ❖ Three or more organisms grown in urine culture are not taken into account and considered as contaminated specimen.

9. Ans. (d) Blood culture

[*Ref.:* Ananthnarayan, 8th ed., page no. 295]

- ❖ **Blood culture is a very useful procedure for diagnosis of enteric fever in the first week of fever.**
- ❖ It is positive in approximately 90 per cent of cases in the first week of fever, 75 per cent of cases in the second week, 60 per cent in the third week and 25 per cent thereafter till the subsidence of pyrexia.
- ❖ Blood cultures, however, rapidly become negative on treatment with antibiotics. Hence bone marrow culture is recommended in the first week of fever if the patient is on antibiotics.
- ❖ Antibodies appear only at the end of 1st week, hence Widal test is recommended in the 2nd and 3rd week of fever.

Week wise diagnosis of choice:

- ❖ 1st week – Gold standard is blood culture
  - Blood culture sensitivity – 90% in 1st week,75% in 2nd week, 60% in 3rd week
  - Clot culture – higher sensitive than blood culture.
- ❖ End of 1st week – Widal test.
- ❖ 2nd and 3rd week – Widal test.
- ❖ 3rd and 4th week – stool and urine culture.
- ❖ *Stool culture:*
  - +ve in both case/carrier.
  - +ve even after start of antibiotics.

10. Ans. (a) Alkaline peptone water

[*Ref.:* Ananthnarayan, 8th ed., page no. 288]

- ❖ Alkaline peptone water is an enrichment media are used for isolation of vibrio cholerae.
- ❖ For other options, refer Q. No. 4.

11. Ans. (b) Widal test

[*Ref.:* Ananthnarayan, 8th ed., page no. 296]

- ❖ Widal test is the traditional serologic test used for the diagnosis of typhoid fever.

Detection of Antibodies (Widal Test):

- ❖ The test measures agglutinating antibodies against flagellar (H) and somatic (O) antigens of S. typhi for typhoid and paratyphoid bacilli in the patient's sera.
- ❖ Antibodies – appear by end of 1st week, peaks 3rd week then falls.
- ❖ 4 fold rise – between 1st and 3rd week is highly significant than single high titer.
- ❖ *Significant titre:*
  - Titer of 1:100 of O agglutinins → significant.
  - 1:200 of H agglutinins → significant.
- ❖ H agglutinins appears late, goes late.
- ❖ O agglutinins appears early, goes early, rise in O antibody indicates recent infection.

- Anamnestic reaction – false +ve in unrelated infection.
- Patients treated with chloramphenicol – false –ve.
- However, Widal test is not used to detect carriers (Vi antibody is determined to detect carriers).

12. Ans. (c) 3rd week and (d) 4th week

[*Ref.:* Harrison, 18th ed., page no. 1276, 17th ed., page no. 955-56]

Gastrointestinal bleeding (10–20%) and intestinal perforation (1–3%) most commonly occur in the third and fourth weeks of illness and result from hyperplasia, ulceration, and necrosis of the ileocecal Peyer's patches at the initial site of Salmonella infiltration. *–Harrison*

13. Ans. (d) All of the above

[*Ref.:* Ananthnarayan, 8th ed., page no. 293]

- **Enteric fever is caused by S. typhi, S. paratyphi A and S. paratyphi B**
- Enteric fever is endemic in many countries of the world. S. typhi is the most common cause throughout the world including India.
- *S. paratyphi* A is prevalent in India and other Asian countries, Eastern Europe and South America, *S. paratyphi* B in North America, Britain and Western Europe, and S. paratyphi C in Eastern Europe and Guyana.

14. Ans. (d) All of the above

[*Ref.:* Ananthnarayan, 8th ed., page no. 274]

- E. coli is the most common cause of urinary tract infection (UTI) in catheterized patient. Proteus and pseudomonas are also the other agents that can cause UTI in catheterized patient.
- Though pseudomonas is more common in catheterized patient because of its ability to produce biofilm but still the most common organism to cause catheter related UTI is E. coli.

Organisms causing UTI:

- *E. coli*
- Proteus
- Klebsiella
- Pseudomonas.

15. Ans. (a) Flea

[*Ref.:* Ananthnarayan, 8th ed., page no. 322]

- *Plague is an acute, contagious, febrile illness transmitted to humans by the bite of an infected rat flea Xenopsylla cheopis.*
- Other form of transmission includes by close contact with infected tissue or body fluids or by directs inhalation of the bacterium (Pneumonic plague).

Plague:

- Zoonotic disease in rodents.
- Three types:
  - Bubonic Plague
  - Septicemic Plague,
  - Pneumonic Plague.
- Vector – Rat flea.

❖ **Incubation Period:**
  - Bubonic and Septicemic (2-7 days)
  - Pneumonic (1-3 days).

❖ **Mode of Infection:**
  - Bubonic (flea bite > contact with rodent)
  - Pneumonic (Man – Man by Inhalational).

❖ Most common variety – *Bubonic.*

❖ Highly infectious and fatal – *Pneumonic.*

PRACTICE MCQ's

1. Hemolytic uremic syndrome is due to:

(a) Enterotoxigenic E. coli (b) Enterohemorhagic E. coli
(c) Citrobacter (d) Salmonella.

2. The mechanism of action of enteropathogenic *E. coli* is:

(a) Stimulates adenyl cyclase (b) Adherance to enterocytes
(c) Increase cAMP (d) Inhibit protein synthesis.

3. Following are true to Widal test except:

(a) Diagnostic in first week (b) Maximum titre in third week
(c) 'H' antibody is more immunogenic (d) O antibody indicates recent infection.

4. Growth factor needed for *Salmonella*: [*March 2005*]

(a) Niacin (b) Tryptophan
(c) Folic acid (d) Bile.

5. All of the following are true regarding typhoid except: [*Sept. 2010*]

(a) Urinary carriers are more dangerous (b) Vi Ab is used for detecting carrier
(c) Vi is seen is normal population
(d) Chronic carrier carry the bacilli for > 6 month.

6. Yersinia pseudotuberculosis causes: [*Sept. 2007*]

(a) Plague (b) Diphtheria
(c) Appendicitis (d) Tetanus.

7. Pneumonic plague is transmitted to humans by: [*March 2009*]

(a) Rat flea (b) Droplet infection
(c) Ingestion (d) Inoculation.

ANSWERS TO PRACTICE MCQ's

1. Ans. (b) Enterohemorhagic E. coli

[*Ref.:* Ananthnarayan, 8th ed., page no. 277]

❖ *Hemolytic uremic syndrome is a complication of Enterohemorhagic E. coli and Shigella dysentriae type 1.*

BACTERIOLOGY IV

2. Ans. (b) Adherance to enterocytes

[*Ref.*: Ananthnarayan, 8th ed., page no. 277]

- Enteropathogenic *E. coli* cause infection by adhering to epithelial cells of the small intestine followed by destruction of the microvillus.
- The bacteria initially form microcolonies on the epithelial cell surface, in which the bacteria are attached to the host cells with help of cup-like pedestals.
- Subsequently the attached bacteria multiply and causes microvilli destruction resulting in diarrhea due to malabsorption.

3. Ans. (a) Diagnostic in first week

[*Ref.*: Ananthnarayan, 8th ed., page no. 296]

- Widal test is used for diagnosis only after end of the first week.

4. Ans. (b) Tryptophan

[*Ref.*: Ananthnarayan, 8th ed., page no. 284]

- S. typhi and S. paratyphi however do not grow in Simmon's citrate media as they need tryptophan as the growth factor.

5. Ans. (d) Chronic carrier carry the bacilli for > 6 month

[*Ref.*: Ananthnarayan, 8th ed., page no. 294]

- Chronic carrier of typhoid fever carries the bacilli for > 1 year.
- Chronic carrier of Hepatitis B infection carries the virus for > 6 months.

6. Ans. (c) Appendicitis

[*Ref.*: Ananthnarayan, 8th ed., page no. 325]

- Y. pseudotuberculosis primarily causes gastroenteritis.
- Gastroenteritis is characterized by a self-limited mesenteric lymphadenitis simulating acute appendicitis.
- Fever, abdominal pain (often right lower quadrant location) and rash are a major triad of *Y. pseudotuberculosis* infection. Diarrhea is not common.

7. Ans. (b) Droplet infection

[*Ref.*: Ananthnarayan, 8th ed., page no. 323]

- Pneumonic plague is transmitted from infected humans to other susceptible human hosts following ***direct inhalation of the bacilli by droplet infection due to close contact*** with infected hosts, or from inhalation of aerosolized bacteria such as may occur if used as a biological weapon.
- The bacilli spread through the lungs producing a severe and rapidly progressive multilobar bronchopneumonia, subsequently leading to bacteremia and septicemia.

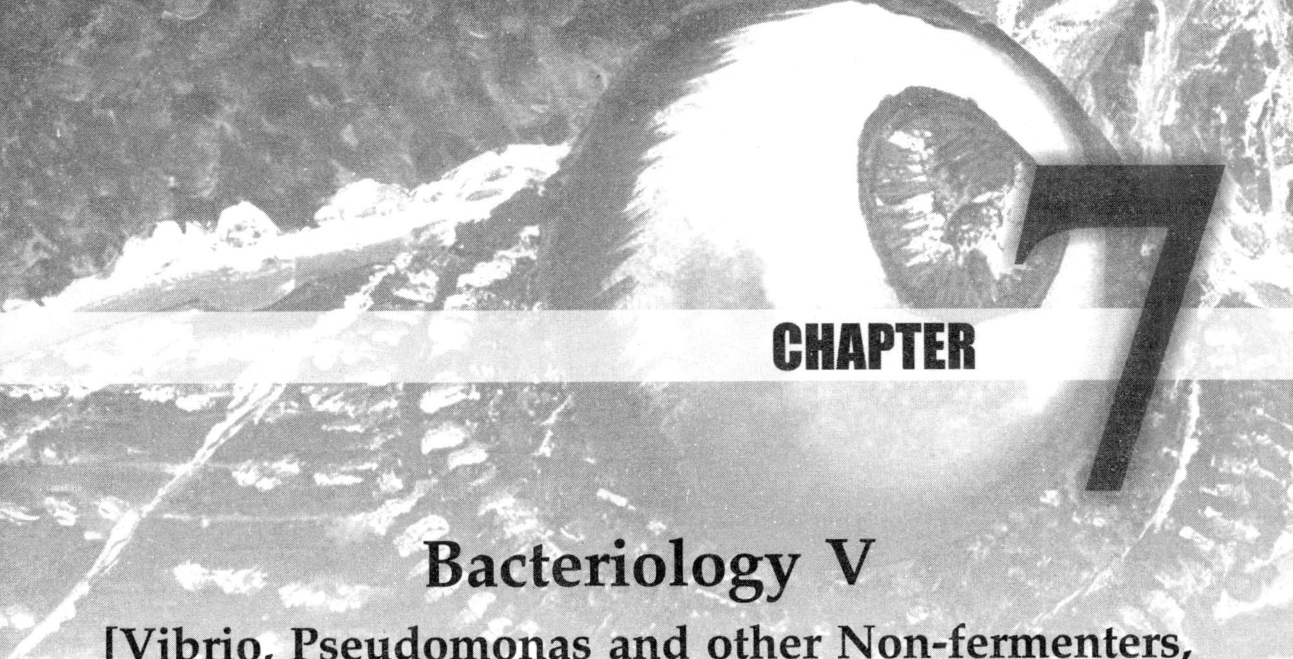

Bacteriology V

[Vibrio, Pseudomonas and other Non-fermenters, Haemophilus, Bordetella, Brucella (HBB)]

VIBRIO

Vibrio cholerae:

- Gram-negative curved rods (comma shaped).
- All Vibrio are halophilic except *V. cholerae, V. mimicus.*
- They possess single polar flagella (shows characteristic ***darting motility***). Also shown by Campylobacter.
- Oxidase positive.
- Non/late lactose fermenter.
- Shows both Indole +ve and Nitrate +ve (***Cholera red reaction***).
- String test +ve with Na deoxycholate.

Culture Media

Transport media: Alkaline pH

- Venkatraman Ramakrishnan (VR) medium.
- Cary Blair medium.
- Autoclaved sea water.

Enrichment

- APW (alkaline peptone water).
- Monsur's taurocholate tellurite peptone water.

Selective

- Bile salt agar (BSA).

- ➢ Monsour's gelatin taurocholate trypticase tellurite agar (GTTA).
- ➢ Thiosulphate citrate bile salt sucrose (TCBS) agar. Yellow colony (*V. cholerae*), Green colony (*V. parahemolyticus*).

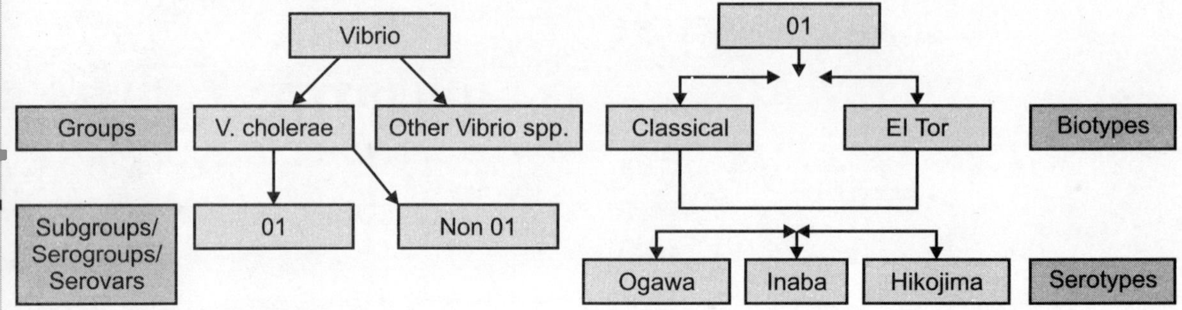

❖ **Cholera Pandemics:**

- 1st 6 pandemics – started in Indian subcontinent and mediated by classical Vibrio.
- 7th pandemic:
  - Started in Indonesia
  - Caused due to ElTor Vibrio
  - Characterized by less severe illness with more carriers.

❖ **ElTor Vs Classical Vibrio:**

- ➢ ElTor is much hardier/resistant than classical
- ➢ ElTor produces less severe cholera
- ➢ ElTor infection is associated with more carrier than cases.

❖ Most common Serotype: Ogawa > Inaba > Hikojima (agglutinated by both ogawa and inaba antisera).

O139 Vibrio (Bengal strains) – 1st in 1992 from Chennai.

- ➢ Capsulated, might be invasive.
- ➢ Arise from ElTor by horizontal transfer of gene.
- ➢ Clinically and epidemiologically indistinguishable from O1.
- ➢ Not neutralized by O1 antisera.
- ➢ Currently – both O1 ElTor and O139 coexist. Classical Vibrio still reported in Bangladesh.

Biotypes of V. cholerae O1	Classical strain	El Tor
Sheep RBC hemolysis	–ve	+ve
Chick erythrocyte agglutination	–	+ve
Polymyxin B (50 iu)	Sensitive	Resistant
Group IV phage susceptibility	Susceptible	Resistant
ElTor Phage V susceptibility	Resistant	Susceptible
VP Test	–ve	+ve
CAMP Test	–ve	+ve

Cholera

- **Cholera:** Occurs only in man (rice water stools).
- *Maintained:*
  - Interepidemics – in sea water.
  - During epidemic – In carriers.
- Acid labile (alkali stable), so require high infective dose of 10^6.
- *Age:*
  - Interepidemics – all age equally.
  - During epidemic – More children.
- Heat labile, but can resist refrigeration.

Pathogenicity

- TCP – toxin co-regulatory pilus- helps in adhesion.
- Cholera Toxin (CT) – resembles heat labile toxin of *E. coli* (LT).
- *Mechanism of Cholera toxin:*
  - A unit – ADP ribosylation of G protein→↑ Adenyl cyclase →↑ cAMP.
  - B unit – Binds to ganglioside receptors.
- LPS – has no role in pathogenesis.

Treatment

- DOC in adult: Doxycycline (if resistant, then ciprofloxacin)
- DOC in children: cotrimoxazole
- DOC in pregnancy: Furazolidone
- DOC for chemoprophylaxis: Tetracycline.

Vaccines

- Parenteral vaccine:
  - Contains – Killed Classical Ogawa and Inaba serotypes.
  - 50-60% protection for 3-6 m.
  - Protection is more in adults than children.
  - No cross protection between Ogawa and Inaba.
  - Cross protection between ElTor and Classical type.
- *Oral vaccine:*
  - Whole cell V. cholerae O1 with recombinant B subunit **(WC/rBS).**
  - Live oral – ***CVD 103- HgR vaccine.***

Halophilic Vibrio:

- Has more NaCl tolerance capacity.
- *Examples:*
  - *V. parahemolyticus.*
  - *V. alginolyticus.*
  - *V. vulnificus.*
- All of them cause food poisoning (sea fish).
- Produce green colony on TCBS (sucrose non-fermenter).

- ***V. parahemolyticus***
    - Shows ***kanagawa phenomenon on wagatsuma agar***.
    - Capsulated.
    - Bipolar staining.
    - Peritrichous flagella.
- ***V. vulnificus*** – lactose fermenter.

PSEUDOMONAS AERUGINOSA

Pseudomonas is the most common nosocomial pathogen because:

- Ubiquitous water and soil organism.
- Resists wide temp. range 5°C to 42°C.
- Produce biofilm.
- Resistant to disinfectant, antiseptics and multidrug resistance (due to resistant plasmids).
- *Virulence factor:*
    - Exotoxin A: Inhibiting protein synthesis (like diphtheria toxin).
    - Exotoxin S: Ribosylation of GTP binding protein.
    - Others: Capsule/slime layer, Exotoxin S, U, Y, protease, elastase, hemolysin, endotoxin.

Distinguishing Characteristics

- Oxidase – positive
- Non-fermenter
- Motile with polar flagella
- Pigments:
    - Pyocyanin (blue-green) by P. aeruginosa
    - Fluorescein (greenish yellow – by all species)
    - Pyorubin (red)
- Pigmentation is produced in **King**'s media
- Selective media – **cetrimide** agar
- Grape-like fruity odor
- Some strains produce slime layer (alginate)
- Non-lactose fermenting colonies on MacConkey agar.

Infections caused by *Pseudomonas*

- Burn patients infection.
- Malignant otitis externa.
- Shanghai fever.
- Blue-green pus.
- Chronic Granulomatous Disease (CGD).
- Ecthyma gangrenosum.
- UTI in catheterized patients.
- Cystic fibrosis – by high slime producing strains (alginate).

Anti Pseudomonal Drugs:

- Penicillin – Piperacillin, Mezlocillin, Ticarcillin.
- Cephalosporin – Ceftazidime, cefoperazone, cefipime.
- Carbapenems – imipenem, meropenem.
- Monobactam – Aztreonam.
- Aminoglycoside – Tobramycin, Gentamicin, Amikacin.
- Quinolone – Ciprofloxacin, Levofloxacin.
- Other – PolymyxinB, Colistin.

BURKHOLDERIA

- Gram –ve Bacilli, Non-fermenter, Oxidase +ve
- Resistant to polymyxin B
- Bipolar stained
- Zoonotic, agent of bioterrorism
- Occupational spread
- Treatment – Ceftazidime/Carbapenems.

Burkholderia pseudomallei

- Causative agent of ***melioidosis***
- **Motile**
- Zoonotic – ***rodents***
- Humans – Pulmonary infections like TB (most common), multiple abscesses, LN
- Known as Vietnam Time-Bomb.

Burkholderia mallei

- ***Non-motile***
- Zoonotic **–** ***horse***
- Mallein test – like tuberculin test
- Causative agent of:
  - **Glanders:** Nodules in respiratory system.
  - **Farcy:** Involve skin with prominent lymphatics underneath.

HAEMOPHILUS

H. influenzae

- Blood loving
- Known as Pfeiffer's bacillus
- Shows pleomorphism
- Oxidase +, Catalase +
- Killed by refrigeration (i.e., why CSF sample should never be refrigerated)
- H.influenzae is capsulated (Capsular polysaccharide)
- Fastidious, require X and V factor for growth
  - **X** (haemin in blood) and
  - **V** factor (NADP inside RBC)

- **Culture Media**
  - Levinthal's agar
  - Field's agar
  - Chocolate agar
  - **Satellitism on blood agar:** H. influenzae usually does not grow on blood agar but can grow around Staph streak which supplies V factor.
- **H. influenzae is serotyped to 6 serotypes:**
  - Based on Capsular polysaccharide ***(a-f).***
  - Most common is type b.
  - Type b capsule is made up **PRP** – poly ribosyl ribitol phosphate.

Hib Vaccine

- Made up PRP (poly ribosyl ribitol phosphate) antigen
- Available for type b only
- Not effective in <2 years of age
- No vaccine for other *H. influenzae* types.

H. aegyptius

- Koch's – Week's bacillus
- Pink eye
- Brazilian purpuric fever.

H. ducreyi

- ***Causative agent of Chancroid/soft sore.***
- Characterized by painful lymph node, tender non-indurated genital ulcer.
- ***"School of fish" or "rail road track"*** appearance, bipolar staining.
- Culture medium used: chocolate agar with 1% isovitalex, Vancomycin.

BORDETELLA

- Gram-negative coccobacilli, oxidase +ve.
- Gram staining – ***Appear as Thumbprint appearance.***
- **Culture**
  - Fastidious organism.
  - Bordet Gengou (glycerol, potato extract).
  - Produces ***bisected pearls or mercury drop colonies.***

Virulence Factors

Pertussis toxin-acts by ↑cAMP	Heat labile toxin	LPS
Agglutinogen	Tracheal Cytotoxin	Pertactin (OMP)
Filamentous hemagglutinin	Adenylate cyclase	

Pathogenesis

- Source of infection – patient in early stage.

- No healthy carrier.
- Secondary attack rate of more than 90%.
- Whooping cough or 100 days cough.
- **Three stages:**
  - Catarrhal – nonspecific symptom, highly infectious, culture and smear +ve.
  - Paroxysmal – whooping cough, vomiting, usually culture and smear –ve.
  - Convalescent stage.
- Specimen of choice – per nasal swab for nasopharynx.
- Whooping cough is also produced by ***Mycoplasma, Adenovirus.***
- *B. pertussis causes more severe infection than B. parapertussis.*

Vaccine

DPT: Pertussis component acts as adjuvant increases immunogenicity of DT and TT.

DTaP: Contains acellular pertussis component hence devoid of neurological complications.

BRUCELLA

- Gram –ve coccobacilli.
- Strict Aerobe.
- Intracellular organism affecting Reticulo Endothelial System.
- Causes Zoonotic infection – different species affect different animal.
  - *B. melitensis* – Sheep, Goat.
  - *B. abortus* – Cattle.
  - *B. suis* – Pig.
  - *B. canis* – Dog.
- Brucellosis is also ***known as Malta/Undulant fever.***
- **Transmitted by:**
  - Raw milk intake (most common)
  - Contact with animal feces/urine
  - ***No person to person spread.***
- B melitensis – most pathogenic.

Diagnosis

- *Culture* – Blood (Castaneda method) and bone marrow culture (↑Sensitive).
- Erythritol – improves growth.
- Catalase +ve.
- Oxidase +ve.
- Urease +ve.
- ***Tbilisi phage*** typing is done.

Serology

- **Standard Agglutination Test (SAT)**
  - For IgM detected using B abortus Antigen.

- **Not** useful for chronic brucellosis.

❖ **CFT and ELISA** – useful for chronic infection.

Animal Brucellosis Diagnosis

❖ Rose Bengal Card Test.

❖ *Milk Ring Test.*

❖ Whey Agglutination Test.

Treatment – WHO regimen:

❖ Adult – Doxycycline + Rifampicin (6 weeks).

FMGE MCQ's

1. **Best method to prevent nosocomial infections:** [*September 2011*]
   (a) Antibiotic chemoprphylaxis
   (b) Frequent fumigation of the ward
   (c) Wearing masks before any invasive procedure in ICU
   (d) Washing of hands before and after attending the patients.
2. **Which has an incubation period of less than a week:** [*March 2010*]
   (a) Cholera (b) Measles
   (c) Filaria (d) Kala-azar.
3. **All the following statements are true for *Pseudomonas aeruginosa* except:** [*September 2010*]
   (a) Non-motile (b) Are oxidase positive
   (c) Are non-fermenters (d) Blue green pigment.
4. **Mechanism of action of cholera toxin:** [*September 2009, 2007*]
   (a) Increase in c-AMP (b) Decrease in c-AMP
   (c) Activates Na+ K+ ATPase (d) Inhibit Na+K+ATPase.
5. **Undulant fever is caused by:** [*March 2009*]
   (a) Bartonella (b) Brucella melitensis
   (c) Bordetella (d) Borellia recurrentis
6. **Milk ring test is seen in:** [*September 2008*]
   (a) Brucellosis (b) Bacteroides
   (c) Tuberculosis (d) Salmonellosis.
7. **Gene that encodes the toxin for cholera is transmitted by:** [*September 2007*]
   (a) Protozoa (b) Bacteria
   (c) Bacteriophage (d) Fungus.
8. **Drug of choice of cholera in adult:** [*March 2005*]
   (a) Tetracycline (b) Doxycycline
   (c) Cotrimoxazole (d) Furazolidone
9. **Venkataraman-Ramakrishnan media is used for:** [*March 2005*]
   (a) Sterptococcus pneumoniae (b) Staphylococcus aureus

(c) Vibrio cholerae (d) Clostridium tetani.

10. Oral cholera vaccine is effective for: [*September 2005*]

(a) 12 months (b) 2 years

(c) 3 years (d) 6 months.

11. Meliodiosis is caused by: [*September 2004*]

(a) Burkholderia pseudomallei (b) Burkholderia mallei

(c) Pseudomonas aeruginosa (d) Brucella melitensis.

ANSWERS TO FMGE MCQ's

1. Ans. (d) Washing of hands before and after attending the patients

[*Ref.:* Ananthnarayan, 8th ed., page no. 683]

- ❖ Most common way of spread of infection in hospital – through the ***hands of hospital staff.***
- ❖ Most effective way to prevent the hospital infection – ***hand washing.***

2. Ans. (a) Cholera

[*Ref.:* Ananthnarayan, 8th ed., page no. 306]

- ❖ V. cholerae causes cholera, an acute diarrhoeal disease. The incubation period is short and varies from 2 days to 3 days after ingestion of the bacteria.

3. Ans. (a) Non-motile

[*Ref.:* Ananthnarayan, 8th ed., page no. 315-16]

- ❖ Pseudomonas are obligatory aerobic **non-fermentative** and mostly **oxidase positive** bacteria. Most of them are **motile** by presence of one or two flagella. They are ubiquitous bacteria mostly saprophytic and are found in soil, water and in other moist environment.

Characteristics of Pseudomonas Aeruginosa

- ❖ Oxidase – positive
- ❖ Non-fermenting
- ❖ Motile with polar flagella
- ❖ *Pigments:*
  - Pyocyanin (blue-green) by P. aeruginosa
  - Fluorescein (greenish yellow – by all spp)
  - Pyorubin
- ❖ Pigmentation is produced in **King**'s media
- ❖ Selective media – **Cetrimide** agar
- ❖ Grape-like fruity odor
- ❖ Some strains produce slime layer (alginate)
- ❖ Non-lactose fermenting colonies on MacConkey.

4. Ans. (a) Increase in c-AMP

[*Ref.:* Ananthnarayan, 8th ed., page no. 306]

- The A (active) subunit of Cholera toxin is responsible for the biological activity of the toxin, it stimulates adenyl cyclase which in turn stimulates cAMP in the intestines of epithelial cells of the gut.
- This inhibits the absorption capacity and activates the excretory chloride transport in the intestinal enterocytes eventually leading to loss of sodium chloride in the intestinal lumen.

Virulence Factors of V. cholerae:

- TCP – toxin co-regulatory pilus – helps in adhesion.
- Cholera Toxin (CT) – resembles heat labile toxin of *E. coli* (LT).
- Mechanism of Cholera toxin:
    - A unit – ADP ribosylation of G protein→↑Adenyl cyclase→↑cAMP.
    - B unit – Binds to ganglioside receptors.
- LPS – has no role in pathogenesis.
- Accessory colonization.
- Neuraminidase.
- Siderophores.

5. Ans. (b) Brucella melitensis

[*Ref.:* Ananthnarayan, 8th ed., page no. 342]

- In acute brucellosis, patients usually complain of non-specific symptoms such as anorexia, fatigue, weakness, malaise or joint pains. Fever is an important symptom and is seen in almost all patients. The fever is intermittent and undulant (hence known as **undulant fever**) and can be associated with a relative bradycardia.
- Brucellosis is primarily a zoonotic infection caused by the organism and wild animals. The disease continues to be a major public health problem worldwide. The condition is also known by various names such as, ***Malta fever, Mediterranean fever, undulant fever***, etc.

6. Ans. (a) Brucellosis

[*Ref.:* Ananthnarayan, 8th ed., page no. 345]

- Milk ring test is a frequently used serological test for demonstration of antibodies in the milk of infected animal. This is a screening test used to detect the presence of Brucella infection in infected cattle.

Animal Brucellosis Diagnosis

- Rose Bengal Card Test
- ***Milk Ring Test***
- Whey Agglutination Test.

7. Ans. (c) Bacteriophage

[*Ref.:* Ananthnarayan, 8th ed., page no. 768-69]

- The genes encoding cholera toxin are part of the genome of a bacteriophage, CTX. The receptor for this phage on the V. cholerae surface is the intestinal colonization factor TCP.
- Since ctxAB is part of a mobile genetic element (CTX), horizontal transfer of this bacteriophage may account for the emergence of new toxigenic V. cholerae serogroups.

8. Ans. (b) Doxycycline

[*Ref.:* Harrison, 18th ed., page no. 1293, 17th ed., page no. 970]

- The WHO recommends administration of antibiotics to cholera patients only if they are severely dehydrated, although wider use is often justifiable.
- ***Doxycycline*** (a single dose of 300 mg, four times a day for 3 days) may be effective in adults but is not recommended for children <8 years of age because of possible deposition in bone and developing teeth.

Treatment for Cholera *–Harrison*

DOC in adult	Doxycycline (if resistant, then ciprofloxacin)
DOC in children	Cotrimoxazole
DOC in pregnancy	Furazolidone
DOC for chemoprophylaxis	Tetracycline

9. Ans. (c) Vibrio cholerae

[*Ref.:* Ananthnarayan, 8th ed., page no. 303]

- ***Venkat raman-Ramakrishnan (VR) medium*** is a transport medium used for Vibrio cholerae.
- It is a simple liquid medium prepared by dissolving 20 g crude sea salt and 5 g peptone in one litre of distilled water (pH of 8.6-8.8).

10. Ans. (c) 3 years

[*Ref.:* Park, 21st ed., page no. 211; 20th ed., page no. 206]

- The oral vaccines for Vibrio cholerae gives an average protection of 50-60% atleast for 3 years.
- Whereas the injectable vaccine confers protection of 50% for a period of 3-6 months.

Vibrio Cholerae Vaccines

- *Parenteral vaccine*
  - Contains – Killed Classical Ogawa and Inaba serotypes
  - 50-60% protection for 3-6 m
  - Protection is better in adult than children
  - No cross protection b/t Ogawa and Inaba
  - Cross protection b/t ElTor and Classical type
- *Oral Vaccine*
  - Whole cell V. cholerae O1 with recombinant B subunit (WC/rBS)
  - Live attenuated oral – **CVD 103-HgR vaccine.**

11. Ans. (a) Burkholderia pseudomallei

[*Ref.:* Ananthnarayan, 8th ed., page no. 318]

- Burkholderia pseudomallei also known as Whitmore's bacillus and it is the causative agent of malleiodiosis (from greek word meaning resemblance to distemper of asses) in rodents.

Burkholderia pseudomallei

- Causative agent of meliodiosis
- Characterized by – Pulmonary infections resembling TB (most common), Multiple abscesses, LN↑

BACTERIOLOGY V

- Motile
- Zoonotic – rodents
- Known as Vietnam Time-Bomb

Burkholderia mallei:

- Causative agent of:
  - **Glanders:** Nodules in Respiratory system
  - **Farcy:** Involve skin with prominent lymphatics underneath
- *Non-motile*
- Zoonotic – ***horse.***

PRACTICE MCQ's

1. All the following Vibrio species are halophilic except:

(a) Vibrio cholerae (b) Vibrio parahemolyticus
(c) Vibrio vulnificus (d) Vibrio alginolyticus.

2. International Reference Center for Vibrio phage typing in India is located at:

(a) Mumbai (b) Kolkatta
(c) Chennai (d) Kasauli.

3. All the following statements are true for *Burkholderia mallei* except:

(a) Causes Glanders in horses (b) Non-motile
(c) Causes Farcy in horses (d) Causes Meliodiosis.

4. The selective medium used for culture of *Pseudomonas aeruginosa* is

(a) MacConkey agar (b) Cetrimide agar.
(c) TCBS agar (d) XLD agar.

5. Satellitism is seen in culture of:

(a) Haemophilus (b) Streptococcus
(c) Klebsiella (d) Proteus.

6. Which sample should never be refrigerated?

(a) CSF (b) Urine
(c) Sputum (d) Pus.

7. Haemophilus ducreyi is causative agent of:

(a) Hard chancre (b) Soft chancre
(c) LGV (d) Granuloma inguinale.

8. Standard agglutination test is done for:

(a) Brucella (b) Bordetella
(c) Haemophilus (d) Leptospirosis.

ANSWERS TO PRACTICE MCQ's

1. Ans. (a) Vibrio cholerae

[*Ref.:* Ananthnarayan, 8th ed., page no. 312]

- Vibrio that require a higher concentration of sodium chloride are known as halophilic vibrios. They are natural inhabitants of sea water and marine life. Vibrio parahaemolyticus, Vibrio alginolyticus and Vibrio vulnificus are three important halophilic vibrios species known to cause infection in humans.
- Vibrio cholerae and Vibrio mimicus are non halophilic Vibrio.

2. Ans. (b) Kolkatta

[*Ref.:* Ananthnarayan, 8th ed., page no. 310]

- International Reference Center for Vibrio phage typing in India is located at – Kolkatta (named as **NICED**- National Institute of Cholera and other Enteric Transmitted Disease).
- National Reference Center for Salmonella typhi phage typing in India is located at Delhi (Maulana Azad Medical College).
- National Reference Center for Staphylococcus aureus phage typing in India is located at Delhi (Lady Harding Medical College).

3. Ans. (d) Causes Melidiosis

[*Ref.:* Ananthnarayan, 8th ed., page no. 318]

- Melidiosis is caused by Burkholderia pseudomallei.

4. Ans. (b) Cetrimide agar

[*Ref.:* Ananthnarayan, 8th ed., page no. 317]

- Laboratory diagnosis of pseudomonal infection is based on isolation of *P. aeruginosa* from clinical specimens containing mixed microbial flora by culture on selective medium such as cetrimide agar.

5. Ans. (a) Haemophilus

[*Ref.:* Ananthnarayan, 8th ed., page no. 330]

- Blood agar with *S. aureus* streak is routinely used for culture and identification of *H. influenzae.*
- The colonies of *H. influenzae* nearer to the *S. aureus* are larger than those colonies which are away from *S. aureus*. This phenomenon is known as ***"Satellitism"***.
- This demonstrates that V factor is available in increased concentration near the staphylococcal colony and in the lower concentration away from it.

6. Ans. (a) CSF

[*Ref.:* Ananthnarayan, 8th ed., page no. 332]

- *H. influenzae dies on refrigeration, hence CSF sample of a suspected pyogenic meningitis case should not be refrigerated* *–Ananthnarayan*

7. Ans. (b) Soft chancre

[*Ref.:* Ananthnarayan, 8th ed., page no. 333]

- **Hard chancre:** Due to Treponema pallidum (primary syphilis) – characterized by painful indurated lymphnode and painful indurated genital ulcer.

- **Soft chancre:** Due to Haemophilus ducreyi – characterized by painless non-indurated suppurative lymph node and painless non-indurated genital ulcer.

8. Ans. (a) Brucella

[*Ref.:* Ananthnarayan, 8th ed., page no. 344]

- Standard agglutination test is done for diagnosis of acute brucellosis.

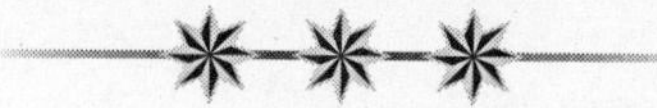

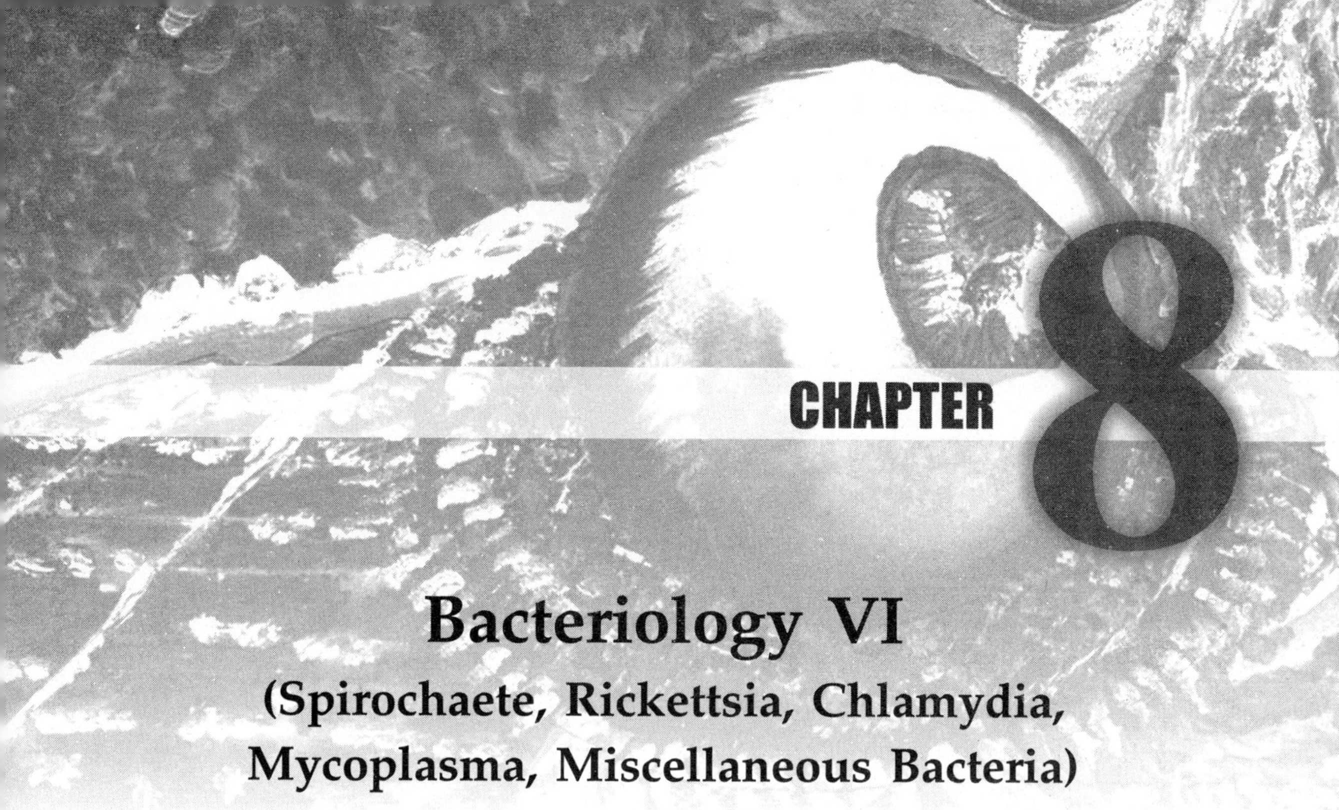

CHAPTER 8

Bacteriology VI

(Spirochaete, Rickettsia, Chlamydia, Mycoplasma, Miscellaneous Bacteria)

SPIROCHETE

- ❖ Spirally coiled and hair like thin bacilli.
- ❖ Pathogenic spirochetes:
  - Treponema
  - Leptospira
  - Borrelia
- ❖ Possess- endoflagella.

Treponema

T. pertenue	:	Yaws
T. endemicum	:	Endemic Syphilis (Bejel)
T. pallidum	:	Syphilis
T. carateum	:	Pinta

Syphilis

- ❖ Incubation Period – 9-90 days.
- ❖ ***Primary syphilis:***
  - Most common genitalia > mouth, nipple.
  - Hard/Hunterian chancre (painless LN↑) + painless ulcer.
  - Dark ground microscopy of ulcer discharge – diagnostic.
- ❖ ***Secondary syphilis***
  - Skin rashes – roseolar or papular

- Condyloma lata at Mucocutaneous junction
- Mucosal patches in orpharynx
- Highly infectious
- All the serological tests are 100% sensitive.

❖ ***Latent syphilis***
- No symptoms
- Diagnosis by serology only.

❖ ***Tertiary syphilis***
- CVS (aortic regurgitation, aneurysm)
- Gummata
- CNS (General paralysis of insane and tabes dorsalis).

Diagnosis

❖ Dark ground microscopy – detection limit 10^4/ml

❖ Direct Fluorescent Antibody test (DFA):
- ↑Sensitive and Specific
- Uses monoclonal antibody to T pallidum).

❖ Light microscopy – not useful.

❖ **Staining:** Silver impregnation stains like Levaditi (tissue), Fontana (smear).

❖ **Culture**
- Pathogenic species cannot be cultivated on artificial media
- Maintained in ***rabbit testes***
- Non-pathogenic spp (Reiter Treponema) culture tried on – ***Smith Noguchi*** medium.

Serology

(A) Non-treponemal Test:

❖ Non-specific Cardiolipin antigen is used (derived from bovine heart).

❖ Older Non-treponemal test:
- Wasserman (CFT)
- Kahn Test (Tube Flocculation)

❖ Newer Non-treponemal Test:
- VDRL (Veneral Disease Research Laboratory Test)
- RPR (Rapid plasma regain).

VDRL

❖ Slide Flocculation test (Type of precipitation test)

❖ VDRL Antigen used – Cardiolipin + Lecithin+ Cholesterol

❖ VDRL Antigen reacts with antibody in patient's serum

❖ Preheating of patient's serum is required – to remove inhibitors

❖ Result is read microscopically – Clumps are formed

❖ Biological false +ve (1%) seen in unrelated infections.

❖ Prozone phenomena seen

BACTERIOLOGY VI

VDRL	RPR
➢ Result read microscopically	➢ Read macroscopically – carbon particle added to Cardiolipin Antigen
➢ Once reconstituted, should be used in 24 hour	➢ Can be stored – EDTA used as stabilizer
➢ Preheating of serum is required to remove inhibitors	➢ Preheating of serum not required – as choline chloride used to remove inhibitors
➢ Sample – blood, plasma, serum, CSF	➢ Cannot be used for CSF sample
➢ Rotation for 4 min	➢ Rotation for 8 min
➢ 78% sensitive in primary syphilis	➢ 86% sensitive in primary syphilis

(B) Specific/Treponemal Test: Specific Treponemal antigen is used.

- ❖ TPI (T. pallidum Immobilization) – using live Nichol's strain.
- ❖ TPA (T. pallidum Particle agglutination) test – Killed *T. pallidum* used.
- ❖ TPHA (T. pallidum haem agglutination) test – using antigenic extract of *T. pallidum.*
- ❖ FTA-ABS (Flouroscent Treponemal Antibody Absorption Test).

☞ **Points to Remember:**

- ➢ **For monitoring the treatment:** VDRL is done.
- ➢ **Primary – Most Sensitive:** TPPA and FTA-ABS.
- ➢ **Secondary syphilis:** All serological tests equally sensitive (100%).
- ➢ **Latent and late:** Most sensitive – TPPA and FTA-ABS.
- ➢ **Overall most specific:** TPPA and FTA-ABS.
- ➢ First test to be positive: FTA-ABS.
- ➢ For rapid and mass screening: VDRL is done.

Congenital syphilis: Diagnosed by

- ❖ 19s IgM FTA ABS test
- ❖ VDRL of mother and baby simultaneously.

Table: Comparison of all the STDs

	Syphilis	Chancroid	LGV	Donovanosis	Herpes
Ulcer	Single painless indurated	Painful, non-indurated irregular	Painless	Painless	Multiple painful ulcers with vesicle
LN	Painless	Painful	Painful	Not enlarged	Not enlarged
IP	9-90 days	<1 week	3 days to 3 weeks	1-4 week	<1 week (2-3 days)

Borrelia

1. Relapsing fever

- ❖ *Epidemic relapsing fever:*
  - Caused by *B recurrentis.*
  - Louse borne.
  - Exclusively human disease.

- ❖ *Endemic relapsing fever:*
    - Caused by other Borrelia species like *B. duttoni, B. hermsii.*
    - Tick borne.
    - Natural host is rodent.
- ❖ *B. recurrentis* shows antigenic variation – reason for relapse of fever.

2. Lyme's disease

- ❖ *B. burgdorferi* – Tick borne.
- ❖ *Clinical Feature:*
    - Erythema migrans
    - Dissemination
    - Persistent infection.
- ❖ *Lab Diagnosis:*
    - Diagnosis mainly on clinical ground.
    - Culture – modified ***Kelley's medium.***
    - *Microscopic detection:*
      Dark ground, phase contrast, immunfluroscence, **silver staining**
    - Antigen detection in urine.

3. Borrelia vincentii:

- ❖ Commensal of mouth.
- ❖ **Causes Vincent's angina**
    - Ulcerative gingivostomatitis.
    - Predisposing conditions such as malnutrition, viral infection.
- ❖ Vincent's angina is also caused by **fusiform bacillus** (*Fusobacterium fusiformis).*

Leptospira

- ❖ Obligate aerobes
- ❖ *Leptospira has two species:*
    - *L. interrogans:*
        - Pathogenic species
        - Further typed to >23 serogroup and >230 serovars
    - *L. biflexa* – free living saprophytic species.
- ❖ Causes Zoonotic disease **(rat)**
- ❖ Transmission – direct contact with animal (occupational)
- ❖ India – Most common in TN, Andaman, Kerala
- ❖ Leptospirosis is associated with – (3R)
    - Rain
    - Rat
    - Rainfall.

Clinical Stage

- ❖ Anicteric (90%) – Fever, conjunctival stuffiness followed by meningitis, uveitis, rash.
- ❖ Icteric stage – (10%) – (known as ***Weil's/Hepato renal hemorrhagic syndrome).***

BACTERIOLOGY VI

Diagnosis

❖ **Dark field microscopy:** Detection limit 10^4/ml, phase contrast, silver impregnation.

❖ **Culture:**
- EMJH media
- Fletcher, Korthoff
- Incubation at 28-30°C for 13 week
- Tedious, sensitivity is less than serology.

❖ **Serology**
- Genus specific – CFT, ELISA.
- ***Microscopic Agglutination Test (MAT):***
  - Gold standard.
  - Sero group and serovar specific.

RICKETTSIA

❖ Obligate intracellular pathogen.

❖ Transmitted by arthropod – except Coxiella.

❖ Not cultivable in cell free media – except Bartonella.

Group	Species	Disease	Vector
Typhus group	*R. prowazekii*	**E**pidemic **T**yphus and Brill Zinsser	**L**ouse Code **(LET)**
	R. typhi	**En**demic typhus	**F**lea Code **(FEN)**
Spotted fever group	*R. rickettsii*	**R**ocky mountain spotted fever (RMS)	**T**ick Code **(TRI)**
	R. conori	**I**ndian tick typhus (ITT)	**T**ick
	R. akari	Rickettsial **p**ox	**M**ite (gamasid) Code **(PSM)**
Scrub typhus	*O. tsutsugamushi*	**S**crub typhus	**M**ite (trombiculid)

☞ **Points to Remember:**

❖ Most severe form – RMS

❖ Mildest form – R pox

❖ Eschar and Lymphadenopathy seen in – Scrub Typhus

❖ Vesicular/vericelliform rash seen – Rickettsial pox

❖ Transovarial transmission occurs only in tick and mite

❖ **Rash:**
- Epidemic (all over except palm and sole)
- Endemic (trunk > extremities)
- RMS, ITT (palm sole)
- No rash – Q fever

❖ Systemic involvement – Rocky mountain spotted fever.

Lab Diagnosis

- Isolation – in lab animals, hens egg (yolk sac) and cell cultures.
- Direct detection of the organisms and their antigens – Giminez, Machiavello and Giemsa stain.
- **Neil Mooser Reaction**
  - Male guinea pig intraperitoneal inoculation leads to:
    - *In Endemic Typhus* – Produces fever and ***positive tunica reaction*** (testicular inflammation).
    - *In Epidemic typhus* – Produces only fever, but negative tunica reaction.
    - *In Rocky mountain spotted fever* – Produces scrotal necrosis.
- **Serology – Weil Felix Reaction**
  - Rickettsial alkali stable polysaccharide Ag cross reacts with non-motile strains of P. vulgaris (OX2, X19) and P. mirabilis (OXK).
  - Rise in titer is more meaningful.
  - False +ve if Proteus infection is present.

Weil Felix Reaction	Antibody to OX2	Antibody to OX19	Antibody to OXK
Epidemic typhus	+	++++	–
Endemic typhus	+	++++	–
RMS fever	+ to ++++	++++	–
Scrub typhus	–	–	+++

Scrub typhus

- Mite and chigger borne.
- Affect rats in deserts, rain forest.
- Eschar at site, rash, LN↑.
- ↑OXK titer in Weil Felix.

Coxiella burnetii

- Transmitted without arthropod vector (respiratory mode).
- It survives **holders method** of pasteurization of milk but killed by flash back method.
- No skin rash in Q fever.
- Zoonotic (wild animal).
- Produces ***interstitial pneumonia.***

Bartonella

- Involve RBC.
- *B. bacilliformis* – causes Oroya fever.
- *B. quintana:*
  - *Causes* – Trench fever
  - Louse borne
  - Also known as 5 days fever.
- *B. hensalae*:
  - Causes Cat scratch disease
  - Bacillary angiomatosis in HIV patients.

CHLAMYDIA

- Obligate intracellular gram negative bacteria.
- Possess modified peptidoglycans.
- Posses both RNA and DNA.
- Can not produce their own ATP ***(Energy parasite).***
- Shows tropism for squamous epithelium and LN.

Species	Character	Serotype	Disease
C. trachomatis	➢ Form compact inclusions with glycogen matrix ➢ Sensitive to sulfonamide ➢ Natural parasite of human ➢ Leave the host cell with a scar	Biovar TRIC – A, B, Ba, C	➢ Trachoma
		Biovar TRIC – D-K	➢ Inclusion conjunctivitis ➢ Infant pneumonia ➢ Genital chlamydiasis
		Biovar LGV – L1,L2,L3	➢ LGV
C. psittaci	➢ Form diffuse vacuolated inclusions without glycogen matrix ➢ Resistant to sulfonamide ➢ Natural parasite of birds ➢ Leave host cell by lysis	Many	➢ Psittacosis (Pneumonia) ➢ Inhalational route ➢ Poultry ingestion – no role ➢ Occupational spread to human
C. pneumoniae TWAR agent	➢ Exclusively human pathogen ➢ Inclusions without glycogen matrix ➢ Resistant to sulfonamide	Only 1	➢ Atypical pneumonia ➢ Associated with • Atherosclerosis • Asthma • Sarcoidosis ➢ Hep2 cell most affective cell line

Life Cycle

Elementary body: Extracellular, Infectious form, Possess rigid cell wall, Smaller size.

Reticulate body: Intracellular, Replicating form (Metabolically active form) possess fragile cell wall, Larger size.

Antigen

- ***LPS:*** Genus specific, used for *CFT.*
- ***Envelop surface Antigen:*** Species specific.
- ***Major OMP:*** Serovar serotype specific – used for *Micro Immuno Flouroscent (microIF) test.*

Diagnosis of Chlamydial Infection

1. **Microscopy**
   - Lugol's I2 – used only for C. trachomatis (stains the glycogen inclusion body).
   - IF using monoclonal antibody.
2. **Culture**
   - Mice (infective by only C. psittaci and LGV)
   - Yolk sac

BACTERIOLOGY VI

- Cell culture (McCoy Cells and HeLa)
- Hep2 for *C. pneumoniae.*

3. **Serology**
   - Micro-IF (serovar specific)
   - CFT (genus specific)
   - High titer seen in – LGV, infant pneumonia, salpingitis.
4. **PCR:** More sensitive and specific.

Treatment of Chlamydial Infections

- C. trachomatis – Azithromycin.
- C. psittaci – Tetracycline.
- C. pneumoniae – Erythromycin/tetracycline.

C. trachomatis

- Most common cause of STD worldwide.
- Most common cause of ophthalmic neonatorum.
- Most common cause of NGU (Non-gonococcal urethritis).
- **Causes inclusion conjunctivitis** in neonate (inclusion blenorrhea).
- In adult – it causes ***swimming pool conjunctivitis***
- *Complications:*
  - Reiter syndrome (conjunctivitis + urethritis + polyarthritis).
  - Fitz Hugh Curtis syndrome – perihepatitis.

LGV

- Most common Serotype-by L2>L1, L3.
- LGV serovars are more invasive than others.
- Most common LN involved – pararectal and intrapelvic nodes.
- *Clinical feature:*
  - *Pain less ulcer*
  - *Painful LN*↑
- Esthiomone (elephantiasis of vulva) rectal stricture.
- Skin test done for diagnosis – **Frie test** (e.g., of Type IV hypersensitivity reaction).

Inclusion Body

- LCL body (Levinthal-Cole-Lillie) body – seen in Psittacosis.
- Miyagawa corpuscle – seen in LGV.
- HP (*Halberstaedter – Prowazek)* body – seen in trachoma.

Non-gonococcal Urethritis (NGU)

- *Chlamydia trachomatis* (most common)
- *Mycoplasma genitalium*
- *Ureoplasma urealyticum*
- *Herpes simplex virus*
- *Trichomonas vaginalis*
- *Candida albicans.*

BACTERIOLOGY VI

Comparison of the Genera Rickettsia, Chlamydia, and Mycoplasma

	Chlamydia	Rickettsia	Mycoplasma
Obligate intracellular parasite	Yes	Yes	No
Make ATP	***No ATP***	Limited ATP	Normal ATP
Peptidoglycan layer	Modified	Normal Peptidoglycan	Absent
Growth on artificial media	No	No	Yes

MISCELLANEOUS BACTERIA

Mycoplasma

- Smallest free living organism.
- Pleomorphism, poorly gram-negative.
- Show ***gliding motility.***
- Lack rigid cell wall – Peptidoglycan layer is absent.
- Peptidoglycan layer is replaced by ***sterols.***
- *Mycoplasma pneumoniae* is also Called ***PPLO*** – Pleuro pneumonia like organism.
- Produces ***Fried egg*** colonies
- ***Mycoplasma pneumoniae*** causes – primary atypical pneumonia (PAP)
- **Lab Diagnosis – Detection of Antibody**
  - Cold agglutination test
  - Streptococcus MG test
  - CFT (complement fixation test)
  - ELISA.

Campylobacter Jejuni

- Curved gram-negative bacilli (***gullwing shaped***).
- Single polar flagellum ***(shows darting motility).***
- **Microaerophilic** – requires 5% O_2.
- *C. jejuni* is ***Thermophilic*** **(42°C).**
- Zoonotic.
- Mode – ingestion of contaminated food (raw milk).
- Selective media: ***Skirrow's media.***

Helicobacter Pylori

- Curved gram-negative bacilli.
- **Microaerophilic.**
- Produces abundant **urease.**
- Prevalence of H. pylori:
  - 30% of population (Developed country)

- 80% of population (Developing country)
- 50% of population (World).

❖ **Disease:**
- Acute gastritis (Antrum)
- Peptic ulcer disease
- Chronic atrophic gastritis
- Autoimmune gastritis
- Adenocarcinoma of stomach and esophagus
- MALT.

❖ **Diagnosis:**
- *Invasive* – Following endoscopic guided biopsy
  - Warthin starrey silver staining.
  - Culture – media for campylobacter and chocolate agar – most specific, but not specific.
  - Biopsy urease test.
- *Noninvasive*
  - ***Urea breath test:*** Most sensitive, Quick, simple.
  - Serology: ELISA.
  - Copro antigen in stool.

Legionella

❖ Pleomorphic rods
❖ Poorly gram – negative
❖ Most common type – L. pneumophila serogroup – SG1
❖ Culture – Fastidious requiring iron and cysteine (**BCYE medium**, buffered charcoal Yeast Extract)
❖ Transmission – ***Aerosols from contaminated AC***
❖ *No human – to human transmission*
❖ *No carrier stage*
❖ Facultative intracellular pathogen
❖ Milder form (flu like) – known as **Pontiac Fever**
❖ Sever form known as – **Legionnaires' disease:**
- *Community acquired* Atypical Pneumonia
- *Numerous PMN, but no organism in sputum.*

❖ **Treatment**
- DOC – Macrolide (Azithromycin) and Quinolone
- β lactams and Aminoglycoside – not affective.

Calymmatobacterium Granulomatis

❖ Produce ***granuloma inguinale, Granuloma venereum or Donovanosis.***
❖ *Shows bipolar staining, safety pin appearance.*
❖ ***Donovan bodies*** – Bacillus within the cytoplasmic vacuoles of large macrophages.
❖ *Clinical feature* – ***Painless ulcer without Lymphadenopathy.***

Rat Bite Fever

- *Streptobacillary moniliformis.*
- *Spirillum minus.*

Gardnerella Vaginalis

- Causes bacterial vaginosis.
- Gram variable (mostly – Gram-negative coccobacilli)
- Bacterial vaginosis is characterized by:
  - Thin profuse vaginal discharge
  - pH > 4.5
  - Fishy odor (Whiff test – addition of 10% KOH enhances the odor)
  - ***Clue cells – epithelial cell studded with organism.***

FMGE MCQ's

Spirochete

1. VDRL is a: [*March 2008, 2010*]

(a) Slide flocculation test
(b) Tube flocculation test
(c) Gel precipiation test
(d) Indirect hemaglutination test.

2. Erythema chronicum migrans is seen in: [*September 2009*]

(a) Relapsing fever
(b) Syphilis
(c) Lyme's disease
(d) Weil's diseaese.

3. Leptospirosis is transmitted by: [*March 2004*]

(a) Bats
(b) Rats
(c) Birds
(d) Dogs.

4. True about Borrelia recurrentis are all except: [*March 2004*]

(a) Causes epidemic relapsing fever
(b) It is transmitted by ixodes tick
(c) No other known animal reservoir of *B. recurrentis* exists
(d) It infects the person via mucous membranes.

Rickettsia

5. True about Endemic Typhus [*March 2008*]

(a) Caused by rickettsia prowazekii
(b) Vector is flea
(c) Reservior is man
(d) Tetracycline is not useful.

6. Disease spread by hard tick is: [*September 2005, 2007*]

(a) Rocky mountain spotted fever
(b) Epidemic typhus
(c) Murine typhus
(d) Scrub typhus.

7. Scrub typhus is spread by: [*September 2003, 2007*]

(a) Ticks
(b) Fleas
(c) Trombiculid mite
(d) Louse.

8. Q fever is caused by: [*March 2005*]

(a) Rochaemelia quintana
(b) Mycoplasma bovis
(c) Coxiella burnetti
(d) Mycoplasma hominis.

9. Mite transmits: [*September 2004*]

(a) Scrub typhus
(b) Trench fever
(c) Endemic typhus
(d) Epidemic typhus.

Chlamydia

10. Drug of choice of LGV: [*September 2007*]

(a) Tetracycline
(b) Doxycycline
(c) Erythromycin
(d) Penicillin.

Miscellaneous Bacteria

11. Urea breath test is done for: [*March 2005*]

(a) H. pylori
(b) Proteus
(c) Corynebacterium
(d) Salmonella.

ANSWERS TO FMGE MCQ's

1. Ans. (a) Slide flocculation test

[*Ref.:* Ananthnarayan, 8th ed., page no. 375]

- VDRL test is a slide flocculation test used widely for diagnosis of syphilis. The test is so named because it was developed first in the Venereal Disease Research Laboratory, USPHS, and New York.

VDRL Test

- Slide flocculation test (Type of precipitation test).
- VDRL antigen used- mixture of ***Cardiolipin + Lecithin + Cholesterol.***
- VDRL antigen reacts with antibody in patient's serum.
- Clumps are formed, result is read microscopically.
- Preheating of patient's serum is required – to remove inhibitors.
- Biological false +ve (1%) seen in unrelated infections.
- Prozone phenomena seen.

2. Ans. (c) Lyme's disease

[*Ref.:* Ananthnarayan, 8th ed., page no. 381]

- Erythema chronicum migrans is the typical skin lesion present at the site of bite in two-third of the patients with lyme disease.

- ❖ This skin rash may be a confluent patch of erythema or may have central clearing. The lesion begins as a small macular papule and becomes larger over the next many weeks and forms a large area of lesion of 5-50 cm in diameter.

Lyme's Disease

- ❖ *Causative agent – B. burgdorferi*
- ❖ Tick borne
- ❖ *Clinical Feature:*
  - ***Erythema chronicum migrans***
  - Dissemination
  - Persistent infection.
- ❖ **Lab Diagnosis**
  - Diagnosis mainly on clinical ground.
  - Culture – modified ***Kelley's medium.***
  - Microscopic detection:
    - Dark ground, phase contrasts, immunfluroscence, **silver staining.**
    - Antigen detection in urine.

3. Ans. (b) Rats

[*Ref.:* Ananthnarayan, 8th ed., page no. 382]

- ❖ Leptospirosis is a zoonotic disease. Wild mammals are the primary reservoirs of infection. Rodents are most important reservoirs and rats are the most common source of infection worldwide.
- ❖ Leptospirosis is associated with (3R)
  - Ricefield
  - Rat
  - Rainfall.

4. Ans. (b) It is transmitted by ixodes tick

[*Ref.:* Ananthnarayan, 8th ed., page no. 379]

- ❖ **Option (b):** Borrelia recurrentis is the causative agent of epidemic relapsing fever, whereas other Borrelia spp like B. duttoni, B. hermsii are the agent of endemic relapsing fever.
- ❖ **Option (a):** Epidemic relapsing fever is transmitted by louse while endemic relapsing fever is tick borne.
- ❖ **Option (c):** Epidemic relapsing fever is an exclusively human disease (no animal reservoir) whereas endemic relapsing fever affects rodents also.
- ❖ **Option (d):** Humans get infection when infected lice are crushed and their fluids contaminate bite wounds, or wounds made by scratching, or other abrasions in the skin and in the mucous membrane.

Relapsing Fever

- ❖ ***Epidemic relapsing fever:***
  - Caused by *B. recurrentis*
  - Louse borne
  - Exclusively human disease.

- ***Endemic relapsing fever:***
    - Caused by other Borrelia species like *B. duttoni, B. hermsii*
    - Tick borne
    - Natural host is rodent.
- *B. recurrentis* shows antigenic variation – reason for relapse.

5. Ans. (b) Vector is flea

[*Ref.:* Ananthnarayan, 8th ed., page no. 407]

- Rat flea (Xenopsiella cheopis) or cat flea (Ctenocephalides felis) are the main vectors responsible for the transmission of disease **(endemic typhus).**

About Other Options:

- **Option (a):** Rickettsia typhi is the causative agent of endemic or murine typhus. The murine typhus occurs in many parts of the world particularly in subtropical temperate costal areas.
- **Option (c):** Rat (Rattus rattus) mice and cats are the natural hosts. Humans are the accidental hosts.
- **Option (d):** Tetracycline, doxycycline and chloramphenicol are highly effective in the treatment of endemic typhus.

6. Ans. (a) Rocky mountain spotted fever

[*Ref.:* Ananthnarayan, 8th ed., page no. 408]

- **Option (a):** Rocky mountain spotted fever is transmitted by hard tick.
- **Option (b) and (c):** Epidemic typhus or Murine typhus – transmitted by louse.
- **Option (d):** Scrub typhus – transmitted by mite (its ***larval form chiggers***).
- **Spotted fever group of rickettsial diseases include:**
    - Rocky mountain spotted fever caused by *Rickettsia rickettsiae*
    - Rickettsial pox caused by *Rickettsia akari*
    - Indian tick typhus – caused by *Rickettsia conori.*
    - **All are transmitted by Tick except Rickettsial pox (Mite borne).**

7. Ans. (c) Trombiculid mite

[*Ref.:* Ananthnarayan, 8th ed., page no. 408]

- *Orientia tsusugamushi formerly R. tsusugamushi is the causative agent of scrub typhus.*
- *The condition is transmitted to humans by the* ***Trombiculid mite****, Leptothromidium akamushi.*
- *Only larval stage (****chigger****) of mite is infectious to humans and other mammals because these stages require blood meal for further development.*

8. Ans. (c) Coxiella burnetti

[*Ref.:* Ananthnarayan, 8th ed., page no. 410-11]

- Coxiella burnetti is the causative agent of Q fever, a zoonotic disease transmitted from animals to humans.

Coxiella burnetii

- Causative agent of Q fever.
- Transmitted without arthropod vector (respiratory mode).

- It survives holders method of pasteurization of milk but killed by flash method.
- No skin rash in Q fever.
- Zoonotic (affects wild animal).
- Produces interstitial pneumonia.

9. Ans. (a) Scrub typhus

[*Ref.:* Ananthnarayan, 8th ed., page no. 408-09]

Scrub typhus

- Transmitted by mite (chigger borne)
- Affect rats in deserts, rain forest
- **Eschar at site, rash, LN↑**
- Weil Felix test shows ↑OXK titer.

10. Ans. (a) Tetracycline

[*Ref.:* Parija's, Microbiology, 1st ed., page no. 533]

- Tetracyclines are usually recommended for treatment of patients with LGV for at least 3 weeks.
- Treatment of children below 9 years, pregnant women and patients unable to tolerate tetracyclines are treated with a macrolide such as erythromycin or azithromycin.
- Azithromycin is the drug of choice for treatment of genital chlamydial infections.

11. Ans. (a) H. pylori

[*Ref.:* Ananthnarayan, 8th ed., page no. 400]

The most consistently accurate non-invasive test H. pylori infection is the urea breath test.

Urea Breath Test

- This test is based on detection of the products of urea degraded by H. pylori.
- In this method, patients drink solution containing urea labelled with a carbon isotope such as C^{14}.
- After a shorten period of time the concentration of labeled carbon is measured in the breath.
- The concentration is high only when urease present in H. pylori found in the stomach breaks down the urea.
- In normal human host the concentration of the labelled carbon in breath won't be high because the human stomach does not contain any urease.
- Positive urea breath test indicated H. pylori infection.
- Disadvantages of the test are that it may show false negative results in:
  - Infections with coccoid forms of H. pylori that do not produce more urease enzymes.
  - In patients receiving antibiotics such as bismuth and histamine 2 blockers.

Diagnosis of H. pylori

- *Invasive* – Following endoscopic guided biopsy:
  - Warthin starrey silver staining.
  - *Culture* – Media for campylobacter and chocolate agar – most specific, but not specific.
  - Biopsy urease test.

❖ *Noninvasive*

- ***Urea breath test:*** Most sensitive, Quick, simple.
- *Serology* : ELISA.
- Copro antigen in stool.

PRACTICE MCQ's

1. The spirochete that cannot be cultured is:

(a) Treponema pallidum (b) Borellia recurrentis
(c) Reitter's treponema (d) Leptospira interrogans.

2. The following is not true of syphilis:

(a) TPI is a specific test (b) VDRL is negative in secondary syphilis
(c) IgM FTA ABS test is specific for congenital syphilis
(d) Serologically syphilis cannot be differentiated from yaws.

3. Following tests are the examples of standard tests of syphilis:

(a) VDRL test (b) TPHA
(c) FTA ABS (d) TPI.

4. Antigenic variation is seen in which of the following:

(a) Syphilis (b) Relapsing fever
(c) Lymes disease (d) Leptospirosis.

5. All the following diseases are transmitted non-venereally except:

(a) Syphilis (b) Bejel
(c) Pinta (d) Yaws.

6. Which of the following produces Fried-egg – like colonies?

(a) Mycoplasma (b) Chalmydia
(c) Borrelia (d) Campylobacter.

7. The serological test used for diagnosis of atypical pneumonia due to *Mycoplasma* is:

(a) Paul Bunnel test (b) Weil Felix test
(c) Cold agglutination test (d) Anti-streptolysin O test.

8. Atypical pneumonia is caused by all the following bacteria except:

(a) Streptococcus pneumoniae (b) Chlamydia pneumoniae
(c) Legionella pneumophila (d) Mycoplasma pneumoniae.

9. Pontiac fever is caused by:

(a) Leptospira (b) Legionella pneumophilia
(c) Spirrilum (d) Brucella.

10. Cat scratch disease is caused by:

(a) Bartonella henslae (b) Legionella pneumophilia
(c) Bartonella quintana (d) Bartonella bacilliformis.

11. Weil-Felix reaction is positive in all the following diseases except:

(a) Epidemic typhus
(b) Q fever
(c) Endemic typhus
(d) Rocky Mountain spotted fever.

12. The rickettsial disease transmitted by ticks is:

(a) Epidemic typhus
(b) Rocky Mountain spotted fever.
(c) Endemic typhus
(d) Scrub typhus.

13. *Coxiella* differs from rickettsial pathogens in being:

(a) Do not grow on artificial media
(b) Rashes seen
(c) Transmitted by mite
(d) Transmitted by inhalation.

14. Inclusion bodies seen in lymphogranulona venereum is known as:

(a) Halbertaedter Prawazek (HP) bodies
(b) Levinthal-Cole-Lille (LCL) inclusion bodies
(c) Bollinger body
(d) Miyagawa corpuscles.

15. Which serovars of C. trachomatis causes swimming pool conjunctivitis?

(a) A, B, Ba, C
(b) D-K
(c) L1-L3
(d) All the serovars.

16. Frei's test is an intradermal skin test used for the diagnosis of:

(a) Lymphogranulona venereum
(b) Trachoma
(c) Infant pneumonia
(d) Neonatal conjunctivitis.

ANSWERS TO PRACTICE MCQ's

1. Ans. (a) Treponema pallidum

[*Ref.:* Ananthnarayan, 8th ed., page no. 372]

- Pathogenic Treponema (i.e., *T. pallidum)* does not grow in artificial culture media.
- Nichole's strain of *T. pallidum* is a pathogenic strain which has been maintained for several decades by serial passage in rabbit testes.
- Non-pathogenic Treponema like T. phagedenis (Reiter's treponema) can be cultured in Smith Naguchi medium.

2. Ans. (b) VDRL is negative in secondary syphilis

[*Ref.:* Ananthnarayan, 8th ed., page no. 376]

- *In secondary syphilis, all serological tests including VDRL are 100% positive.*
- Specific test for syphilis includes – TPI, TPHA, FTA-ABS. *–Ananthnarayan*
- IgM FTA ABS test is recommended for the diagnosis of congenital syphilis.
- T. pertenuae is morphologically and antigenically similar to that of T. pallidum. So serologically syphilis cannot be differentiated from yaws. *–Ananthnarayan*

3. Ans. (a) VDRL test

[*Ref.:* Ananthnarayan, 8th ed., page no. 375]

- Non-treponemal tests are non-specific serological tests used for diagnosis of syphilis. These tests are also called as ***standard tests of syphilis***.
- This group of tests use non-treponemal antigen known as cardiolipin as antigen in the test to detect *regain antibodies in patient's serum.*

❖ **Examples includes:**
- Wasserman complement fixation test
- Kahn's tube flocculation test
- VDRL test
- Rapid plasma reagin (RPR) Test.

4. Ans. (b) Relapsing fever

[*Ref.:* Ananthnarayan, 8th ed., page no. 379]

❖ *B. recurrentis* shows antigenic variation, i.e., the reason for relapse of fever in relapsing fever.

5. Ans. (a) Syphilis

[*Ref.:* Ananthnarayan, 8th ed., page no. 378]

❖ **Treponema that are transmitted non-venereally:**
- *T. pertenue* – causative agent of Yaws.
- *T. endemicum* – causative agent of Endemic Syphilis (Bejel).
- *T. carateum* – causative agent of Pinta.

❖ **Treponema that are transmitted venereally (sexual route):** *T. pallidum* – causative agent of Syphilis.

6. Ans. (a) Mycoplasma

[*Ref.:* Ananthnarayan, 8th ed., page no. 388]

❖ *Fried-egg* – like colonies produced by- Mycoplasma & Malassezia (fungi).

7. Ans. (c) Cold agglutination test

[*Ref.:* Ananthnarayan, 8th ed., page no. 389]

❖ Cold agglutination test is a non-specific serological tests used for the diagnosis of cases of atypical pneumonia due to mycoplasma pneumoniae.

❖ It based on the principle that auto antibodies that agglutinate human O group cells at low temperatures appear in most of the cases of atypical pneumonia.

8. Ans. (a) Streptococcus pneumoniae

[*Ref.:* Ananthnarayan, 8th ed., page no. 389]

❖ Streptococcus pneumoniae causes lobar pneumonia affecting the alveoli.

❖ Atypical pneumonia (interstitial pneumonia) – agents includes:
- Mycoplasma pneumoniae
- Legionella pneumophila
- Chlamydia pneumoniae
- Viral pneumonia.

9. Ans. (b) Legionella pneumophilia

[*Ref.:* Ananthnarayan, 8th ed., page no. 400]

❖ Pontiac fever is a mild self-limiting condition caused by Legionella pneumophilia.

❖ The condition presents as fever and myalgia that resolve without treatment.

10. Ans. (a) Bartonella henslae

[*Ref.:* Ananthnarayan, 8th ed., page no. 412]

- Bartonella henslae is the causative agent of cat scratch disease.

Bartonella

- *B.bacilliformis* – Causes Oroya fever.
- *B. quintana* – Causes Trench fever.
- *B. hensalae* – Causes Cat scratch disease and Bacillary angiomatosis in HIV patients.

11. Ans. (b) Q fever

[*Ref.:* Ananthnarayan, 8th ed., page no. 410]

- Weil-Felix reaction is negative in Q fever and Ricketssial pox.

Weil-Felix Reaction: It is heterophile agglutination detection test that detects anti-rickettsial antibody by using *Proteus antigens*.

Weil-Felix Reaction	Antibody to OX2	Antibody to OX19	Antibody to OXK
Epidemic typhus	+	++++	–
Endemic typhus	+	++++	–
RMS/Indian tick typhus	+ to ++++	++++	–
Scrub typhus	–	–	+++

12. Ans. (b) Rocky Mountain spotted fever

[*Ref.:* Ananthnarayan, 8th ed., page no. 408]

Rickettsial disease transmitted by tick are:

- Rocky mountain spotted fever caused by *Rickettsia rickettsiae.*
- Indian tick typhus – caused by *Rickettsia conori.*
- Kenya tick bite fever.
- African tick typhus.
- Mediterranean spotted fever.

13. Ans. (d) Transmitted by inhalation

[*Ref.:* Ananthnarayan, 8th ed., page no. 408]

14. Ans. (d) Miyagawa corpuscles

[*Ref.:* Ananthnarayan, 8th ed., page no. 420]

Inclusion body in chlamydial infections:

LCL body (Levinthal Cole Lillie) body	Seen in Psittacosis
Miyagawa corpuscle	Seen in LGV
HP (*Halberstaedter – Prowazek)* body	Seen in Trachoma

15. Ans. (b) D-K

[Ref.: Ananthnarayan, 8th ed., page no. 417]

Chlamydia Trachomatis Biovars and Serotypes:

Biovar	Serotype	Disease
Biovar TRIC (Trachoma – Inclusion conjunctivitis Biovar)	Serotype – A, B, Ba, C	➢ Trachoma
	Serotype – D-K	➢ Inclusion conjunctivitis – ***swimming pool conjunctivitis*** and ophthalmia neonatorum ➢ Infant pneumonia ➢ Genital chlamydiasis
Biovar LGV	Serotype – L1, L2, L3	➢ LGV (Lymphogranuloma venereum)

16. Ans. (a) Lymphogranuloma venereum

[*Ref.:* Ananthnarayan, 8th ed., page no. 420]

❖ Frei's test is an intradermal skin test (delayed hypersensitivity reaction) used for the diagnosis of Lymphogranuloma venereum.

❖ **Frei's Test:**

- It is an intradermal skin test used for the diagnosis of LGV.
- 0.1 ml of A heat inactivated *C. trachomatis* LGV antigen is injected intradermally in the forearm.
- It is a delayed hypersensitivity reaction.
- Positive reaction is shown by development of an inflammatory macule measuring >7mm in diameter on the test arm after two days.
- The nodule reaches maximum size in 4 days to 5 days.
- The skin test becomes positive 2-6 weeks after infection and remains positive for several years. However, now a day's skin test is rarely used for diagnosis.

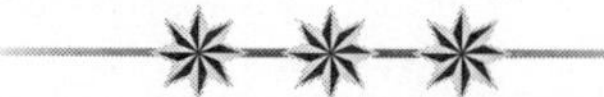

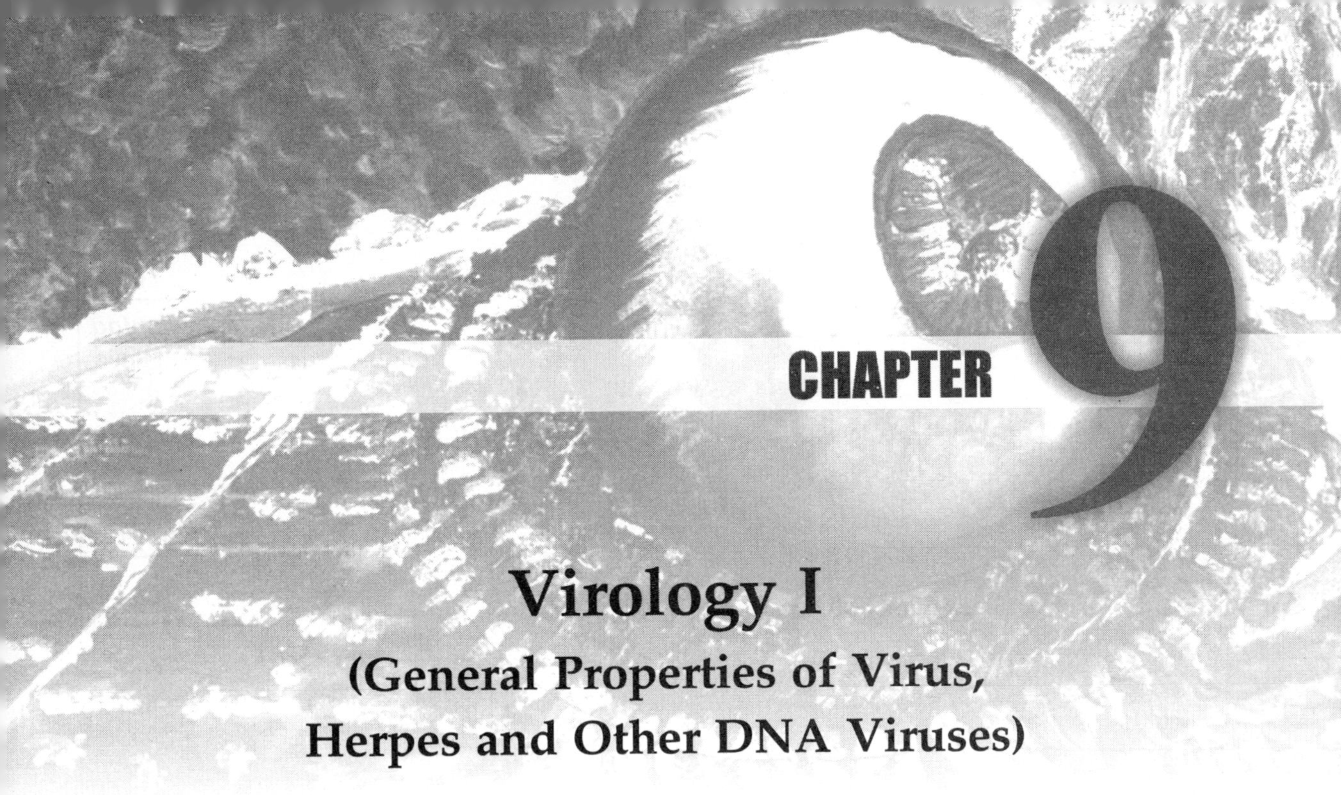

Virology I
(General Properties of Virus, Herpes and Other DNA Viruses)

INTRODUCTION AND DNA VIRUSES

General Properties of Virus

Virus Vs Bacteria

Property	Virus	Bacteria
Nucleic acid	DNA or RNA	Both
Binary fission	No	Yes
Cellular organelle	Absent	Absent (only ribosome present)
Cellular organization	No	Present
Location	Intracellular	Intra/Extra
Resistant to	Antibiotics (exception- Rifampicin to Pox)	Sensitive
Culture in artificial media	No	Can be grown (except – Rickettsia, Chlamydia, M. leprae, Treponema pallidum)
Ribosome	Absent	Present

Size of Viruses

- Size determines by:
  - Ultrafiltration in gradcol membrane of graded porosity.
  - Ultracentrifugation.
  - Electron microscopy.

- Largest – Pox virus (300 nm) – Possess Elementary body.
- Smallest – Parvo virus (20 nm).

Shape of Viruses

- *Structure* – Consists of nucleocapsid (Nucleic acid and protein layer capsid).
- Capsid is made up capsomere units.
- Most of the viruses are roughly spherical except:
    - Rabies – Bullet.
    - Pox virus – Brick.
    - Ebola virus – Filamentous.
    - Tobaco mosaic virus – Rod.
    - Space vehicle – Adenovirus.

Nucleic Acid

- Made up of either DNA or RNA.
- DNA viruses – Herpes, HBV, Adeno, Papova, Parvo, Pox and Bacteriophage.
- RNA viruses – Others.
- All the RNA viruses are single stranded except Reoviruses (double stranded RNA).
- All the DNA viruses are double stranded except Parvoviruses (single stranded DNA).

Symmetry

- Icosahedron – All DNA, most of the RNA virus possess icosahedron symmetry.
- Helical – Few RNA viruses – Bunya, Myxo, Rhabdo, Filoviridae **(MRF – BAT).**
- Pox – Complex symmetry.

Envelop

Enveloped Virus

- Made up lipoprotein subunits called peplomere.
- Lipid part is host cell membrane derived and protein part is virus derived.
- Envelop provides chemical, physical and biological properties to cell.
- Ether sensitive, heat labile, pleomorphic.
- *Example* – Other than few nonenveloped virus, most of the viruses are enveloped (See below).

Non-enveloped Virus:

- Ether resistant, heat stable and non-pleomorphic.
- DNA – Parvo, Adeno, Papova ***(PAP).***
- RNA – Picorna, Astrovirus, Calcivirus, Reovirus ***(PARC).***

Segmented RNA (*BIRA*):

- Bunya
- Influenza
- Rota
- Arena (Causative agent of LCM – lymphocytotrophic meningitis).

Replication

1. **Adsorption**
    - Most specific step requires respective receptors.
    - If bypassed then any virus can attack any cell.

2. **Penetration**
3. **Uncoating**
4. **Biosynthesis:**
   - *DNA Viruses* – Replicates in nucleus (except – Pox)
   - *RNA Virus* – Replicates in Cytoplasm (except – Myxo and Retro virus)
   - Viral protein is synthesized only in cytoplasm
   - ***+ve sense RNA virus:***
     - Viral RNA itself acts as mRNA
     - Infectious and translated directly to protein
     - *Example:* Picorna, Togaviruses.
   - ***–ve Sense RNA virus:***
     - Have polarity opposite to mRNA
     - Non-infectious and possess their own RNA polymerase for transcription to form mRNA.
     - *Example:* Myxo, Rabies,
   - ***Retroviruses:***
     - Viral reverse transcriptase converts viral ssRNA to dsDNA
     - Then dsDNA integrates with host DNA.
5. **Maturation**
6. **Assembly**
7. **Release:**
   - Bacteriophage – by host cell lysis
   - Animal virus – usually without lysis (Myxo – by budding)
   - *Exception* – Picorna – releases by host cell lysis.

Viral Cultivation

Animal Inoculation in Mice

- *Coxsackie:*
  - By intracerebral inoculation into suckling mice.
  - Coxsackie A produces – Flacid paralysis, Coxsackie B produces – spastic paralysis.
- Arbovirus.

Egg Inoculation

- Chorioamniotic membrane – Produce pocks, e.g., Vaccinia, Variola, HSV.
- Yolk sac – Arbovirus, Chlamydia, Rickettsia.
- Amniotic membrane – Influenza culture.
- Allantoic cavity – vaccine preparation for Influenza, Yellow (17D), Rabies (Flury).

Tissue Culture

- **Organ culture –** Tracheal ring (corona)
- **Explant culture –** Adenoid (Adeno).

- **Cell line:**
  - ***Primary cell line:*** Undergo limited division (5-10), diploid karyosome.
    - *Example:* Rhesus Kidney cell line, Human amniotic cell line, Chick embryo fibroblast.
  - ***Secondary cell line:*** Undergo moderate cell division (10-50), diploid karyosome.
    - *Example:* Human fibroblast used for CMV.
  - ***Continuous cell line:*** Indefinite divisions, haploid karyosome
    - *Example:* HeLa, Hep2, BHK.
- **Cytopathic effect**
  - Crenation of cells and degeneration of entire cell sheet : Enterovirus.
  - Syncytium formation: Measles virus, RSV, Herpes, Parainfluenza.
  - Large granular clumps like grapes: Adenovirus.
  - Cytoplasmic vacuolation – SV40.
  - Diffuse roundening of cells – Herpes.

Inclusion Bodies

Intracytoplasmic

- Negri body – Rabies.
- Guarnieri body – Vaccinia.
- Paschen body – Variola.
- Bollinger body – Fowl pox.
- Molluscum body – Molluscum contagiosum virus.

Intranuclear

- Cowdry A (*HAY*) – Herpes (*Lipschultz* body), Yellow fever (*Torres body*).
- Cowdry B (*BAP*) – Adeno, Polio.
- Both – Measles, CMV.

Viral Interference

- When two viruses infect a cell, one inhibits the multiplication of the other virus.
- Seen in Rubella, Polio.

Viral Hemagglutnation

- Shown by Myxovirus, Rabies, Arbo, Pox.
- Elution (due to neuraminidase) – shown only in Myxovirus (except – RSV and Measles).

Latent Virus

- Herpes – HSV 1, 2, VZV – nerve
- CMV – Kidney, secretory gland
- EBV – Lymphoid
- HIV – CD4 T cell
- Slow virus – Neuron

Teratogenic Virus Transfer through Placenta

- CMV
- Rubella
- Coxsackie B
- Hepatitis B, C

- Herpes
- Varicella
- Parvo B19.
- HIV
- Measles, Mumps

Viral Vaccine

Inactivated Vaccine	Live Vaccine
• Salk polio • Influenza • Japanese B – (Nakayama) formalinized mouse brain • Hepatitis B (subunit – HBsAg cloned in yeast) • Rabies: – Neural – BPL, Semple and infant mouse brain – Non neural (PVC, PCEC, HDC)	• Sabin Polio • Influenza – egg • Japanese B – (14-14-2) • MMR • Yellow (17D) – chick embryo • Small Pox • Oka Strain – Varicella • Towne and AD – CMV • Jerryl Lynn – Mumps • Edmonston – Zagreb : Measles • RA 27/3 – Rubella

HERPES

Characters	Alpha	Beta	Gamma
Replicative cycle	Fast (12-18 hrs)	Slow (>24 hrs)	Slow
Host range	Wide	Narrow	Narrow
Cytopathology	Rapid, Cytolytic	Slow, Cytomegaly	Lympho-proliferative
Virus	HSV1, 2, VZV	CMV, HHV6,7	EBV, HHV8
Latency	Neuron	CMV-Secretary glands, kidney, HHV6, 7-Lymphoid tissue	Lymphoid tissue

Herpes Simplex Virus

Clinical Feature

Mucosal

- Most common site – buccal mucosa.
- Most frequent primary lesion – gingivostomatitis, pharyngitis.
- Most frequent recurrent lesion – herpes labialis.
- Most common cause of ulcerative stomatitis – HSV.
- Secondary bacterial infection is common with – Streptococcus, Pneumococcus.

CNS

- Most common sporadic acute viral encephalitis.
- Molaret meningitis.

- Most common site – temporal lobe.
- Most important diagnosis – brain biopsy.
- Transverse Myeltis, GBS.

Cutaneous

- Most common site – Face.
- Herpetic whitlow – seen in doctor, nurse.
- Erythema multiforme – Most common cause – HSV.

Ophthalmic

- Acute keratoconjunctivitis.
- Dendritic ulcer – Rx: Topical acyclovir, IFN C/I – steroid.

Genital

- HSV 2 MC than HSV 1.

Diagnosis

- TZANCK smear of keratinocyte.
- Toludine blue staining of base of vesicle reveals multinucleated giant cell with faceted nuclei and homogenously stained ground glass appearance.
- Type A intranuclear inclusion body in Giemsa stain.
- Isolation – CAM, primary human kidney cell line.

HSV 1 and 2 differentiated by

- HSV1 : lesion around mouth
- HSV2 : lesion around genital infection
- *Latency*
  - HSV1: in trigeminal ganglia
  - HSV2: in sacral ganglia.
- *Transmission*
  - HSV1: contact droplet inhalation
  - HSV2: sexual mode.
- HSV2 larger pocks in chorioallantoic membrane
- HSV2 more temperature sensitive
- HSV2 more neurovirulent
- HSV2 more drug resistance
- Antigen detection and PCR also can differentiate HSV 1 and 2.

Varicella Zoster

- Causes chicken pox in childhood and zoster in adult due to reactivation of latent virus in later life.
- Most common site of Latency:
  - Spinal cord – D3 to L2 (chicken pox)
  - Trigeminal N-Ophthalmic branch (Zoster).
- Chicken pox is a disease of childhood.
- When occur in adult, it is more severe with bullous and hemorrhagic rash.

- Contact with either chicken pox or zoster patient leads to only chicken pox but not zoster.
- One attack gives life long immunity.
- *Source* – Patients.
- Portal of entry – respiratory tract or conjunctiva.
- Incubation period – **2 weeks.**
- Infectious during initial stage: **–2 to +5 days** of onset of rash.
- **Rash:** Usually start in trunk, rapid evolution, appears in crops, centripetal distribution.
- *Complication:*
  - Varicella pneumonia.
  - Myocarditis, nephritis, encephalitis, cerebellar ataxia.
  - Reye's syndrome – fatty liver after salicylate.
- *Vaccine:* **Oka strain** (live attenuated) and VZIG (immunoglobulin).
- *Treatment:*
  - Acyclovir
  - Steroid is contraindicated.
- *Zoster:*
  - Reactivation of latent virus in adulthood
  - Site of Latency – Trigeminal N (Ophthalmic branch)
  - Rashes are always segmented and unilateral.
  - When it affects Geniculate ganglia – causes ***Ramsay hunt syndrome*** characterized by *facial N palsy and vesicle on tympanic membrane, external auditory meatus and tongue.*

Chicken Pox in Pregnancy:

- For mother – high risk for pneumonia.
- 1st half of pregnancy – asymptomatic.
- 2nd half of pregnancy: Fetal varicella syndrome – skin lesion, limb hypoplasia, chorioretinitis and CNS defects.
- *Infection near delivery:*
  Develops Congenital/neonatal Varicella.

Chicken pox	Herpes Zoster (Shingles or Zona)
Primary infection	Reactivation of latent virus
Most common site of Latency – Spinal cord – D3 to L2	Site of Latency – Trigeminal N (Ophthalmic branch)
Rashes- Generalized and bilateral	Rashes – Segmented and unilateral.
Child > adult (severe)	Old age
Persist and reactivate as zoster	Act as source of chicken pox

CMV

- Largest member of Herpes virus family.
- Causes enlargement of the virus infected cell.

- Both intranuclear and cytoplasmic inclusion body are formed – Owl's eye apperance.
- It spreads slowly and requires close contact.
- Route – via secretions, sexual, blood transfusion and vertical transmission.
- Exhibit strict host specificity.

Congenital – Cytomegalic inclusion disease

- Hepatosplenomegaly (most common).
- Microcephaly.
- Mental retardation.
- 3Cs – chorioretinitis, cerebral calcification, convulsion.
- Infants are highly infectious.
- Transmit the virus in urine for 3-5 year.

Acquired CMV Infection

- Mononucleosis like syndrome:
  - Occurs in adult (following blood transfusion)
  - Atypical lymphocytosis seen
  - Paul Bunnel test (heterophile antibody) is negative.
- CMV is the most common organism to cause post kidney transplant infection.
- In HIV patient – causes chorioretinitis (Opportunistic pathogen).

Lab Diagnosis:

- Specimen – urine, saliva, cervix secretion, semen.
- Culture – ***human fibroblast cell line.***
- **IgM** antibody detection.
- Fourfold rise of IgG.
- PCR detecting CMV DNA.

Treatment: Anti CMV drugs are:

- Gancyclovir
- Valgancyclovir
- Foscarnet
- Cidofovir.

EBV (Epstein Barr Virus)

- Attach to CD21/CR2 receptor on B cell.
- B cell become immortalized and polyclonally activated leading to hypergammaglobulinemia.
- In response to this, ***atypical lymphocytosis*** occurs with T cell.
- EBV is not highly contagious, spread slowly.
- Intimate oral contact required.
- Most common source – Saliva (Kissing disease).
- Commonly found in hyperendemic malaria areas
- *Disease:*
  - Hodgkin lymphoma
  - Burkit lymphoma
  - Nasopharyngeal Ca-

- Duncan syndrome (X linked lymphoproliferative disorder)
- Hairy cell leukemia
- Infectious mononucleosis.

Infectious Mononucleosis

- Glandular fever
- Seen in nonimmune young adults following primary infection with EBV
- Incubation period – 4-8 weeks
- Characterized by:
  - Atypical T cell (IM)
  - LN ↑
  - Hepatosplenomegaly
  - Rash (after ampicillin).
- Heterophile antibody to sheep RBC – detected by Paul Bunnel test.
- Confirmed by monospot test/differential absorption test – by using Ox RBC and guinea pig kidney cells.

HHV 6

- Causes sixth disease.
- Also known as Exanthem subitum, Roseola infantum.

HHV 8

- Kaposi sarcoma.
- Primary effusion lymphoma.

OTHER DNA VIRUSES

Pox Viruses

- Largest virus, possess dsDNA.
- Only DNA virus which replicates in cytoplasm.
- Brick shaped.

Small Pox

- Caused by Variola virus.
- Small pox Eradicated from world – 1980.
- Still can be a potential agent of bioterrorism.

Small Pox Eradication is successful because:

- Exclusively human pathogen, no reservoir.
- *Source* – Patient only, no carriers.
- Highly affective live vaccine:
  - Prepared from live vaccine using Vaccinia virus.
  - Freeze dried vaccine (↑stability) and multiple puncture technique.
  - Jenner has used Cowpox vaccine (not used later).

Molluscum Contageosum

- Seen in children and young adult.
- Pearly white wart like nodule on skin composed of eosinophilic inclusion bodies.
- Human are the only host.
- Cannot be grown in egg or tissue culture and animal.
- Sexually transmitted.

Adenovirus

- DNA, non-enveloped, space vehicle shaped.
- *Manifestation*
  - *Hemorrahgic cystis* – Adeno 11 and 21 (also by cyclophophamide).
  - *Infant diarrhoea* – Adeno 40, 41.
  - Epidemic conjuntivitis – Adeno 8, 19, 37 (shepard eye, industrial worker).
  - *Swimming pool conjunctivitis* – Adeno 3, 7, 14.
  - Pharyngitis and Pneumonia.
  - STD.
- *Adeno-associated virus* – Defective virus, requires adenovirus for multiplication.

Parvovirus

- Smallest virus.
- Only DNA virus that has ***single stranded DNA.***
- Causes 5th disease.
- Also known as ***Erythema infectiosum*** is characterized by:
  - Rash – ***Slapped cheek*** appearance – rash 1st on cheek.
  - Arthralgia.
  - Lymphadenopathy.
- Causes ***Aplastic crisis*** in sickle cell anemia patients.
- *In pregnancy* – Causes nonimmune fetal hydrops.
- *Transmission* – Respiratory route, via blood and vertical spread.

Papovavirus

Human Papillomavirus

- Ca cervix
  - Low risk – type 6,11 – CIN.
  - High risk – type 16,18,31,33 – Ca Cx.
  - Risk factor – early sex, multiple sex, multiparous, OCP users.
- Condyloma acuminata/genital wart – by Type 6,11.
- Common wart/verruca vulgaris – by Type 1,2,3,4.
- Epidermodysplasia verrucoplasia.

Other Papovaviruses

- JC virus – Causes Hodgkin disease and PML (progressive multifocal leukoencephalopathy).
- BK virus – Causes renal infection.
- Polyoma virus – affects mice.
- Simian Vacuolating virus 40 (SV40) – affects monkeys.

Bacteriophage

- Viruses that attack bacteria
- Made up dsDNA surrounded by protein coat
- Bacteriophage consists of head, neck and tail
- 2 cycles – Lytic and lysogenic phage
- *Uses:*
  - ***Phage typing:*** *Staphylococcus*, Vi antigen typing of *S. typhi, V. cholerae.*
  - ***Phage assay:*** Depending on the number, size, shape and nature of the plaque produced by the bacteriophage on a lawn culture of bacteria.
  - ***Transduction (transfers bacterial DNA from one bacteria to other).***
  - Used as a ***cloning vector (used in DNA recombination technology).***
  - Used in diagnosis, e.*g., Mycobacteriophage.*
  - ***Codes for Bacterial Toxin:***
    - Cholera toxin
    - Verocytotoxin (VT) of Enterohemorrhagic E. coli (EHEC)
    - Botulinum toxin C, D
    - Diphtheria toxin
    - Streptococcal pyrogenic toxin A, C.

FMGE MCQ's

1. Which of the following is not a live vaccine? [*September 2011*]

(a) Oral polio vaccine (b) MMR vaccine
(c) Yellow fever vaccine (d) Hepatitis B vaccine.

2. Paul Bunnel test is done for: [*March 2011*]

(a) Malta fever (b) Typhus fever
(c) Enteric fever (d) Infectious mononucleosis.

3. All the following are the examples of intracytoplasmic inclusion bodies except: [*September 2009*]

(a) Molluscum bodies (b) Guarneri bodies
(c) Bollinger bodies (d) Owl's eye.

4. EBV (Epstein barr virus) causes all except: [*September 2005*]

(a) Glandular fever (b) Burkitt lymphoma
(c) Pancreatic carcinoma (d) Nasopharyngeal carcinoma.

5. **Carriers for Herpes simplex virus is:** [*September 2005*]

(a) Man
(b) Monkey
(c) Both
(d) None.

ANSWERS TO FMGE MCQ's

1. **Ans. (d) Hepatitis B vaccine**

[*Ref.:* Ananthnarayan, 8th ed., page no. 450-451]

- ❖ Hepatitis B vaccine is a recombinant vaccine where the subunit HBsAg is cloned in baker's yeast.

Inactivated Viral Vaccine:

- ❖ Salk polio
- ❖ Influenza
- ❖ Japanese B (Nakayama)
- ❖ ***Hepatitis B*** *(subunit –HBsAg cloned in yeast)*
- ❖ *Rabies:*
  - Neural – BPL, Semple and infant mouse brain
  - Non neural – PVC, PCEC, HDC.

Live Viral Vaccine

- ***Sabin Polio***
- Influenza
- Japanese B (14-14-2)
- ***Yellow (17D)***
- Small Pox
- Oka Strain – Varicella
- Towne and AD – CMV
- ***MMR***
  - Jerryl Lynn – Mumps
  - Edmonston – Zagreb : Measles
  - RA 27/3 – Rubella.

2. **Ans. (d) Infectious mononucleosis**

[*Ref.:* Ananthnarayan, 8th ed., page no. 476]

- ❖ Paul Bunnell test is a heterophile agglutination test used for diagnosis of infectious mononucleosis by using sheep RBC as antigen.

Paul Bunnell test

- ❖ This heterophile antibody (IgM) is not directed against EBV or EBV infected cells, but is produced due to polyclonal activation of B cells by EBV.
- ❖ The patient's serum is inactivated at 56°C for 30 minutes and in doubling dilution of serum is mixed with equal volume of a 1% suspension of sheep RBC's. The test is incubated at 37°C for 4 hours.

VIROLOGY I

❖ A serum titre of 100 or greater is considered a positive test and is suggestive of infectious mononucleosis.

3. Ans. (d) Owl's eye

[*Ref.:* Ananthnarayan, 8th ed., page no. 473, 444; Parija's, Microbiology, 1st ed., page no. 611]

❖ The presence of an enlarged cell that contains a dense central **Owl's eye appearance basophilic intranuclear inclusion body** is the characteristic feature of the cell infected by CMV.

❖ These cells are found in most tissues of the body and in the urine.

Inclusion Bodies

❖ Inclusion bodies are the characteristic histological feature in virus infected cells reflecting the change in the appearance of the target cells.

❖ Inclusion bodies may result from virus induced changes in the membrane or chromosomal structure. It also represents the sites of viral replication or accumulation of viral capsids.

Intracytoplasmic

- Negri body – seen in Rabies
- Guarnier body – seen in Vaccinia
- Paschen body – seen in Variola
- Bollinger body – seen in Fowl pox
- Molluscum body – seen in Molluscum contagiosum virus

Intranuclear

- Cowdry A
  - Herpes (*Lipschultz* body)
  - Yellow fever (*Torres body*)
- Cowdry B
  - Adenovirus
  - Poliovirus

Intracytoplasmic and Intranuclear

❖ Measles

❖ CMV – intranuclear form is called as Owl's eye appearance.

4. Ans. (c) Pancreatic carcinoma

[*Ref.:* Ananthnarayan, 8th ed., page no. 475]

Disease caused by EBV

❖ Hodgkin lymphoma

❖ Burkit lymphoma

❖ Nasopharyngeal Ca-

❖ Duncan syndrome (X linked lymphoproliferative disorder)

❖ Hairy cell leukemia

❖ Infectious Mononucleosis.

5. Ans. (a) Human

[*Ref.:* Ananthnarayan, 8th ed., page no. 469]

❖ HSV infections are exclusively human disease. Humans are the only natural reservoirs. No vectors are involved in transmission of the disease. **An infected person is a lifelong source and reservoir of the virus.** Vesicle fluid, saliva and vaginal secretions are the important sources of infection for both types of HSV.

PRACTICE MCQ's

1. Double stranded RNA is seen in:

(a) Reovirus (b) Rhabdovirus

(c) Parvovirus (d) Retrovirus.

2. Which of the following does not possess both DNA and RNA:

(a) Bacteria (b) Fungus

(c) Virus (d) Spirochete.

3. The viruses show all the following features except:

(a) They are filterable agents (b) They are obligate intracellular parasites

(c) They contain either DNA or RNA, but not both

(d) Multiply by binary fission.

4. All the followings are the examples of enveloped viruses except:

(a) Polio virus (b) Rubivirus

(c) Adenovirus (d) Herpes virus.

5. Syncitium formation is the typical CPE produced by:

(a) Adenovirus (b) Herpes virus

(c) Measles virus (d) SV40.

6. The polyomavirus that causes progressive multifocal leukoencephalopathy (PML) in humans is:

(a) BK virus (b) JC virus

(c) SV 40 vius (d) Polyomavirus of mice.

ANSWERS TO PRACTICE MCQ's

1. Ans. (a) Reovirus

[*Ref.:* Ananthnarayan, 8th ed., page no. 439]

- ❖ All RNA viruses possess single stranded RNA: except Reoviridae, e.g., Rotavirus (dsRNA).
- ❖ All DNA viruses possess double stranded DNA: except Parvovirus (ssDNA).

2. Ans. (c) Virus

[*Ref.:* Ananthnarayan, 8th ed., page no. 425-26]

- ❖ Viruses possess either DNA or RNA but never both.

3. Ans. (d) Multiply by binary fission

[*Ref.:* Ananthnarayan, 8th ed., page no. 425-26]

- ❖ Bacteria multiply by binary fission whereas viruses divide by a complex process.
- ❖ The viruses are too small to be seen with a light microscope. Their small size allows them to pass through filters that are used to retain back bacteria in contaminated fluids. Hence, they were first described as filterable agents.

The viruses show the following features:

- ❖ They are filterable agents.

- They are obligate intracellular parasites.
- They contain a single type of nucleic acid either DNA or RNA, but not both.
- The virion of the virus particle consist of a nucleic acid genome packaged into a protein coat (capsid), sometimes itself enclosed by an envelope of lipid, proteins and carbohydrates known as envelope.
- They multiply inside the living cells by using the synthesizing machinery of the host cell.
- They replicate by the assembly of the individual components and do not replicate by division such as binary fission.
- They have a few or no enzymes for their own metabolism. They always use host cell machinary to produce their components such as viral messenger RNA, protein and identical copies of the genome.

Property	Virus	Bacteria
Nucleic acid	DNA or RNA	Both
Binary fission	No	Yes
Cellular organelle	Absent	Absent (only ribosome present)
Cellular organization	No	Present
Location	Intracellular	Intra/Extra
Culture in artificial media	No	Can be grow (except – Rickettsia Chlamydia)

4. Ans. (a) Polio virus

[*Ref.:* Ananthnarayan, 8th ed., page no. 426-27]

Non-enveloped virus

- Non-enveloped DNA viruses – Parvo, Adeno, Papova ***(PAP).***
- Non-enveloped RNA viruses – Picorna, Astrovirus, Reovirus, Calcivirus ***(PARC).***

5. Ans. (c) Measles virus and (b) Herpes

[*Ref.:* Ananthnarayan, 8th ed., page no. 435]

- Some viruses such as ***Mealses, Varicella zoster, Respiratory syncitial vitus and Herpes simplex*** virus cause formation of syncitia containing several (upto 100) nuclei in infected cells.

6. Ans. (b) JC virus

[*Ref.:* Ananthnarayan, 8th ed., page no. 550]

- *JC virus is isolated from patients with progressive multifocal leukoencephalopathy (PML).*

Polyomavirus	Manifestation
BK virus	Renal diseases (haemorrhagic cystitis and urethral stenosis)
JC virus	Progressive multifocal leukoencephalopathy

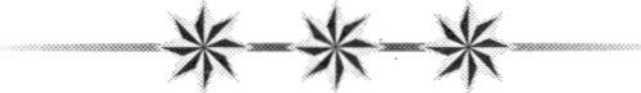

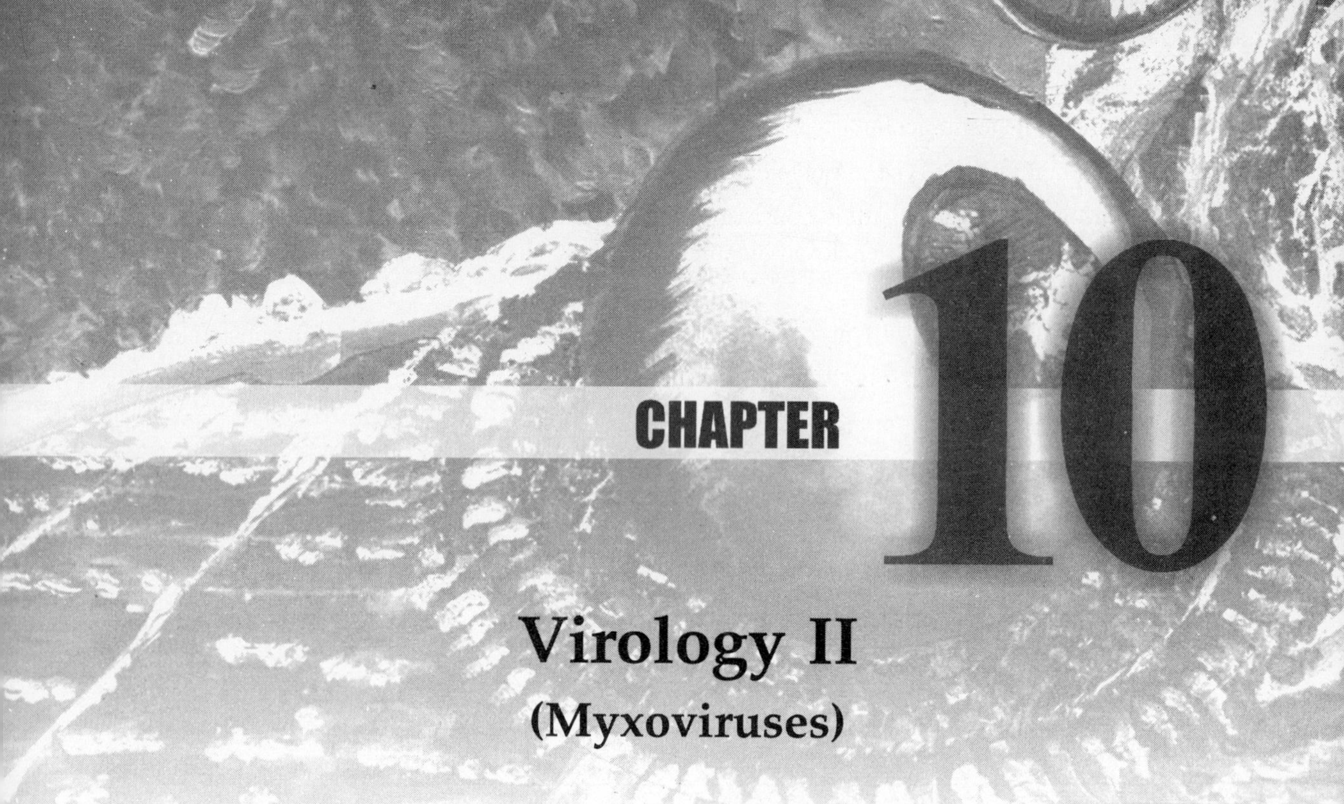

CHAPTER 10

Virology II
(Myxoviruses)

MYXOVIRUSES

Orthomyxo

- Influenza A, B, C.
- Segmented RNA, unstable.
- Both hemagglutinin (HA) and Neuraminidase (NA) spikes present. So Hemagglutination is reversible (elution).

Paramyxo

- Para influenza, Measles, Mumps, RSV, Metapnemuovirus.
- HA spike present in – Parainfuenza, Mumps, Measles.
- NA spike present in – Parainfuenza, Mumps.
- Single RNA, stable.

INFLUENZA

- Influenza – A (most common), B, C.
- Antigenic shift – Results in Pandemic – Most common seen in Type A.
- Antigenic drift – Results in Epidemic – Most common seen in Type A, B.
- HA Ag – H1 to H15, – protective.
- NA antigen – N1 to N9, less protective.
- Most common manifestation: URTI.

- Most common complication:
  - Bacterial pneumonia > viral pneumonia
  - Reye's syndrome with ***Type B*** (following aspirin).

Diagnosis

- Egg inoculation – Amniotic cavity, isolation by A, B, C Allanotic cavity by only A.
- Hemagglutination with Fowl and Guinea pig RBC.

  Type A – agglutinates with Guinea pig, Type B – both, Type C – agglutinates with fowl RBC at 4c.
- Ag detection from nasopharyngeal cells by immunfluroscence.
- Four fold rise of antibody by – Hemagglutination inhibition test (HAI).
- *Vaccine* – Killed, Live, Recombinant.

Avian Flu

- H5N1.
- Seen from 2003 onwards.
- Only bird to human transmission seen, but no human – human transmission seen.
- Highly virulent (as PB1F2 targets host mitochondria, induces apoptosis).

H1N1 2009 Flu

- April 2009
- Pandemic – Including India
- Recombination of 4 strain – (1 Human + 2 Swine + 1 Avian)
- Human to human transmission seen
- Less virulent (as it lacks PB1F2 gene)
- *Diagnosis* by RT PCR detecting HA and NA genes
- *Treatment* – NA Inhibitor: Oseltamivir (Tamiflu), Zanamivir
- Resistant to amantadine
- *Vaccine*:
  - Injectable killed – HA Protein
  - Live nasal spray – HA protein.

MUMPS

- Most common cause of Parotitis (non-suppurative enlargement).
- *Complication*:
  - Epididymo – Orchitis (U/L > B/L) seen in 1/3rd of post pubertal male patients.
  - Aseptic meningitis.
  - Pancreatitis.
  - Diabetes – Mumps, Rubella, Cox Sackie B4.
- Resolve except deafness.
- Secondary attack – 85%.
- Human – only host.
- *Source* – Only patients, no carriers.

- Most common seen in children.
- Once infected, gives lifelong immunity.
- Transmission – Droplet, saliva, direct contact, Fomite borne, urine.
- Saliva is infectious from –1 to +2 weeks of parotitis.
- Specimen – Urine, saliva, CSF.
- *Lab diagnosis*:
  - Isolation: Egg, MKC.
  - IgM Antibody by ELISA.
  - CFT using S antigen.
  - Antibody to S antigen (internal Ag) appear early, goes early – indicates acute infection.
  - Antibody to V antigen (surface Ag) appear late, goes late.
- *Vaccine*: Jeryl Lynn strain (at 9 months) and MMR.

MEASLES

- Rubeola
- Most common childhood rash
- *Source* – Cases only, no subclinical/carrier stage
- Highest secondary attack rate – 90%
- Period of communicability – 4 to +5 days of rash
- *Incubation Period* – 10 days
- *Koplik's spot* – Pathognomic, appear before rash
- *Rash* – Appear at 4th day, fades after 4 day, most common site is face and neck
- *Diagnosis*
  - Antigen detection by IF (also +ve before rash).
  - Warthin finkeldy giant cell.
  - Isolation from nose, throat, conjunctiva and blood – Amniotic route and PKM cell line.
- *Complication*
  - Diarrhea
  - Pneumonia
  - Otitis media
  - Encephalitis
  - ***SSPE*** (Subacute Sclerosing Panencephalitis) – high titer antibody in CSF is diagnostic
  - Suppressed delayed hypersensitivity (false –ve Mantoux test and worsening of TB)
  - Recovery from measles leads to – recovery from asthma, lipoid nephrosis.
- *Vaccine*
  - Prepared – chick embryo or human diploid cell line (no egg vaccine available)
  - Age – given at 9 months (maternal antibody disappears)
  - Can be given at 6 months if measles outbreak seen (2nd dose to be given at 9 month)
  - *Type*: Live attenuated – Edmonston-Zagreb strain or combined (MMR, MR, MMRV)

- *Side effect*: Toxic shock syndrome (due to contamination of vial), mild measles like illness
- Vaccination to contacts – given within 3 days is affective (IP of vaccine strain is 7 days and wild strain is 10 days)
- Immunoglobulin – Can also be given 3days (in this case live vaccine is given after 8-12 week).

RESPIRATORY SYNCYTIAL VIRUS

- No HA and NA spike
- ***Most common cause of bronchiolitis in children***
- Also causes pneumonia and otitis media
- Age – ***6 wk-6 – months***, new borne are protected due to maternal antibody
- Reinfection – milder illness
- Causes epidemics in winter (temperate) and rainy (tropics)
- Culture – ***Giant cell and Syncytial formation***
- T/T – Rivabirin.

PARA INFLUENZA VIRUS

- Para influenza type 1 and 2 – causes ***Croup*** (acute laryngotracheobronchiolitis)
- Para influenza type 3 – LRTI
- Type 3 – more endemic and affects <1 year, causes shipping fever in cattle
- Type 1 and 2 – affect preschool children.

RUBELLA

- German measles
- Belongs to family Togaviridae, not a Myxovirus
- Identified by interference with Echovirus
- *Source* – Cases
- Period of communicability: –1 wk to +1 wk
- IP – 2-3 wk
- Transmission – droplet, contact, sexual
- Rash on day 1 (face), Lymphadenopathy
- **Forchheimer spots** seen
- ***Congenital Rubella***
  - 1st Trimester – Risk is maximum, after 5th month– risk negligible.
  - Classical Congenital Rubella syndrome – Triadcataract (most common), deafness, cardiac (PDA).
  - Expanded Congenital Rubella syndrome – myocarditis, hepatosplenomegaly, bone lesion.
- **Vaccination – *RA 27/3 live attenuated***
  - Prepared from human diploid cell line
  - Given after 1 year
  - If later then, pregnancy should be avoided for 3 months.

Vaccine storage

- Deep freezer – Polio, Measles.
- Vaccine stored at 4°C : DPT, Typhoid, TT, DT, BCG diluent.

FMGE MCQ's

1. **Incubation period of measles is:** [*September 2011*]
   (a) 7 days (b) 10 days
   (c) 14 days (d) 21 days.
2. **Koplik spots are seen in:** [*September 2011*]
   (a) Chicken pox (b) Measles
   (c) Mumps (d) Diphtheria.
3. **All are true about measles except:** [*September 2011*]
   (a) Infective period is 5 days after appearance of rash
   (b) Infection gives life long immunity
   (c) SSPE is a common complication (d) Koplik spots are seen.
4. **A two year old unimmunized child presents to a primary health centre with fever since 5 days. Mother also gives a history of rash starting behind ear-pinna a day before coming OPD. On examination, child is having running nose and congested eyes. Most probable diagnosis is:** [*September 2011*]
   (a) Measles (b) Mumps
   (c) Rubella (d) Chicken pox.
5. **An 8 year old female child following URTI developed maculopapular rash on the jaw spreading onto the trunk which cleared on the 3rd day without desquamation and tender post-auricular and sub-occipital lymphadenopathy. The diagnosis is:** [*March 2011*]
   (a) Kawasaki disease (b) Erythema infectiosum
   (c) Rubella (d) Measles.
6. **2009 Swine flu is due to:** [*September 2010*]
   (a) H1N1 (b) H5N1
   (c) H2N2 (d) H3N2.
7. **SSPE (Subacute sclerosing panencephalitis) is associated with:** [*March 2010; September 2008*]
   (a) Tetanus (b) Meningitis
   (c) Cholera (d) Measles.
8. **Influenza shows which type of trend:** [*September 2009*]
   (a) Antigenic variation (b) Person to person transmission
   (c) Seasonal – in winter it is more common (d) All of the above.
9. **MMR vaccine is a type of:** [*September 2009*]
   (a) Killed vaccine (b) Toxoid
   (c) Live attenuated vaccine (d) Immunoglobulin.
10. **Post exposure vaccination for measles should be done in:** [*September 2009*]

(a) 1 day of exposure
(b) 2 day of exposure
(c) 3 day of exposure
(d) 7 day of exposure.

11. Which of the following is not a complication of mumps? [*March 2009*]
(a) Orchitis
(b) Oophoritis
(c) Encephalitis
(d) Hepatitis.

12. Measles is infective for: [*March 2009*]
(a) One day before and 4 days after rash
(b) Four days before and five days after rash
(c) Entire incubation period
(d) Only during scabs falling.

13. Koplik spot seen in: [*September 2008*]
(a) Mumps
(b) Rubella
(c) Measles
(d) Enteric fever.

14. All of the following vaccine shows herd immunity except: [*September 2008*]
(a) Measles vaccine
(b) Rabies vaccine
(c) Rubella vaccine
(d) OPV.

15. Which of the following vaccine should not be given in pregnancy? [*September 2008*]
(a) Rabies vaccine
(b) Salk Polio vaccine
(c) Killed influenza vaccine
(d) OPV.

16. Most serious complication of measles is: [*September 2008*]
(a) Croup
(b) Meningoencephalitis
(c) Otitis media
(d) Pneumonia.

17. Vaccine contraindicated in pregnancy: [*March 2008*]
(a) IPV
(b) MMR
(c) Rabies
(d) DPT.

18. Chronic carrier state is seen in all except: [*September 2007*]
(a) Typhoid
(b) Hepatitis B
(c) Measles
(d) Gonorrhoea.

19. How many doses of MMR are given? [*September 2007*]
(a) 1
(b) 5
(c) 3
(d) 4.

20. After the appearance of rash, prophylactic isolation of measles case is necessary for a minimum of: [*September 2007*]
(a) 2 days
(b) 5 days
(c) 7 days
(d) 9 days.

21. Infectivity period of measles is: [*March 2007*]
(a) 5 day before and 4 days after appearance of rash
(b) 4 days before and 5 day after appearance of rash
(c) 4 days before and 1 day after appearance of rash
(d) Entire incubation period.

22. Which of the following vaccine should not be kept in freezer? [*March 2005*]
(a) DPT
(b) Measles

(c) OPV (d) All of the above.

23. Vaccine and immunoglobulins can be given together in all except: [*September 2002*]

(a) Tetanus (b) Rabies

(c) Measles (d) HBV.

ANSWERS TO FMGE MCQ's

1. Ans. (b) 10 days

[*Ref.:* Ananthnarayan, 8th ed., page no. 509; Park, 21st ed., page no. 137; 20th ed., page no. 136]

- **Incubation period of measles varies from 9 - 11 days (average 10 days).**

Incubation Period of Important Diseases

- 1 weak – Diphtheria (2-6d),
- 1-2 weaks – Measles (10d), Small Pox (12d), Pertussis (7-14d), Polio (7-14d), Tetanus (6-10d)
- 2-3 weak – Chicken pox (14-16d), Mumps (18d), Rubella (18d).

Arboviruses:

- Dengue – 5-6 days
- Chikungunya – 5-6 days
- Japanese – B-5-15 days
- Yellow Fever – 3-6 days
- KFD – 4-8 days.

Hepatitis Viruses

- Hepatitis A, D, E – 15-45 days
- Hepatitis B – 45-180 days
- Hepatitis C – 15-180 days.

Others:

- Meningococcal meningitis – 3-4 days
- Gonorrhoea – 2-8 days
- Syphilis – 9-90 days
- HIV – months to 10 years
- Rabies – 1-3 months
- Plague:
  - Bubonic and septicemic – 2-7 days
  - Pneumonic – 1-3 days.

2. Ans. (b) Measles

[*Ref.:* Ananthnarayan, 8th ed., page no. 509]

- Koplik's spot is the typical pathogenic lesion found in the mucous membrane of measles patients.

Koplik's Spots:

- They are pathognomic of measles. Their presence establishes the diagnosis of measles.
- These are bluish grey specks or grain substance on a red base which usually appear on the buccal mucosa opposite the second molar.
- They appear at the end of the prodrome, just before the appearance of the rash.
- Koplik's spots usually appear after 2 days of illness and last for 24-48 hours.
- May also appear on the mucous membrane of the conjunctiva and the vagina.

Also remember:

- ❖ Koplik's spot – Pathognomic of measles.
- ❖ Forchheimer spots – Pathognomic of rubella.

3. Ans. (c) SSPE is a common complication

[*Ref.:* Park, 21st ed., page no. 138, 20th ed., page no. 137; Ananthnarayan, 8th ed., page no. 510]

- ❖ The most common complications of measles are – diarrhea, pneumonia, other respiratory complications and otitis media.
- ❖ Subacute sclerosing panencephalitis is not a common complication. SSPE occurs in about 1 in every 300,000 natural cases of measles.

  Also remember:

  - Pneumonia is the most common life threatening complication of measles and accounts for >90% measles related death.

Epidemiology of Measles:

- ❖ Measles is exclusively a human disease.
- ❖ Infected respiratory droplets are the primary source of infection.
- ❖ The infection is transmitted from person-to-person by inhalation of large droplet aerosols.
- ❖ **Patients are infectious from 4 days before to 5 days after the onset of rash.**
- ❖ Infectivity is maximum at the prodrome and diminishes rapidly with the onset of the rash.
- ❖ High risk – Children (1-5 years), person with immunodeficiency due to leukemia, corticosteroid therapy or HIV.
- ❖ Epidemics occur every 2-3 years and usually seen in late winter and early spring.
- ❖ **Once infected (natural or by vaccine) gives lifelong immunity.**

4. Ans. (a) Measles

[*Ref.:* Ananthnarayan, 8th ed., page no. 510; Park 21st ed., page no. 138, 20th ed., page no. 136]

- ❖ **Points in favour of Measles:**
  - History of unvaccination.
  - 2 year old child.
  - Maculopapular rashes which begins behind the ears.
  - Fever, running nose and congested eyes.

Clinical Feature of Measles:

- ❖ Incubation period of measles varies from 9-11 days (average – 10 days).
- ❖ **Prodromal phase** – Characterized by fever, coryza with sneezing, nasal discharge, cough and redness of eye.
- ❖ **Eruptive phase:** is characterized by typical dusky red Maculopapular rashes which begins behind the ears and spreads rapidly in few hours over the face and trunk.
- ❖ The most common complications of measles are – diarrhea, pneumonia, other respiratory complications and otitis media.
- ❖ Pneumonia is the most common life threatening complication of measles and accounts for >90% measles related death.

- **Subacute sclerosing panencephalitis** is a rare, degenerating disease of the CNS, occurs after years after persistent measles infection.

5. Ans. (c) Rubella

[*Ref.:* Ananthnarayan, 8th ed., page no. 551; Park, 21st ed., page no. 140-41, 20th ed., page no. 139]

- **Points in favor of Rubella:**
  - Maculopapular rash on the face spreading onto the trunk.
  - Rash is cleared on the 3rd day without desquamation.
  - Tender post–auricular and sub-occipital lymphadenopathy.

Clinical Feature of Rubella

- Incubation period of rubella varies from 2 to 3 weeks (average 18 days).
- Rubella is a milder and subtle disease than measles.
- Rubella has more asymptomatic cases (50-65%) than measles.
- Maculopapular rash – starts within 24 hrs of fever on the face and progresses downwards to involve the trunk and extremities. The rash typically lasts three days.
- Rubella rashes spread much faster and clears more rapidly and less confluent than measles rashes.
- Tender lymphadenopathy – that affects all the nodes but most commonly post-auricular, posterior cervical nodes and sub-occipital is the hallmark of rubella.

6. Ans. (a) H1N1

[*Ref.:* Internet]

- The **2009 flu pandemic** or **swine flu** was an influenza pandemic caused by **H1N1** and the second of the two pandemics involving H1N1 influenza virus (the first was the 1918 flu pandemic).

H1N1 2009 Flu

- Started in April 2009.
- Pandemic – affects the whole world including India.
- It is made by recombination of 4 strain (1 Human + 2 Swine + 1 Avian strain).
- Human to human transmission seen – hence more infectious
- But less virulent (as it lacks PB1F2 gene).
- *Diagnosis* – by RT PCR detecting Hemagglutinin and Neuraminidase genes.
- *Treatment* – Neuraminidase inhibitor – Oseltamivir (Tamiflu), Zanamivir.
- Resistant to Amantadine.
- *Vaccine* – Injectable killed and live nasal spray are available.

7. Ans. (d) Measles

[*Ref.:* Ananthnarayan, 8th ed., page no. 510; Park 21st ed., page no. 138, 20th/page no. 137]

Subacute sclerosing panencephalitis

- The SSPE is a degenerating disease of the central nervous system occurs after years after persistent measles infection.
- This is a serious and late neurological sequelae of measles that affect CNS characterized by the development of behavioral and intellectual deterioration and seizures.

- **SSPE occurs in about 1 in every 300,000 natural cases of measles.**
- High risk – occurs most commonly in children < 2 years.
- Diagnostic – extremely high measles antibody titre in CSF and blood.
- Mortality – 10-20%.

8. Ans. (d) All of the above

[*Ref.:* Ananthnarayan, 8th ed., page no. 496]

- Influenza virus causes epidemics and occasionally, pandemics mainly due to inherent ability of the virus to undergo antigenic variations.
- In temperate climates, the epidemics of influenza typically occur in the winter and cause considerable morbidity in all age groups.
- Infected humans are the main reservoir of infections for influenza virus. Respiratory secretions of infected person are the important source of infection.

Antigenic variation seen in influenza virus:

Antigenic shift	Major abrupt drastic discontinuous change in genome	Results in Pandemic	Most common seen in Type A
Antigenic drift	Minor gradual sequential antigenic change in genome	Results in Epidemic	Seen in Type A, B

9. Ans. (c) Live attenuated vaccine

[*Ref.:* Ananthnarayan, 8th ed., page no. 511; Park 21st ed., page no. 141, 20th ed., page no. 141]

- **MMR vaccine is a live attenuated vaccine composed of:**
  - Measles vaccine – Edmonston-Zagreb strain.
  - Mumps vaccine – Jeryl Lynn strain.
  - Rubella vaccine – RA 27/3 strain.

10. Ans. (c) 3 day of exposure

[*Ref.:* Park, 21st ed., page no. 139, 20th ed., page no. 136]

- Incubation period of measles vaccine strain is 7 days and measles wild strain is 10 days.
- So vaccination to contacts (post exposure) can be given within 3 days.

Measles Vaccine

- Live attenuated – Edmonston-Zagreb strain.
- Prepared – chick embryo or human diploid cell line.
- *Age* – Given at 9 months (because maternal antibody disappears).
- Can be given at 6 months if measles outbreak seen (2nd dose to be given at 9 month).
- *Type* – Given single or combined (MMR, MR, MMRV).
- *Side effect* – Toxic shock syndrome (due to contamination of vial), mild measles like illness.
- **IP of vaccine strain is 7 days and wild strain is 10 days.**
- Vaccination to contacts – given with in 3 days is affective.
- **Immunoglobulin can also be given 3 days of contacts (in this case live vaccine is given after 8-12 weak).**

11. Ans. None or (d) Hepatitis

[*Ref.:* Ananthnarayan, 8th ed., page no. 506; Park 21st ed., page no. 142, 20th ed., page no. 141]

Common Complications of Mumps

- Orchitis – Mostly unilateral (75%)
- Aseptic meningitis
- Pancreatitis and diabetes
- Oophoritis.

Rare Complications of Mumps

- Encephalitis
- Hepatitis
- Thyroiditis
- Myocarditis
- Nerve deafness.

12. Ans. (b) Four days before and five days after rash

[*Ref.:* Park, 21st ed., page no. 137, 20th ed., page no. 136-37]

- Measles patients are infectious from 4 days before to 4 days after the onset of rash.

Period of Communicability

- Chicken pox patients are infectious from 2 days before to 5 days after the onset of rash.
- Mumps patients are infectious from 1 week before to 2 weeks after the onset of parotitis.
- Measles patients are infectious from 4 days before to 4 days after the onset of rash.
- Rubella patients are infectious from 1 week before to 1 week after the onset of rash.

13. Ans. (c) Measles

[*Ref.:* Ananthnarayan, 8th ed., page no. 509]

See Q. No. 2.

14. Ans. (b) Rabies vaccine

[*Ref.:* Ananthnarayan, 8th ed., page no. 89; Park, 21st ed., page no. 97]

- Herd immunity does not with Rabies vaccine. Rabies vaccine is a killed inactivated vaccine and there is no subclinical cases of Rabies.

Herd Immunity

- Refers to an overall level of immunity in a community.
- Eradication of an infectious disease depends on development of a high level of herd immunity against the pathogen.
- Epidemics of a disease is likely to occur when herd immunity against that disease is very low, indicating the presence of a large number of susceptible people in the community.

Elements that contributes to Herd immunity are:

- Occurrence of clinical and subclinical cases in herd
- Ongoing immunization programme
- Herd structure – includes population.

Herd immunity occurs with the following vaccines:

- ❖ OPV
- ❖ Diphtheria
- ❖ Pertussis
- ❖ Measles, Mumps, Rubella
- ❖ Small Pox.

15. Ans. (d) OPV

[*Ref.:* Park, 21st ed., page no. 98]

- ❖ Live vaccines are contraindicated in pregnancy as there is risk of fetal damage.
- ❖ Among the options, only oral polio vaccine is a live vaccine.

16. Ans. (b) Meningoencephalitis

[*Ref.:* Park 20th ed., page no. 136-37; Harrison, 18th ed., page no. 1603]

Rare but serious complications of measles involve the central nervous system (CNS) like:

- Postmeasles encephalomyelitis
- Measles inclusion body encephalitis (MIBE)
- Subacute sclerosing panencephalitis (SSPE)

Also remember

Pneumonia is the most common life threatening complication of measles and accounts for >90% measles related death.

17. Ans. (b) MMR

[Ref.: Park 21st ed., page no. 98]

- ❖ Live vaccines are contraindicated in pregnancy as there is risk of fetal damage.
- ❖ Among the options, only MMR vaccine is a live vaccine.

18. Ans. (c) Measles

[*Ref.:* Ananthnarayan, 8th ed., page no. 509-10]

- ❖ Measles is highly contagious and is spread from person-to-person by aerosols.
- ❖ Humans are the only host. Cases are the source of infection.
- ❖ There is no carriers neither any subclinical cases.

19. Ans. (a) 1

[*Ref.:* Ananthnarayan, 8th ed., page no. 506]

- ❖ MMR vaccine given single dose subcutaneously after 1 year of age.
- ❖ Remember, all live vaccines are given single dose mostly except OPV.

20. Ans. (c) 7 days

[*Ref.:* Park, 21st ed., page no. 139, 20th ed., page no. 138]

Control measures recommended for post exposure measles:

- ❖ Isolation of cases for 7 days after onset of rash
- ❖ Immunization of contacts within 3 days of exposure.

- ❖ Immunoglobulin is given within 3-4 days of exposure if vaccine is contraindicated.
- ❖ Immunoglobulin and vaccine are never given together, given 8-12 weeks later.

21. Ans. (b) 4 days before and 5 day after appearance of rash

[*Ref.:* Ananthnarayan, 8th ed., page no. 510; Park, 21st ed., page no. 137]

- ❖ Measles patients are infectious from 4 days before to 5 days after the onset of rash.

22. Ans. (a) DPT

[*Ref.:* Park, 21st ed., page no. 101]

- ❖ Vaccines that has to be kept in freezer compartment (–20°C) – Polio and Measles.
- ❖ Vaccines that has to be kept in cold but never allowed to freeze – DPT, BCG, TT, DT, Diluent.

23. Ans. (c) Measles

[*Ref.:* Park, 21th ed. page no. 139]

- ❖ Measles immunoglobulin and vaccine are never given together, given 8-12 weeks later.

PRACTICE MCQ's

1. The influenza virus responsible for pandemics is:

(a) Influenza virus A (b) Influenza virus B
(c) Influenza virus C (d) Any of the above.

2. Which of the following is an RNA virus?

(a) Hepatitis B virus (b) Parainfluenza virus
(c) Adenoviruses (d) Herpes simplex virus.

3. All the following statements are true for influenza viruses except:

(a) Helical symmetry (b) Single stranded unsegmented RNA
(c) Haemagglutinin and neuraminidase spikes present
(d) RNA dependent RNA polymerase.

4. The paramyxovirus virus that lacks both haemagglutinin and neuraminidase activities is:

(a) Mumps virus (b) Measles virus
(c) Respiratory syncitial virus (d) Parainfluenza virus.

5. The most likely cause of bronchiolitis in a 6 month old infant is:

(a) Measles virus (b) Mumps virus
(c) Respiratory syncitial virus (d) Parainfluenza virus.

6. The genome of paramyxoviruses consist of:

(a) Single stranded segmented RNA (b) Single stranded non-segmented RNA
(c) Double stranded segmented DNA (d) Double stranded non-segmented DNA.

7. All the following statements are true for mumps virus except:

(a) Involves all salivary gland (b) Mumps orchitis is bilateral
(c) Complication – Aseptic meningitis and pancreatitis
(d) Vaccine – Jery Lynn strain.

VIROLOGY II

ANSWERS TO PRACTICE MCQ's

1. Ans. (a) Influenza virus A

[*Ref.:* Ananthnarayan, 8th ed., page no. 496]

Pandemic	Most common seen in Influenza Type A
Epidemic	Seen in Influenza Type A, B

2. Ans. (b) Parainfluenza virus

[*Ref.:* Ananthnarayan, 8th ed., page no. 504]

- Parainfluenza virus belongs to paramyxoviridea family and contains unsegmented single stranded RNA.
- **DNA viruses includes**
  - Hepatitis B virus and Herpes
  - Papova, Pox and Parvovirus
  - Adenoviruses.
- The remaining viruses are RNA viruses.

3. Ans. (b) Single stranded unsegmented RNA

[*Ref.:* Ananthnarayan, 8th ed., page no. 494]

- Influenza virus possesses single stranded segmented RNA (8 segments).

4. Ans. (c) Respiratory syncitial virus

[*Ref.:* Ananthnarayan, 8th ed., page no. 505]

- Influenza and mumps possess both haemagglutinin and neuraminidase spikes.
- Measles possesses haemagglutinin but lacks neuraminidase spikes.
- RSV lacks both haemagglutinin and neuraminidase spikes.

5. Ans. (c) Respiratory syncitial virus

[*Ref.:* Ananthnarayan, 8th ed., page no. 508]

- Respiratory syncitial virus is the most common cause of bronchiolitis in infant.

6. Ans. (b) Single stranded non-segmented RNA

[*Ref.:* Ananthnarayan, 8th ed., page no. 504]

- Orthomyxovirus – Single stranded segmented RNA
- Paramyxoviruses – Single stranded non-segmented RNA
- Rotavirus – Possess Double stranded segmented DNA.

7. Ans. (b) Mumps orchitis is bilateral

[*Ref.:* Ananthnarayan, 8th ed., page no. 505-06; Park, 21th ed., page no. 142, 20th ed., page no. 141]

- Mumps orchitis is mostly unilateral (75%).

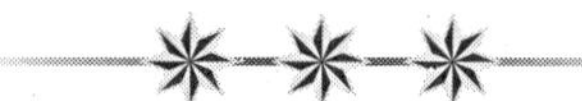

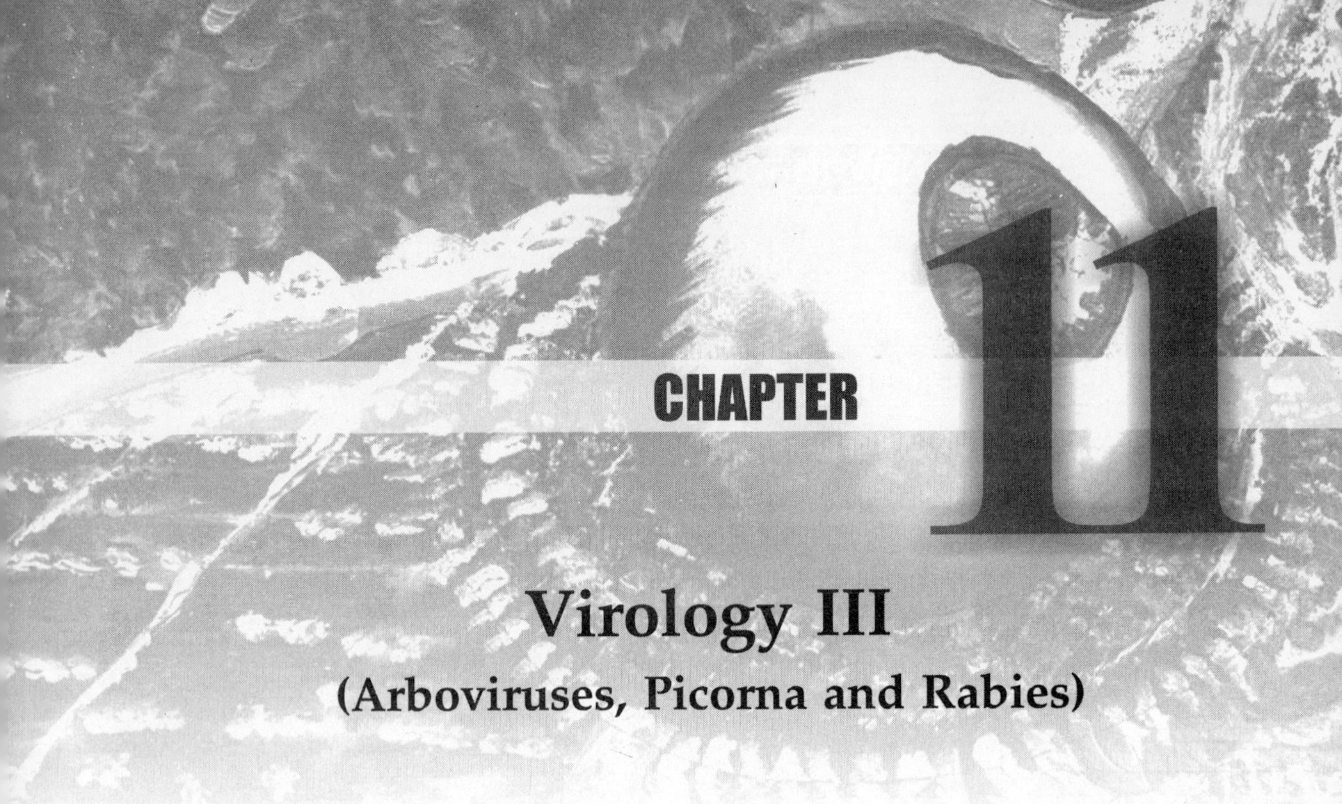

Virology III
(Arboviruses, Picorna and Rabies)

ARBOVIRUSES

Arboviruses common in India:

- *Hemorrhagic:* Dengue, Chikungunya, KFD.
- *Encephalitis:* Japanese B, Westnile, Sindbis.
- *Rare:* Ganjam, Vellore, Chandipura, Bhanja.
- Yellow fever not found in India.

Animal Reservoirs

- In many cases, the actual reservoir is not known.
- Birds: Japanese B encephalitis, St. Louis encephalitis, EEE, WEE.
- Pigs: Japanese B encephalitis (Amplifier host).
- Monkeys: Yellow fever.
- Rodents: VEE, Russian Spring-Summer encephalitis.

Clinical Features

- Fever and rash with athralgia – non-specific.
- Encephalitis, e.g., EEE, WEE, St. Louis encephalitis, Japanese encephalitis.
- Hemorrhagic fever, e.g., Yellow fever, Dengue, Crimean-Congo hemorrhagic fever, Chikungunya, Hanta.
- Hemorrhagic fever with shock – Dengue.

Lab Diagnosis

- **Serology**
  - HAI antibody, CFT antibody, Neutralizing antibody.
  - ELISA – MAC ELISA (IgM), IgG ELISA.
  - *Indicators:*
    - IgM detection.
    - Seroconversion of IgG.
    - Four fold rise in titer of IgG of paired sera.
- *Isolation* – Suckling mice brain, Mosquito inoculation.
- *Culture* – Mosquito cell lines : C3/36 cell line.
- *Detection of antigen* – NS1 Antigen (ELISA and ICT).
- *Detection of RNA* – (rt-PCR).

Japanese Encephalitis

- 1st seen in Japan as "Summer encephalitis" epidemics – but now uncommon in Japan.
- Called 'B' – to distinguish from encephalitis A (encephalitis lethargica/Von Economo disease).
- Affect from Korea to India and Malayasia.
- Vector – *C. tritaeniorhynchus,* C. vishnui (India).
- India – Vellore, Tamil Nadu – A.P. – Karnataka border, now world wide.
- Reservoir – Ardeid (wading) birds.
- Amplifying hosts – Pigs, bats.
- Incidental hosts – Horses, humans, others.
- The most common cause of epidemic encephalitis.
- *Seasonal variation:*
  - Temperate area (June-September)
  - Subtropical areas (March-October).
- Live attenuated vaccine (14-14-2).
- Inactivated vaccine (Nakayama strain).

Dengue

- DEN 4 serotypes – 1, 2, 3, 4 – Type 3 most common.
- Vector – Aedes aegypti mosquito.
- Mixed infection – Antibody dependent enhancement (ADE).
- *Clinical feature:*
  - Dengue fever (DF) – Biphasic (Saddle back), Break bone fever, LN↑, Maculopapular rash.
  - Dengue Hemorrhagic Fever (DHF).
  - Dengue Shock Syndrome (DSS).

Chikungunya

- Fever, rash, LN↑, arthralgia (name derived – doubled up due to joint pain).

- Differ from Dengue:
  - Hemorrhagic manifestations rare
  - Chikungunya outbreaks are shorter.
- Vector – Aedes aegypti.
- 1964 outbreak – Africa, India (Vellore, Pondicherry, Chennai).
- 1973-2005 – No outbreaks.
- Re-emerged in 2005 – Hyderabad, Karnataka, Maharastra.
- Reason of re-emergence:
  - New vector – Aedes albopictus.
  - Viral factor – E1 glycoprotein mutation of virus.
  - More rural involvement.

Yellow Fever Virus

- *Endemic* – West Africa and Central South America.
- *Reservoir:*
  - Forest – Monkey and forest mosquito.
  - Urban – Cases urban mosquito.
- *Two major forms:*
  - Jungle YF – Cycle involving primates and forest mosquitoes.
  - Urban YF is – Cycle involving human to human by Aedes aegypti mosquito.
- **Do not exist in India,** because
  - Aedes aegypti is present in East cost area in India (whereas YF is endemic in West Africa)
  - Strict vigilance and Quarantine for the travelers.
  - Cross reacting Dengue antibody provides protection.
  - But YF immunization does not protect from dengue.
- *Incubation period* **– 3-6 days.**
- *Clinical feature* – Hemorrhages, Fever, Platelet dysfunction, Relative bradycardia, Jaundice.
- Liver – Midzonal necrosis, Councilman bodies.
- ***Torres*** bodies (intranuclear inclusion body).
- Darkar vaccine – Mouse brain vaccine, risk of encephalitis.
- 17D live attenuated vaccine
  - Prepared in India (CRI, Kasuli)
  - Chick embryo, no risk of encephalitis
  - Single dose given sc
  - 95% effective within 10 days of inoculation
  - Reimmunization required every 10 years for travelers
  - Cholera and YF vaccine should not be given together
  - Measures in airport:
    - Unprotected travelers – 6 days quarantine
    - Aedes aegypti index <1 400 mt surrounding airport.

Kyasanur Forest Disease

- Hemorrhagic fever
- Tick borne
- Seen in Kyasanur Forest in Shimoga District, Karnataka.

Incubation Period

- Dengue – 5-6days
- Chikungunya – 5-6d days
- Japanese B – 5-15 days
- Yellow fevr – 3-6 days
- KFD – 4-8 days.

Hemorrhagic Virus (Non-arthropod borne)

Hantavirus:

- HF with renal syndrome.
- Rodent borne (Most common route – inhalation from rodent excreta).
- Hanta pulmonary syndrome – by Sin Nombre virus.

Others: Marbug, Ebola, Lassa.

PICORNAVIRIDAE

Include two major groups of human pathogens:

- Enteroviruses – Polio and Coxsackie
- Rhinoviruses.

Poliovirus:

- **Three subtypes:**
  - Type 1 – Most common wild type
  - Type 2
  - Type 3 – Most common cause of vaccine associated paralysis.
- **CFT detects:**
  - C Ag (coreless)
  - D Ag (dense Ag, type specific).
- **Risk factors:**
  - Following Tonsillectomy
  - Pregnancy
  - IM injection
  - Muscular activity
  - Coxsackie A
  - Genetic predisposition.
- **Pathogenesis:**
  - Mode if transmission – Faeco oral > Inhalation > Conjunctiva
  - Spread – Hematogenous spread (Most common), also direct neural spread (Following Tonsillectomy)

- Site of action – Anterior horn of spinal cord
- Earliest change in neuron – ***Nissl body*** degeneration
- Pathological changes always more extensive than distribution of paralysis.

Clinical Types

- In apparent infection – 90-95%,
- Abortive infection – 5-10%
- Aseptic meningitis (non paralytic) – 0.1%
- Paralytic (<0.1%) – Ascending flaccid paralysis (AFP).

Lab Diagnosis

- Blood, throat swab, CSF, feces (till 6 weeks).
- Isolation – Monkey kidney tissue culture followed by Neutralization test.
- Neutralizing antibody – comes early, stay long.
- CFT Antibody- Anti C- comes early, goes early, Anti D- comes late, goes late.

Polio vaccine	Salk (Injectable)	Sabin (Oral)
Preparation	Formalin killed preparation of all three types in MKC (monkey kidney cell line)	Each dose contains: ❖ Type 1 – 10 lakh, Type 2- 2 lakh ❖ Type 3 – 3 lakh of TCID50 ❖ Stabilized in $MgCl_2$, *pH<7*
Safety	Relatively more safer	Safer except in immunocompromised pt.
Efficiency	80-90% by full course	90-100% by 1 or 2 doses Efficacy decreases: ❖ Interference by other enteroviruses ❖ Frequent diarrheal disease ❖ Breast feeding
Economy	Relatively expensive	Economical
Duration of protection	Need booster doses periodically	Long lasting
In epidemics	Cannot be used	Can be used
Herd immunity	Not provided	Provided
Local mucosal immunity	Not provided	Provided (IgA antibody)

Coxsackie Virus

Group A Coxsackie virus	Group B Coxsackie virus
Suckling mouse inoculation ❖ Flaccid paralysis ❖ Generalized myositis	**Suckling mouse inoculation** ❖ Spastic paralysis ❖ Focal myositis ❖ Necrosis of brown fat ❖ Pancreatitis, hepatitis, myocarditis, encephalitis
❖ Herpangina (vesicular Pharyngitis) ❖ Hand-foot-and-mouth disease (Also by Enterovirus-71) ❖ Acute hemorrhagic conjunctivitis (Cox-A24 and Enterovirus 70) ❖ Pneumonitis of infants ❖ Diarrhea ❖ URTI ❖ Fever with rash	❖ Pleurodynia (epidemic myalgia)/ Bornholm disease – B1,B5 ❖ Myocarditis, pericarditis ❖ Diabetes mellitus – B4 ❖ Pneumonia **Both Cox A and B – can cause** ❖ Aseptic meningitis (Most common – A7) ❖ Encephalitis ❖ Cold ❖ Hepatitis

RABIES VIRUS

- Bullet shaped, –ve sense RNA virus.
- *Reservoir:*
  - Urban Rabies – Dog 99%, cat.
  - Wild life Rabies – Fox, Jackal, Wolf.
- *Source* – Saliva of Rabid animal.
- *Mode of transmission* – Bite (Most common), Lick on abrasion, corneal transplant, air borne.
- Speed of rabies progress in sensory nerve – ***3 mm/hr.***
- Earliest symptom – Neuritic pain at bite site.
- Sensory N → UMN → sympathetic → mental system.
- *Incubation period* – 1-3 month.
- IP is shorter in children and upper limb bite (than leg bite).
- *Mechanism* – Neural apoptosis, ↓Acetyl choline.

Street virus	Fixed virus
❖ Freshly isolated	❖ After serial passage
❖ Produce Negri body	❖ Does not produce Negri body
❖ Affect salivary gland	❖ Does not affect salivary gland

Furious Rabies	Dumb Rabies
80% of all cases	20% of all cases
Hydrophobia,	No hydrophobia
Absent – Fever, Fasciculation, Percussion edema	Present – Fever, Fasciculation, Percussion edema
Paralytic, Proximal muscle	Paralytic, Proximal muscle
Seen in unvaccinated individuals	Associated with partial vaccine course

Antemortem Diagnosis

- Direct Florescent Antibody Test
  - corneal impression smear (30% Sn, in late stage)
  - hair follicle of nape of neck.
- Isolation – Mice, cell line followed by IF.
- Antibody in CSF.
- RNA detection by RT-PCR.

Post mortem Diagnosis

- Negri body
  - Pathognomic – 3-27μ
  - Hippocampus most common site (next-cerebellum)
  - Absent in 20% cases
  - Seller technique – methylene blue and basic fuchsin
- Mouse inoculation
- Isolation
- DFA on brain smear.

Vaccine

- ***Neural:***
  - Semple, BPL (Konnor), Infant brain.
  - Poor immunogenic, encephalogenic.
- ***Non-neural:***
  - Purified chick embryo cell (PCEC)
  - Purified vero cell (PVC)
  - Human diploid cell (HDC)
  - Protection for 6 m.
- Preexposure – 3 doses, at day 0, 7, 28.
- Post exposure – 6 doses, at day 0, 3, 7, 14, 28 and 90 days.

FMGE MCQ's

Arboviruses

1. **KFD is transmitted by:** [*September 2011, March 2010*]
   (a) Mite (b) Louse
   (c) Tick (d) Mosquito.
2. **Yellow fever is transmitted by:** [*September 2011*]
   (a) Culex (b) Anopheles stephensi
   (c) Aedes aegypti (d) Mite.
3. **Amplifier host in Japanese encephalitis is:** [*September 2011*]
   (a) Man (b) Culex mosquito
   (c) Pig (d) Horse.
4. **In dengue infection, number of petechial spot per square inch in cubital fossa should be:** [*September 2007, 2010*]
   (a) >5 (b) >10
   (c) >15 (d) >20.
5. **Certificate of Yellow fever vaccination is valid upto:** [*September 2010*]
   (a) 10 days (b) 1 year
   (c) 5 years (d) 10 years.
6. **Which is true of KFD?** [*March 2010*]
   (a) Transmitted by tick (b) It is a arboviral infection
   (c) Also known as Monkey Disease (d) All of the above.
7. **All are features of Dengue hemorrhagic fever except:** [*September 2010*]
   (a) Thrombocytopenia (b) Narrow pulse pressure
   (c) Hematocrit elevated (d) Positive torniquet test.
8. **Dengue hemorrhagic fever is caused by:** [*March 2010*]
   (a) Alphavirus (b) Flavivirus
   (c) Bunyavirus (d) Orbivirus.
9. **Dengue is transmitted by:** [*March 2010; September 2006*]
   (a) Anopheles (b) Culex
   (c) Mansonia (d) Aedes.
10. **False statement regarding Japanese encephalitis is:** [*March 2010*]
    (a) It is caused by flavivirus (b) Transmitted by aedes mosquito
    (c) Endemic in India (d) Man is dead-end host.
11. **All of the following belong to arboviruses group except:** [*September 2009*]
    (a) Bunyavirus (b) Paramvxovirus
    (c) Flavivirus (d) Alphavirus.
12. **Culex mosquito spreads all of the following disease except:** [*March 2008*]
    (a) Viral arthritis (b) West Nile fever
    (c) Yellow fever (d) Bancroftian filariasis.

13. Natural reservoir of Chikungunya virus in India is: [*March 2007*]

(a) Monkey
(b) Guinea pig
(c) Aedes
(d) Dog.

14. Which of the following is spread by Aedes mosquitoes? [*September 2007*]

(a) Loa Loa
(b) Malaria
(c) Dengue
(d) Japanese encephalitis.

15. Quarantine period for yellow fever is: [*September 2005*]

(a) 1 day
(b) 2 days
(c) 6 days
(d) 10 days.

Picornavirdae

16. Polio is transmitted by: [*March 2010*]

(a) Feco oral
(b) Blood
(c) Skin contact
(d) Inhalational.

17. True statement regarding poliomyelitis is: [*March 2010*]

(a) Poliovirus is resistant to pasteurization
(b) For every clinical case, there may be 1000 subclinical cases in adults
(c) Commonly spreads by faeco-oral route
(d) Most outbreaks of polio are due to type-3 poliovirus.

Rabies

18. Incubation period of Rabies depends on: [*September 2010*]

(a) Severity of bite
(b) Number of bite
(c) Site of bite
(d) All of the above.

19. Rabies vaccine is prepared from: [*September 2010*]

(a) Live virus
(b) Street virus
(c) Fixed virus
(d) None of the above.

20. Best specimen for Rabies diagnosis in living person: [*March 2009*]

(a) Corneal smear
(b) CSF
(c) Biopsy of hair follicle of neck
(d) Saliva.

21. Which of the following is not a part of management in grade III dog bite infected with rabies? [*March 2009*]

(a) Vaccination
(b) Stitch the wound with antibiotic coverage
(c) Wash with soap and water
(d) Administration of antirabies serum and vaccination.

22. Which of the following is best for ante-mortem diagnosis of rabies? [*March 2009*]

(a) Antirabies antibodies in blood
(b) Immunofluorescence of corneal impressions
(c) Immunofluorescence of LN biopsy
(d) Isolation of virus from saliva.

23. Post exposure prophylaxis in Rabies: [*March 2008*]

(a) Day 0, 3, 7
(b) Day 0, 7, 28
(c) Day 0, 3, 7, 14, 21, 90
(d) Day 0, 3, 7, 14, 28, 90.

24. Negri body seen in: [*September 2003, 2007, 2008*]
(a) Measles
(b) Rabies
(c) Tatanus
(d) HIV.

25. For post-exposure prophylaxis, dose of human rabies immunoglobulin is: [*September 2007*]
(a) 10 IU/kg
(b) 20 IU/kg
(c) 30 IU/kg
(d) 40 IU/kg

26. Virus that spreads by neural route is: [*September 2007*]
(a) Rabies virus
(b) Polio virus
(c) EB virus
(d) Enterovirus.

27. Cell culture Rabies vaccine is given at: [*September 2005*]
(a) Medial part of thigh
(b) Deltoid muscle
(c) Anterior abdomen
(d) Lateral part of thigh.

28. Virus causing rabies in man is: [*March 2005*]
(a) Wild virus
(b) Mild virus
(c) Fixed virus
(d) All of the above.

ANSWERS TO FMGE QUESTIONS

Arboviruses

1. Ans. (c) Tick

[*Ref.:* Ananthnarayan, 8th ed., page no. 514]

- **Kyasanur Forest Disease (KFD) is an example of tick-borne hemorrhagic fever.**

Arboviruses and their Vectors

Vector	Arboviruses
Aedes Aegypti	Dengue Chikungunya Yellow fever virus
Culex tritaeniorhynchus	Japanese encephalitis
Tick	Kyasanur Forest Disease (KFD) Russian spring summer encephalitis Powassan virus Omsk hemorrhagic fever Crimean Congo hemorrhagic fever Colorado tick fever

2. Ans. (c) Aedes aegypti

[*Ref.:* Ananthnarayan, 8th ed., page no. 514]

- Yellow fever is a mosquito (Aedes aegypti) borne acute febrile illness that occurs in Africa and South America. The disease is not reported in India.

3. Ans. (c) Pig

[*Ref.:* Ananthnarayan, 8th ed., page no. 517]

- Pigs are usually the amplifier host of Japanese encephalitis.
- The high cattle pig ratio in India is a major factor which has been suggested to control infection in India.

Japanese Encephalitis

- Reservoir: Ardeid (wading) birds
- Amplifying hosts – Pigs
- Incidental hosts – Horses, humans, (dead end)
- Mosquito attractant – Cattle and Buffalo
- Horse is the only animal that shows signs of encephalitis.

4. Ans. (d) >20

[*Ref.:* Park, 21st ed., page no. 227, 20th ed., page no. 220]

- Dengue hemorrhagic fever is diagnosed by Positive Tourniquest test which indicates number of petechial spot per square inch in cubital fossa is >20 per 2.5 cm (1 inch) square area.

Tourniquest Test

- Done to detect thrombocytopenia.
- The standard method uses the blood pressure cuff.
- To identify dengue and chikungunya infection.
- Positive Tourniquet test – Number of petechial spot per square inch in cubital fossa is >20.
- Any of the following may be present – petechiae, purpura, ecchymosis, epistaxis, gum bleeding, hemetamesis or melena.

Criteria for Diagnosis of Dengue Hemorrhagic Fever (DHF):

- Fever – acute, high, continuous for 2-7 days
- Positive Tourniquet test
- Enlargement of liver.

5. Ans. (d) 10 years

[*Ref.:* Park, 21st ed., page no. 259; 20th ed., page no. 248]

- In India, Certificate of Yellow fever vaccination starts after 10 days of vaccination and is valid upto 10 years. Revaccination is required every 10 years.
- This certificate is required for all the travellers coming from endemic zone including infants too.
- Travellers without a valid certificate are placed in a mosquito free ward for 6 days.

6. Ans. (d) All of the above

[*Ref.:* Ananthnarayan, 8th ed., page no. 520; Park, 21st ed., page no. 264, 20th ed., page no. 251]

VIROLOGY III

Kyasanur Forest Disease (KFD)

- An example of arboviral infection, belongs to Flaviviridae.
- Transmitted by tick (*Haemaphysalis spinigera*). The tick also acts as the reservoir host because the virus is transmitted transovarially.
- The monkeys appear to act as amplifier host, but not reservoir host, because monkeys die of the infection.
- Cattle also play an important role for maintenance of tick.
- Man- dead end, no role in transmission.
- This disease is so called because this was first reported in Kyasanur forest of shimoga district Karnataka in 1957.
- Incubation period of 4-8 days.
- Haemorrhagic fever.
- No specific antiviral treatment is available. Prevention of the disease is based primarily on control of ticks and personal protection by using adequate clothings and insect repellants.
- A killed KFD vaccine is also available for use against the KFD.

7. Ans. (b) Narrow pulse pressure

[*Ref.:* Park, 21th ed., page no. 227; 20th ed., page no. 220]

- Narrow pulse pressure is measure of shock which is a manifestation of Dengue shock syndrome.

Criteria for Diagnosis of Dengue Hemorrhagic Fever (DHF)

- Fever – acute, high, continuous for 2-7 days
- Positive Tourniquest test
- Enlargement of liver
- Laboratory evidence
- Thrombocytopenia (< 100,000/mm^3)
- Haemoconecerntration (Haematocrit raised by >20%).

Criteria for Diagnosis of Dengue Shock Syndrome (DSS)

- All the above criteria of DHF, plus.
- Shock-manifested with rapid and weak pulse with narrow pulse pressure (<20 mm Hg) or hypotension with presence of cold, clammy skin and restlessness.

8. Ans. (b) Flavivirus

[*Ref.:* Ananthnarayan, 8th ed., page no. 513]

- Dengue virus belongs to flaviviridae family.

Family	Genus	IMP Species
Togaviridae	Alphavirus	Chikungunya, Eastern/Western/Venezuelan Equine encephalitis virus (EEE,) WEE, VEE Sindbis Rose river, Semiliki Forest

Flaviviridae	Flavivirus	Japanese encephalitis B Dengue West Nile Yellow fever Kyasanur Forest Disease (KFD) Virus St. Lous Murray Valley Russian Summer Spring Encephalitis (RSSE) Virus
Bunyaviridae	Bunyavirus	California encephalitis virus
	Phlebo	Sandfly fever virus, Rift Valley
	Nairo	Crimean Congo hemorrhagic virus, Ganjam virus
	Hanta	Hantan, Seoul, Puumala, Prospect Hill
Reoviridae	Orbivirus	Colorado Tick fever

9. Ans. (d) Aedes

[*Ref.:* Ananthnarayan, 8th ed., page no. 519]

- ❖ Dengue is transmitted by Aedes aegypti (tiger mosquito). (see Q. No. 1)

10. Ans. (b) Transmitted by aedes mosquito

[*Ref.:* Park, 21st ed., page no. 262-263, 20th ed., page no. 249; Ananthnarayan, 8th ed., page no. 516-517]

- ❖ JE is transmitted to humans by certain species of Culex mosquitoes widely prevalent in rice fields in Asia. The disease is spread throughout mostly in rural areas of Asia most often by Culex tritaeniorhynchus.
- ❖ Belongs to flavivirridae family (Genus – favivirus).
- ❖ JE is Endemic in India. Reported from various states like TamilNadu, West Bengal, Assam, Karnataka, various areas in Uttar Pradesh.
- ❖ Man is an accidental dead-end host and does not transmit the disease.

11. Ans. (b) Paramvxovirus

[*Ref.:* Ananthnarayan, 8th ed., page no. 514]

- ❖ Paramvxovirus is not an arbovirus.

12. Ans. (c) Yellow fever

[*Ref.:* Ananthnarayan, 8th ed., page no. 518]

- ❖ Yellow fever is transmitted by Aedes aegypti (tiger mosquito). (see Q. No. 1)

13. Ans. (c) Aedes

[*Ref.:* Ananthnarayan, 8th ed., page no. 515]

- ❖ Chikungunya is transmitted by Aedes aegypti (tiger mosquito) which also acts as reservoir of infection.
- ❖ There is no animal reservoir identified so far.

14. Ans. (c) Dengue

[*Ref.*: Ananthnarayan, 8th ed., page no. 519]

❖ Dengue is transmitted by Aedes aegypti (Tiger mosquito). (see Q. No. 1)

15. Ans. (c) 6 days

[*Ref.*: Park, 21st ed., page no. 259; 20th ed., page no. 248]

❖ Travellers without a valid certificate are placed in a mosquito free ward for 6 days.

Picornavirdae

16. Ans. (a) Feco oral

[*Ref.*: Ananthnarayan, 8th ed., page no. 485]

❖ The poliovirus is transmitted primarily by the faecal-oral route by ingestion of food and water contaminated with human faeces. The infection can also be transmitted by inhalation or through fomites contaminated with respiratory secretions.

17. Ans. (c) Commonly spreads by faeco-oral route

[*Ref.*: Ananthnarayan, 8th ed., page no. 484; Park, 21st ed., page no. 184-85; 20th ed., page no. 179]

❖ The poliovirus is transmitted primarily by the faecal-oral route.

About Other Options:

❖ Poliovirus is susceptible to pasteurization, heat. Resistant to low pH and bile and proteolytic enzymes of intestine.

❖ For every clinical case, there may be 1000 subclinical cases in children and 75 in adults.

❖ Most outbreaks of polio are due to type-1 poliovirus whereas vaccine induced poliomyelitis is due to Type 3.

Rabies

18. Ans. (d) All of the above

[Ref.: Ananthnarayan, 8th ed., page no. 528]

❖ Incubation period of Rabies is 1-3 months

❖ **The incubation period is less:**

- If the patient is bitten on the head or neck
- If inoculum is heavy
- Multiple bites
- Deep wounds, or large wounds
- Children.

Pathogenesis of Rabies

❖ Mode of transmission – Bite (most common), lick on abrasion, corneal transplant, air borne

❖ Mode of spread – Sensory N → UMN → sympathetic → mental system

❖ Speed of Rabies progress in sensory nerve – 3 mm/hr

❖ Earliest symptom – Neuritic pain at bite site

❖ Incubation period – 1-3 month

- ❖ IP is shorter in children and upper limb bite (than leg bite)
- ❖ Mechanism – Neural apoptosis, ↓Acetyl choline.

19. Ans. (c) Fixed virus

[*Ref.*: Ananthnarayan, 8th ed., page no. 526]

- ❖ Fixed virus is defined Virus is isolated after several serial intracerebral passages in rabbits and can be used for vaccine production.

Street virus	Fixed virus
Freshly isolated	After serial intracerebral passages in rabbits
Produce Negri body	Does not Produce Negri body
Affect salivary gland	Does not affect salivary gland
Can cause fatal encephalitis	Neurotropic but much less infective
Incubation period – 1-12 weak	Incubation period – 5-6 days
	Used for vaccine

20. Ans. (c) Biopsy of hair follicle of neck

[Ref.: Ananthnarayan, 8th ed., page no. 530]

- ❖ Corneal smears, biopsy from hair follicle form the nape of the neck, and saliva are the usual specimens for antemortem diagnosis of rabies.
- ❖ Corneal impression smear is only 30% sensitive mainly it is positive in late stage.
- ❖ Biopsy of hair follicle of base of neck is more sensitive and considered as the best sample for Direct Florescent Antibody (DFA) test done for antemortem diagnosis of Rabies.
- ❖ The brain of the dead animal is the specimen of choice for postmortem diagnosis of rabies.

Antemortem Diagnosis of Rabies:

- ❖ Direct Florescent Antibody test
  - Corneal impression smear (30% Sn, in late stage)
  - Hair follicle of nape of neck.
- ❖ Isolation – Mice, cell line followed by IF
- ❖ Antibody in CSF
- ❖ RNA detection by RT–PCR.

Postmortem Diagnosis of Rabies

- ❖ Negri body
  - Pathognomic – 3-27 μ
  - Hippocampus most common site (next – cerebellum)
  - Absent in 20% cases
  - Seller technique – methylene blue and basic fuchsin.
- ❖ Mouse inoculation
- ❖ Isolation
- ❖ DFA on brain smear.

21. Ans. (b) Stitch the wound with antibiotic coverage

[*Ref.:* Ananthnarayan, 8th ed., page no. 530]

Wound should never be stitched immediately to prevent additional trauma that may help in spread of the virus in the deeper tissue.

"If suturing is necessary, then it has to be done after 24-48 hr later, applying minimum stitches under the coverage of antirabies serum locally."

–Park

Local Care of Rabies Includes

- *Cleansing* – Wound should be scrubbed well immediately with soap & water – soap kills the virus effectively.
- *Chemical treatment* – Wound is treated with quartenary ammonium compounds (like cetavlon or tincture iodine).
- *Anti rabies serum* – given for grade III bites.
- Antitenaus measures and local antibiotics.
- Observe the animal for 10 days.

22. Ans. (b) Immunofluorescence of corneal impressions

[*Ref.:* Ananthnarayan, 8th ed., page no. 530]

- Direct Florescent Antibody test of corneal impression smear or hair follicle of nape of neck is the ideal method of antemortem diagnosis of Rabies.

23. Ans. (d) Day 0, 3, 7, 14, 28, 90

[*Ref.:* Ananthnarayan, 8th ed., page no. 532; Park, 21st ed., page no. 255]

- **Post exposure prophylaxis for Rabies is given, on days 0, 3, 7, 14, 28 and booster at 90 days.**

Postexposure Prophylaxis

- Requires a course of 6 doses, starting as soon as possible given, on days 0, 3, 7, 14, 28 and booster at 90 days.
- The first dose on the day 0, is combined with an injection of human hyper immunoglobulin (20 IU/kg).
- Vaccination with complete dosages gives virtually complete protection, for at least five years.
- During this period of five years if any further exposure occurs, only one or two booster doses (on days 0, 3) may be given.
- After five year a full course of five injections is given if again exposed to infection.

24. Ans. (b) Rabies

[*Ref.:* Ananthnarayan, 8th ed., page no. 530]

- **Demonstration of Negri bodies by microscopy is the characteristic histopathological feature and pathognomic of rabies.**

Negri bodies

- Negri bodies are made up of a finely fibrillar matrix and rabies virus particles.
- Intracytoplasmic, inclusion body.
- They measure 3 μm to 27 μm in size.
- They are found only in the neural tissues, and are found more in the ***cerebellum and hippocampus.***

- Absent in 20% of human cases of rabies. Therefore failure to demonstrate Negri bodies in neural tissue do not rule out the diagnosis of rabies.
- **Seller's technique:** Used to stain impression smears of the human brain tissue (postmortem)
- The stain contains methylene blue alcohol as fixative and basic fuchsin as staining reagent.

25. Ans. (b) 20 IU/kg

[*Ref.:* Ananthnarayan, 8th ed., page no. 533; Park, 21st ed., page no. 255]

- Both vaccination and immunoglobulin are recommended in Grade III dog bite infected with rabies.
- Human hyper immunoglobulin (20 IU/kg) is recommended.

Risk	Exposure type	Post Exposure Prophylaxis
Category I: No exposure	Touching, feeding of animals or licks on intact skin	None
Category II: Min exposure	❖ Minor scratches or abrasions without bleeding ❖ Licks on broken skin ❖ Nibbling of uncovered skin	Vaccine
Category III: Severe exposure	❖ Single or multiple transdermal bites, scratches or contamination of mucous ❖ Membrane with saliva (i.e., licks) ❖ Bat bite	IG + Vaccine

26. Ans. (a) Rabies virus

[*Ref.:* Ananthnarayan, 8th ed., page no. 527]

- **Rabies:** Virus that spreads by neural route.
- **Poliovirus:** Virus that spreads by hematogenous route.

27. Ans. (b) Deltoid muscle

[*Ref.:* Ananthnarayan, 8th ed., page no. 533; Park, 21st ed., page no. 255]

- Cell culture vaccines like human diploid cell vaccine, purified chick embryo cell vaccine and purified Vero cell vaccines are given intramuscularly or subcutaneously **in the deltoid region in adults and on the anterolateral side of the thigh in children.**

28. Ans. (a) Wild virus

[*Ref.:* Ananthnarayan, 8th ed., page no. 526

- **Wild virus** is defined as – Virus which is present in nature that causes Rabies in humans.
- **Street virus** is defined as – Virus that is isolated from natural human or animal infection. It can cause fatal encephalitis in laboratory animals after a long incubation period of 1-12 weeks.
- **Fixed virus** is defined as – Virus is isolated after several serial intracerebral passages in rabbits and is used for vaccine production. It is neurotropic but much less infective. It can cause fatal encephalitis in laboratory animals after a short and fixed incubation period of 6-7 days.

PRACTICE MCQ's

1. Arbovirus transmittred by tick all except:

(a) Western equine encephalitis
(b) Kyasanur forest disease
(c) Russian spring summer encephalitis
(d) Omsk heemorrhagic fever.

2. All the following viruses are transmitted by arthopod vectors except:

(a) Hantavirus
(b) Chandipura virus
(c) Rift valley fever
(d) Sand fly fever.

3. The vaccine is not available for:

(a) Dengue fever
(b) Japanese encephailitis
(c) Yellow fever
(d) KFD.

4. The prototype strains for Type 1 poliovirus is:

(a) Brunhilde and Mahoney strains
(b) Lansing and MEFI strains
(c) Leonand Saukett strains
(d) None of the above.

5. Which of the following statement is true for Coxsackie A virus?

(a) It has 24 serotypes
(b) It causes juvenile diabetes
(c) It shows predilection for visceral organs
(d) It produces flaccid paralysis.

6. Which of the following Enteroviruses is a hepatitis virus?

(a) Enterovitus 69
(b) Enterovitus 70
(c) Enterovitus 71
(d) Enterovitus 72.

7. All the following statements are true for rabies virus except:

(a) Infection may be prevented by active and passive immunization
(b) The animal reservoir differs from country to country
(c) Rabies vaccine is a live attenuated vaccine
(d) Diagnosed by DFA.

ANSWERS TO PRACTICE MCQ's

1. Ans. (a) Western equine encephalitis

[*Ref.:* Ananthnarayan, 8th ed., page no. 515]

- Western equine encephalitis – transmitted by horse.

Tick borne arboviruses

- Kyasanur Forest Disease (KFD)
- Russian spring summer encephalitis
- Powassan virus
- Omsk hemorrhagic fever
- Crimean Congo hemorrhagic fever
- Colorado tick fever.

2. Ans. (a) Hantavirus

[*Ref.:* Ananthnarayan, 8th ed., page no. 522]

- Hantavirus is transmitted by respiratory route.

3. Ans. (a) Dengue fever

[*Ref.:* Ananthnarayan, 8th ed., page no. 519]

- ❖ The vaccine is not available for: Dengue fever.

4. Ans. (a) Brunhilde and Mahoney strains

[*Ref.:* Ananthnarayan, 8th ed., page no. 484]

- ❖ Brunhilde and Mahoney strains – Polio Type 1 strain
- ❖ Lansing and MEFI strains – Ty Polio Type 2 strain
- ❖ Leon and Saukett strains – Polio Type 3 strain.

5. Ans. (a) It has 24 serotypes and (d) It produces flaccid paralysis

[*Ref.:* Ananthnarayan, 8th ed., page no. 489]

- ❖ Coxsackie A virus – produces flaccid paralysis in mice.
- ❖ Coxsackie B virus – produces spastic paralysis in mice.

6. Ans. (d) Enterovitus 72

[*Ref.:* Ananthnarayan, 8th ed., page no. 536]

- ❖ Enterovitus 72 is known as hepatitis A virus.

7. Ans. (c) Rabies vaccine is a live attenuated vaccine

[*Ref.:* Ananthnarayan, 8th ed., page no. 533]

- ❖ Rabies vaccine is an inactivated attenuated vaccine.

Other Options:

- ❖ Both active and passive immunization is recommended for grade III exposure.
- ❖ The animal reservoir differs from country to country, in India it is Dog.
- ❖ Antemortem Diagnosed is done by **Direct Florescent Antibody (DFA)** test of corneal scrapping.

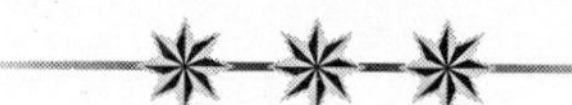

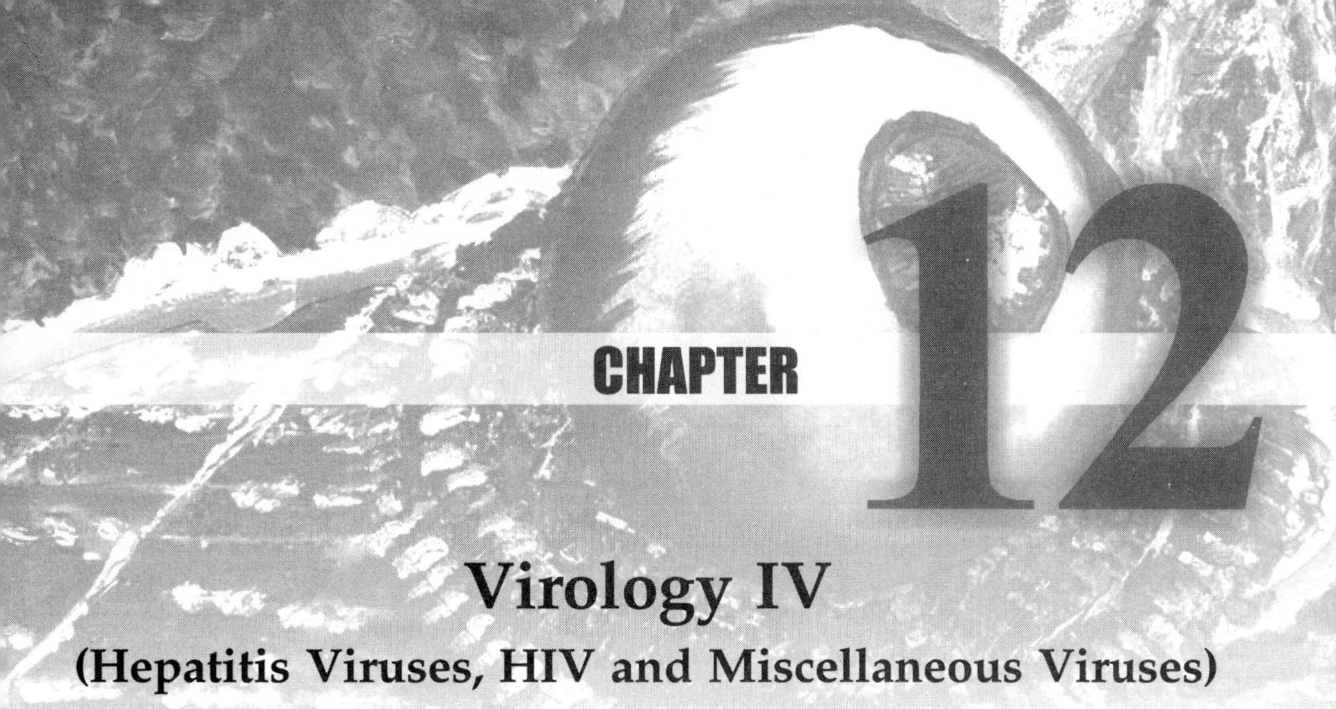

CHAPTER 12

Virology IV

(Hepatitis Viruses, HIV and Miscellaneous Viruses)

HEPATITIS VIRUSES

Viral Causes of Hepatitis

- Hepatitis A, B, C, D, E, G
- Cytomegalovirus
- Herpes simplex virus
- Entero-virus
- Yellow fever virus
- Epstein bar virus
- Rubella virus
- *Others* – Leptospira, Toxoplasma, Coxiella.

	HAV	HBV	HCV	HDV	HEV
Common name	Infectious	Serum	Non A non B Post transfusion	Delta agent	Non A non B Enteric transmitted
Family	Entero 72	Hepadna	Flavi	Viroid like	Calci
Onset	Abrupt	Insidious	Insidious	Abrupt	Abrupt
Age	Children	Any	Adult	Any	Young adult
Route	Feaco-oral	Blood, sexual, vertical	Blood, sexual, vertical	Blood, sexual	Feaco-oral
I.P. (days)	15-50	50-150	15-150	15-50	15-50
Mortality	<0.5%	1-2%	0.5-1%	High	Usually 1-2% and Pregnancy – 20-40%
Chronic carrier	No	Yes	Yes	Yes	No

Oncogenic	Nil	Present (neonate)	Present	Nil	Nil
Associated Other feature	Secondary attack rate 10-20%	HCC, cirrhosis, Autoimmune disorder like AGN, arthritis, PAN	HCC, cirrhosis, Autoimmune-AGN, arthrits, cryoglobuli-nemia	HCC, cirrhosis, fuminant hepatitis	Secondary attack rate 1-2% Not seen in western countries

Laboratory Diagnosis of Hepatitis

HAV	HBV	HCV	HDV	HEV
• IgM HAV • HAV RNA	• HBsAg: Acute, chronic, carrier • HBeAg: Active infection • Anti HBc: – IgM: Acute, window period – IgG: chronic infection • Only Anti HBs – vaccination • HBV DNA: Active infection, viral load (monitoring infection) • Anti HBc: Epidemiological marker	• Antibody by 3rd generation ELISA using NS5 antigen • HCV RNA • Genotyping • 7 subtypes	• HBsAg • Anti HBc – IgM: Coinfection – IgG: Superinfection • HDV Ag • HDV RNA • Anti HD IgM	• Anti HBE Antibody • EM of stool • HEV RNA

VIROLOGY IV

HBV

- ❖ HBV – dsDNA virus (double strand is incomplete)
- ❖ DNA polymerase has double action – DNA depdDNA polymerase + RT activity
- ❖ Has 3 form – spherical (Most common), tubular, Dane particle (complete)
- ❖ > 1/3rd of world population are infected with HBV
- ❖ Pathogenesis – immune mediated
- ❖ Hepatocyte carrying viral antigen subjected to antibody dependent NK cell/CD8 T cell cytotoxicity
- ❖ In absence of affective immune system – leads to carrier state (infants)
- ❖ HBV does not grow in conventional cell line.

HBV Gene

- ❖ S gene (HBsAg)
- ❖ Core gene – HBcAg
- ❖ Pre core – HBeAg
- ❖ P gene – DNA polymerase
- ❖ X gene – Regulatory gene

Mutants

- Precore mutant – unable to form HBeAg, medeterrian
- Escape mutant – unable to form HBsAg –ve (S gene mutation)
- Seen in infant borne to HBeAg +ve mother
- Seen in liver transplant recepient receiving combined HBV vaccine + Immunoglobulin.

HBV Carrier

- Persistent of HBV for >6 months – called as chronic carrier for HBV
- India ranks 2nd (China 1st)
- Populations can be divided to
  - Low endemicity – carrier rate – <2% (North India)
  - Intermediate – 2-8% – India
  - High endemicity – >8% (south India)
- ***Super carriers –*** High HBsAg, HBeAg, HBV DNA, DNA polymerase
- ***Simple carrier –*** Low HBsAg, No HBeAg
- ***Carrier rate*** – Following infection:
  - 5-10% of adult becomes carrier
  - 50% of children becomes carrier
  - 90% of neonate becomes carrier

Transmission

- Blood (most common route in developing) – highly infectious than HIV
- Vertical
  - During delivery (most common)
  - In-utero
  - Breast feeding
  - HBeAg +ve mother – high risk
- Sexual (most common route in developed country)
- Direct skin contact with open skin lesion
- High risk occupation – paramedical workers, sex workers
- Though HBV can survive in mosquito, but no transmission seen.
- Age- Developed country – (young adults), Developing country (younger age)
- No seasonal variation.

Vaccine

- HBsAg subunit – Prepared in Baker's yeast
- Three dose – 0, 1, 6 months
- Booster after 5 yrs if *Anti HBS <10 IU/ml*
- Non responder – 5-10%
- Neonate born to HBV mother – ***HBIG + Vaccine*** *(with in 12 hr)*
- Newer – containing whole HBsAg (i.e., *Pre S1 + Pre S2 + S)*

HCV

- Belongs to flaviviridae

- ssRNA, enveloped
- 50-80% of patients develops – chronic infection
- Carrier rate – 1-20%
- Affect only human
- Most common cause of post transfusion hepatitis
- Mode of transmission – Blood transfusion, IV drug abuser, sexual, vertical
- Antigenic Diversity – 6 genotype (quasi species)
- Hence, affective vaccination is difficult
- 3rd generation ELISA detecting antibody against NS5 Ag
- RNA PCR.

HGV

- Flavivirus
- Also known as GB virus
- ssRNA
- Mode of transmission – Blood transfusion, sexual, vertical
- Associated with – Acute, chronic, fulminant hepatitis.

HIV

Antigen

- *Envelope antigens*
  - Spike antigen – gp120 (principal antigen)
  - Transmembrane pedicle protein – gp41
- *Shell antigen*
  - Nucleocapsid protein – p18
  - Core antigen
  - Principal core antigen – p24
  - Other core antigens – p15, p55
- *Polymerase antigens*
  - p31, p51, p66

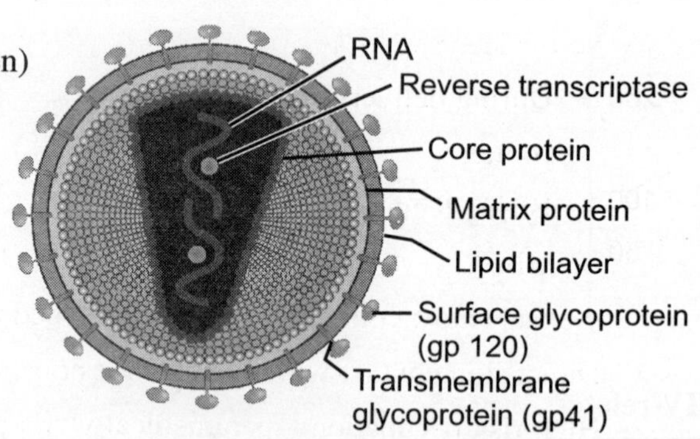

Fig. 12.1: Antigen of HIV

Types of HIV

- HIV-I and HIV-2
- HIV-1-divided to 3 groups: M (major), O (outlier), N (new)
- M group – 10 subtypes or clades (A to J)
- India – Type-1-clade C more common and both type 1 and 2 are seen
- 90% HIV cases in A.P, T.N, Karnataka, Maharashtra, Nagaland and Manipur.

Mode of Transmission

Type of exposure	Risk %
Sexual	0.1-1%
Blood transfusion	>90%
Tissue or donation of organ	50-90%
Injection and injuries	0.5-1%
Mother to baby	**30%**

High viral load found in blood, genital secretion, CSF.

❖ **Receptors** – binds to gp120 of HIV
- All cells expressing CD4 molecules like T helper cells (T tropic strains)
- Macrophages (M tropic strains)
- Dendritic cells
- Glial cells

❖ **Co-receptors** – binds to gp-41 of HIV
- CXCR4 – T tropic strains
- CCR5 – M tropic strains

CD4 T cell Count at which Opportunistic Infection Takes Place

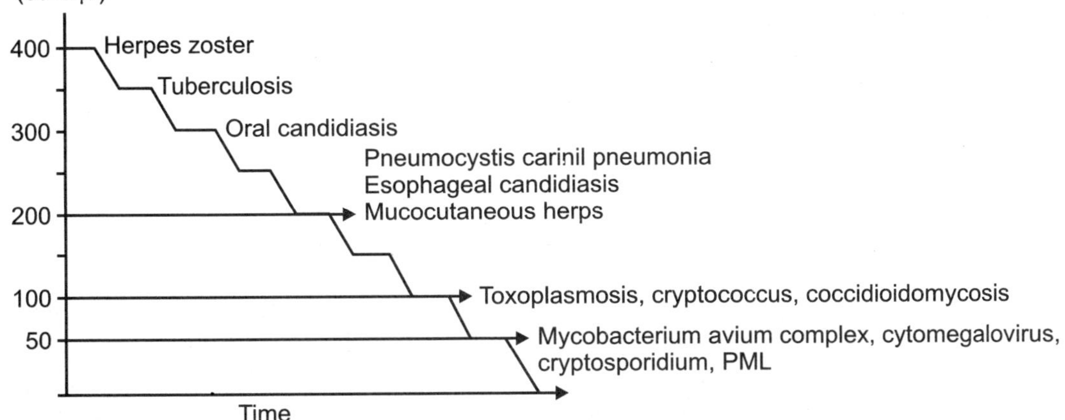

HIV-related infections most frequently encountered in India

Bacterial	Viral	Fungal	Parasitic	Other illnesses
Tuberculosis	Herpes simples virus infection	Candidiasis	Cryptosporidiosis	AIDS dementia complex
Bacterial respiratory infections	Oral hairy leukoplakia	Cryptococcosis	Microsporidiosis	Invasive cervical cancer
	Varicella zoster virus disease	Pneumocystic jiroveci pneumonia	Isosporiasis	Non-Hodgkin lymphoma
Salmonella infection	Cytomegalovirus disease	Penicilliosis	Giardiasisww stongyloides	
	Human papillomavirus infections		Toxoplasmosis	

Rare infections include those due to Bartonella henselae, Rhodococcus equi, Atypical mycobacterioses and Human herpesvirus (HHS) – 8 infections.

Lab Diagnosis of HIV

- ***Screening*** **(E/R/S)**
  - ELISA
  - Rapid
  - Simple

  ELISA:
  - 1st generation ELISA – crude preparation of HIV antigen is used
  - 2nd generation ELISA – recombinant Ag
  - 3rd generation ELISA – synthetic oligopeptide
  - 4th generation ELISA – combination of recombinant and synthetic peptide and detect both HIV antgen (p24) and antibody.
- ***Confirmatory***
  - Antibody detection:
    - Western blot – uses whole virus lysates
    - Immunofluorescence assay
    - Radioimmunoprecipitation assay (RIPA)
    - Line immunoassay (LIA) – recombinant/synthetic antigen used – More specific.
  - HIV RNA
  - Viral culture
- ***Surrogate markers***
  - CD4 count
  - Hypergammaglobulinemia
  - Altered CD4 : CD8 ratio.
- ***Criteria used for HIV 1 by Western Blot:***
  - WHO – Two envelop bands gp41, gp120/160 with or without gag or pol bands.
  - CDC – Any two – p24, gp41, gp120/160.
- ***NACO strategy*** of HIV diagnosis:
  - Strategy I – done for screening for Donor/Blood bank – 1 test.
  - Strategy IIa – done for Seroprevalance/epidemiological purpose – 2 test.
  - Strategy IIb – done for HIV symptomatic patients – 2 test.
  - Strategy III – done for asymptomatic HIV patients – 3 test.
- ***Prognosis/monitoring***
  - CD4 T cell count – most commonly used.
  - HIV RNA – Most consistent.
  - P24 antigen detection.
  - Neopterin.
  - β2 macroglobulin.

- ***Pediatric HIV***
  - HIV DNA – Most recommended
  - p24 antigen detection
  - IgM antibody
  - IgG ELISA at 18 months only.
- ***NACO guidelines to prevent neonatal HIV:*** Single dose Nevirapine to mother during labor and to the baby within 72 hours after birth.
- ***Diagnosis in window period***
  - Initial time when the antibody detection methods are negative
  - p24 antigen detection (30% sensitive)
  - HIV RNA – best
- Guidelines for post exposure prophylaxis (PEP)
  - Body fluid considered at risk – blood, genital secretion, CSF and other body fluid
  - Body fluid not considered at risk – tear, sweat, saliva, feces
  - PEP should be started within 2 hr.
  - **Basic regimen** – Zidovudine or Lamivudine for 4 weeks
  - **Expanded regimen –** Basic + Indinavir for 4 weeks.

MISCELLANEOUS VIRUSES

Rota Virus

- Belong to family Reoviridae
- Double walled virus – looks like a wheel with short spokes
- Segmented dsRNA virus (11 segments)
- Serologic types – A to G (most common – group A, adult rotavirus strains belongs to Group B)
- Commonest cause of diarrhea in infant and children (6-24 months)
- Seasonal variation – Most common in Winter
- Route – Faeco-oral
- Incubation period – 2-3 days
- *Lab diagnosis*:
  - Electron microscopy – Detection limit 106 particle/ml
  - ELISA detecting antigen in stool
  - Culture – Difficult, rolling of tissue culture facilitates growth
  - RT – PCR.

Causes of Viral Gastroenteritis

- Rotavirus
- Enteric adenovirus, type 40,41
- Calcivirus, e.g., Norwalk
  - Outbreaks associated with uncooked ***shellfish*** in older children
  - Calci – means 32 cup shaped depression on virus surface.
- Astroviruses
- Coronavirus
- H1N1

Slow Virus Diseases

- **Definition:** Group of viruses which cause slow, progressive, neuro degenerative disease of CNS with long incubation period and high mortality rate.
- **Character:**
  - Long incubation periods ranging from months to years
  - Predilection to CNS
  - Immune response is either absent or contributes to pathogenesis
  - Fatal termination
  - Slow growth rate
  - Genetic predisposition.
- **Group A Slow viral disease**
  - Slowly progressive infections of sheep
  - Caused by lentivirus
  - Visna – Demyelinating disease of sheep
  - Maedi – Hemorrhagic pneumonia of sheep.
- **Group B – Prion disease of the CNS**
- **Discoverer** – Stanley B Prusiner
- Prions are proteins not virus (protein without nucleic acid)
- The pathogenic mechanism – Normal prion protein PrPc present on chromosome 20 gets mutated to abnormal prion protein (PrPsc) which acumulates— Amyloid Plaques gets deposited in CNS.
- ***Pathology***
  - Progressive vacuolation in dendritic and axonal process of neuron
  - Astroglial hypertrophy
  - Spongiform degeneration.
- ***Animal:***
  - Scrapie (sheep)
  - Mink encephalopathy
  - Bovine spongiform encephalopathy (BSE) (Mad Cow Disease)
- ***Human Prion disease:***
  - Kuru – tremor, due to cannabalism
  - Gerstmann-Straussler-Scheinker (GSS) syndrome
  - Creutzfeldt-Jakob disease
  - Fatal familial insomnia.
- ***Symptoms are related to site:***
  - Cerebral cortex – Loss of memory and mental acuity and visual imparement (CJD).
  - Thalamus – Insomnia (FFI)
  - Cerebellum – Problems to coordinate body movements and difficulties to walk (kuru, GSS).
- **Group C Slow viral disease:**
  - Two unrelated CNS disease of human
  - Subacute sclerosing panencephalitis (defective measles virus)
  - Progressive multifocal leucoencephalopathy (JC virus)

FMGE MCQ's

Hepatitis Viruses

1. **Which of the following is not a live vaccine?** [*September 2011*]
   (a) Oral polio vaccine (b) MMR vaccine
   (c) Yellow fever vaccine (d) Hepatitis B vaccine.
2. **Which vaccine can be given in pregnancy?** [*March 2010*]
   (a) Measles vaccine (b) Rubella vaccine
   (c) BCG vaccine (d) Hepatitis B vaccine.
3. **Perinatal Hepatitis transmission is maximum in:** [*March 2008*]
   (a) 1st trimester (b) 2nd trimester
   (c) 3rd trimester (d) During delivery.
4. **Which Hepatitis virus is associated with highest mortality in pregnancy?** [*September 2007*]
   (a) Hepatitis A (b) Hepatitis B
   (c) Hepatitis C (d) Hepatitis E.
5. **Hepatitis virus that spreads by faeco oral route:** [*March 2007*]
   (a) Hepatitis A (b) Hepatitis B
   (c) Hepatitis C (d) Hepatitis D.
6. **Hepatitis E is transmitted by:** [*September 2007*]
   (a) Feco oral route (b) Blood transfusion
   (c) Needle prick (d) Sexual mode.
7. **Which is known as Australian antigen?** [*September 2006*]
   (a) HBsAg (b) HBeAg
   (c) HBcAg (d) HBV DNA.
8. **Acute hepatitis B is diagnosed by:** [*September 2006*]
   (a) HBsAg (b) HBeAg
   (c) HBcAg (d) Anti HBc antibody (IgM).
9. **Hepatitis B vaccine should be given as per which schedule:** [*September 2005*]
   (a) 0, 1, 6 days (b) 0, 1, 6 weeks
   (c) 0, 1, 6 months (d) 0, 1, 6 years.

HIV

10. **HIV affects which cell mainly:** [*September 2011*]
    (a) CD4 cell (b) CD8 cell
    (c) Microphages (d) Nerve cells.
11. **Average incubation period for AIDS is:** [*March 2011*]
    (a) 6 years (b) 8 years
    (c) 10 years (d) 12 years.
12. **Most common malignancy in AIDS is:** [*March 2011*]

(a) Kaposi sarcoma (b) B-cell lymphoma
(c) Leukemia (d) Burkitts lymphoma.

13. Least affective mode of transmission of HIV: [*September 2010*]
(a) Sexual (b) Blood product
(c) Needle/syringe (d) Mother to fetus.

14. True of HIV all except: [*March 2010*]
(a) Infects CD4 cells (b) Reversal of CD4/CD8 ratio
(c) Also affects macrophages (d) DNA virus.

15. All of the following is true regarding HIV virus except: [*March 2010*]
(a) Belongs to the subgroup lentivirus (b) Double stranded DNA virus
(c) The presence of characteristic reverse transcriptase enzyme
(d) Acts on CD4 cells.

16. Most common opportunistic infection in HIV in India: [*March 2008*]
(a) Tuberculosis (b) Pneumocystis
(c) Candida (d) Histoplasma.

17. Single dose of which drug given in HIV patients during labour, to prevent transmission: [*September 2007*]
(a) Zidovudine (b) Nevirapine
(c) Lamividune (d) Indinavir.

18. Specific laboratory test to diagnose HIV infection: [*March 2007*]
(a) ELISA (b) Western blot
(c) Complement fixation test (d) RIA.

19. Best indicator of HIV prognosis: [*September 2007*]
(a) CD4 count (b) CD8 count
(c) HIV RNA (d) TLC count.

20. HIV predominantly affects: [*March 2007*]
(a) CD4 cells (b) CD8 cells
(c) B cells (d) Any T cells.

21. HIV is associated with which of the following opportunistic infection: [*September 2005*]
(a) M. tuberculosis (b) MAC
(c) Oropharyngeal candidiasis (d) All of the above.

Prions

22. True about prions are all except: [*September 2009*]
(a) Associated with Cruetzfeldt-Jacob disease
(b) Heat labile
(c) Sensitive to proteases
(d) Infectious proteinaceous particles.

ANSWERS TO FMGE QUESTIONS

1. Ans. (d) Hepatitis B vaccine

[*Ref.:* Ananthnarayan, 8th ed., page no. 544]

Hepatitis B vaccine is a recombinant DNA vaccine composed of Hepatitis B surface antigen (HBsAg) prepared in Baker's yeast.

Hepatitis B Vaccine:

- HBsAg recombinant subunit vaccine by cloning the S gene (which codes for non-glycosylated HBsAg particle) in Baker's yeast by recombinant DNA technique.
- 3 dose given at 0, 1, 6 months.
- Site – IM into the Deltoid (adult), anterio lateral thigh (infant).
- Gluteal injection – not recommended because of poor immune response.
- Dose – 10-20 μg/dose.
- Duration of protection – at least 15 years.
- Protection rate – >95% for children and adolescence and falls there after.
- Booster after 5 yrs if Anti *HBS <10 IU/ml.*
- Non responder – 5-10%.
- Neonate born to HBV mother – ***HBIG + Vaccine*** *(with in 12 hr).*
- Indication:
  - All less than 18 years.
  - High risk group – high risk sexual, health care workers, person requiring frequent transfusion/ transplantation, IV drug abusers.
- Plasma derived vaccine:
  - HBsAg is harvested and purified from plasma of human carriers of HBV.
  - Equally affective and same duration of protection and reactogenicity.
  - Drawback – Costlier and difficult to get plasma of carriers.
- **Newer vaccine:** Containing whole HBsAg *(Pre S1 + Pre S2 + S gene derived).*

2. Ans. (d) Hepatitis B vaccine

[*Ref.:* Ananthnarayan, 8th ed., page no. 544]

- All the live attenuated vaccines are contraindicated in pregnancy.

3. Ans. (d) During delivery

[*Ref.:* Ananthnarayan, 8th ed., page no. 542; Park, 21st ed., page no. 194, 20th ed., page no. 188]

- The transmission occurs from infected mother to child more commonly during the time of delivery due to contact with mothers infected blood or ingestion or accidental inoculation. Exposure followed by transplacental passage of the virus is rare.
- Transmission risk is more if mother is HBeAg +ve.
- The HBV virions although found in breast milk, but the role of breast feeding in transmission is unclear.

4. Ans. (d) Hepatitis E

[*Ref.:* Ananthnarayan, 8th ed., page no. 546]

- ❖ HEV causes fulminant hepatitis in pregnant women especially in last trimester of pregnancy and has a high fatality rate of 15-20%. Encephalopathy and DIC are the important causes of death. HEV infection does not appear to cause chronic liver diseases.

5. Ans. (a) Hepatitis A

[*Ref.:* Ananthnarayan, 8th ed., page no. 537]

- ❖ HAV infection is transmitted primarily by fecal oral route. Most commonly, the virus spreads from person-to-person through contaminated water and food including shell fish collected from sewage contaminated water. The virus is rarely transmitted by blood or blood products because the level of viraemia in HAV is low and chronic infection does not occur.

Hepatitis A and E virus	Spreads by faeco oral route
Hepatitis B, C, D	Spreads by blood, vertical and sexual routes

6. Ans. (a) Feco oral route

[*Ref.:* Ananthnarayan, 8th ed., page no. 546]

- ❖ HEV transmitted primarily by fecal oral route due to fecal contamination of water in endemic areas. Fecal contaminated water is the important source of infection. The reservoir of HEV is unknown, but it may be transmitted by animals.

7. Ans. (a) HBsAg

[*Ref.:* Ananthnarayan, 8th ed., page no. 539]

- ❖ Blumberg and his colleagues in 1965 described the **hepatitis B surface antigen (HBsAg)** in the serum of an Australian aboringe and named it as Australian antigen.

8. Ans. (d) Anti HBc antibody (IgM)

[*Ref.:* Ananthnarayan, 8th ed., page no. 543]

- ❖ Demonstration of antibodies (HBcAb) against hepatitis B core antigen can differentiate acute and chronic infection.

  IgM HBcAb is diagnostic of acute HBV infection.

  IgG HBcAb is diagnostic of chronic HBV infection.

Interpretation of common serological markers in HBV infection:

HBsAg appears in blood during incubation period, acute, chronic and carrier state. So, the presence of HBsAg alone does not necessarily indicate replication of virion and patients may not have symptoms of liver damage.

HBcAg is not detectable in the serum, but can be demonstrated in the liver cells by immunofluorescence.

HBeAg and HBV DNA can be present in acute or chronic stage or in carriers. The presence of HBeAg/HBV DNA indicates a high infectivity and transmissibility and activeness of disease.

HBsAb: Hepatitis B surface antibody (HBsAb) is a protective antibody that neutralizes the virus. Presence of only HBsAb indicates immunity following vaccination.

***HBcAb*:** 1st antibody to appear. Demonstration of antibodies (HBcAb) against hepatitis B core antigen can differentiate acute and chronic infection.

IgM HBcAb: is diagnostic of acute HBV infection.

IgG HBcAb is diagnostic of chronic HBV infection.

Interpretation of common serological markers in HBV infection

Viral markers						Interpretation
HBsAg	HBeAg	HbcAb		Anti-HBs	Anti-HBe	
		IgM	IgG			
+	+	–	–	–	–	Late incubation period or early hepatitis
+	+	+	–	–	–	Acute HBV infection, highly infectious
+	±	–	+	–	–	Late/chronic HBV infection
–	–	–	+	+	+	Past infection
+	–	–	–	–	–	Simple carrier
+	+	–	–	–	–	Super carrier
–	–	–	–	+	–	Immunity following vaccination

9. Ans. (c) 0, 1, 6 months

[*Ref.:* Ananthnarayan, 8th ed., page no. 544; Park, 21st ed., page no. 195, 20th ed., page no. 190]

- The HBV vaccine for adult is recommended at **0, 1 and 6 months.**
- In new borne – two schedules followed.
  - 3 dose regimen – 1st dose given at birth, 1st and 3rd given along with 2nd and 3rd DPT dose.
  - 4 dose regimen – 1st dose given at birth, 2nd, 3rd, 4th doses given along with 1st, 2nd and 3rd DPT dose.

HIV

10. Ans. (a) CD4 cell

[*Ref.:* Ananthnarayan, 8th ed., page no. 573]

- HIV affects any cell bearing CD4 molecule like
  - T helper cells (T tropic strains)
  - Macrophages (M tropic strains)
  - Dendritic cells
  - Glial cells.
- **Primary Receptors – *CD4 molecule*** binds to gp120 of HIV
- **Co-Receptors:**
  - CXCR4 (T tropic strains) – binds to gP – 41 of HIV
  - CCR5 (M tropic strains) – binds to gP – 41 of HIV.

11. Ans. (c) 10 years

[*Ref.:* Ananthnarayan, 8th ed., page no. 574]

- The long and variable incubation period of HIV is because of this latency. Clinical latency can be as long as 10 years.

- The median time between primary HIV infection and development of AIDS is approximately 10 years.
- In 5-10% of cases – it may be 15 years (long term non-progressors/survivors).
- This period of clinical latency does not correlate with microbiological latency as virus multiplication goes on throughout.

12. Ans. (a) Kaposi sarcoma

[*Ref.:* Ananthnarayan, 8th ed., page no. 477]

- **Human herpes virus 8-associated Kaposi's sarcoma is the most common malignancy associated with AIDS.**
- Other AIDS associated malignancy conditions include
  - Hodgkin's lymphoma
  - Non-Hodgkin's lymphoma
  - Cervical cancer
  - Anogenital cancer.
  - Burkitt's lymphoma has been shown to be even much more common in AIDS patients than in general population.
- **Kaposi's sarcoma** is condition which is much more common in untreated AIDS patients than in general population. It is a vascular tumor suggested to be of endothelial origin that is found in the skin, mucous membrane, lymphnode and visceral organs.

13. Ans. (a) Sexual

[*Ref.:* Ananthnarayan, 8th ed., page no. 581]

- Though HIV is transmitted primarily through sexual contact and constitutes more than 70% of the HIV transmission, but the risk of transmission is less (0.1-1%).
- Increased risk – ↑sexual partners, sex with commercial sex workers, homosexuals presence of other STD.

Mode of Transmission of HIV

Type of exposure	Risk %
Sexual	0.1-1%
Blood transfusion	>90%
Tissue or donation of organ	50-90%
Injection and injuries	0.5-1%
Mother to baby	30%

- **High viral load found in blood, genital secretion, CSF.**

14. Ans. (d) DNA virus

[*Ref.:* Ananthnarayan, 8th ed., page no. 570]

- HIV is a RNA virus contains two copies of single stranded RNA.

15. Ans. (b) Double stranded DNA virus

[*Ref.:* Ananthnarayan, 8th ed., page no. 570]

- HIV is a RNA virus contains two copies of single stranded RNA.

16. Ans. (a) Tuberculosis

[*Ref.:* NACO, Guideline for HIV Testing, 2007]

- Most common opportunistic infection in HIV in India – Tuberculosis.
- Most common opportunistic infection in HIV in Western World – Pneumocystis jerovecii.

17. Ans. (b) Nevirapine

[*Ref.:* NACO, Guideline for HIV Testing, 2007]

Single dose Nevirapine (NVP) to mother during labor and to the baby within 72 hours after birth.

18. Ans. (b) Western blot

[*Ref.:* NACO, Guideline for HIV Testing, 2007; Ananthnarayan, 8th ed., page no. 576]

Confirmatory/Specific Test for HIV

- *Antibody detection:*
  - Western blot – uses whole virus lysates
  - Immunofluorescence assay
  - Radioimmunoprecipitation assay (RIPA)
  - Line immunoassay (LIA) – recombinant/synthetic Antigen used – More specific.
- HIV RNA – Most specific test.
- Viral culture
  - The most specific test for HIV diagnosis – HIV RNA.
  - The most sensitive test for HIV diagnosis – ELISA.

19. Ans. (c) HIV RNA

[*Ref.:* Ananthnarayan, 8th ed., page no. 59-80]

Prognosis/Monitoring of HIV

- CD4 T cell count – most commonly used
- HIV RNA – most consistent and best method
- P24 antigen detection
- Neopterin
- β2 macroglobulin.

20. Ans. (a) CD4 cells

[*Ref.:* Ananthnarayan, 8th ed., page no. 573]

- ***HIV affects any cell bearing CD4 molecule like***
  - T helper cells (T tropic strains)
  - Macrophages (M tropic strains)
  - Dendritic cells
  - Glial cells.

21. Ans. (d) All of the above

[*Ref.:* Ananthnarayan, 8th ed., page no. 576; Harrison 18th ed., page no. 1507]

Indicator Diseases of AIDS:

Bacterial:

- Mycobacterium avium-intracellulare complex.
- Atypical mycobacterial disease.
- Pyogenic bacterial infections.
- Nocardia infection and actinomycosis.
- Extrapulmonary tuberculosis.
- Salmonellosis.
- Campylobacter infections.
- Legionellosis.

Viral:

- Cytomegalovirus disease.
- Herpes simplex virus infection.
- Hairy leukoplakia by Epstein-Barr virus.
- Progressive multifocal leukoencephalopathy (JC virus).

Protozoal:

- Toxoplasmosis.
- Isosporiasis.
- Pneumocystis carinii pneumonia.
- Cryptosporidiasis.
- Generalized strongyloidiasis.

Fungal:

- Candidiasis.
- Aspergillosis.
- Coccidioidomycosis (disseminated).
- Cryptococcosis (extrapulmonary).
- Histoplasmosis (disseminated).

Malignancies:

- Kaposi's sarcoma.
- Lymphomas: Hodgkin and non-Hodgkin types.

Others:

- HIV wasting syndrome.
- Lymphoid interstitial pneumonia.
- HIV encephalopathy.

22. Ans. (b) Heat labile

[*Ref.:* Ananthnarayan 8th ed., page no. 552]

- Prions are the most resistant structure (heat, disinfectant and radiation) known so far followed by cyst and spore.

About Other Options:

- The prions are small protein – containing infectious particles without detectable nucleic acid.
- Cruetzfeldt-Jacob disease is the most common Prion Disease in humans characterized by a sub-acute progressive encephalopathy. Dementia, myoclonic jerks, behavioural changes and confusion are the common clinical manifestations.
- Scrapie prion protein is protease resistant, however human or other animal prion proteins are sensitive to proteases.

–Parija

Group B – Prion Disease of the CNS:

- Discoverer – Stanley B Prusiner.
- Prions are infectious proteins not virus (protein without nucleic acid).

The Pathogenic Mechanism:

- Normal prion protein PrPc present on chromosome 20 gets mutated to abnormal prion protein (PrPsc) which acumulates – Amyloid Plaques gets deposited in CNS.

Pathology:

- Progressive vacuolation in dendritic and axonal process of neuron.
- Astroglial hypertrophy.
- Spongiform degeneration.

Animal:

- Scrapie (sheep).
- Mink encephalopathy.
- Bovine spongiform encephalopathy (BSE) (Mad Cow Disease).

Human Prion Disease:

- Kuru – tremor, due to cannabalism.
- Gerstmann-Straussler-Scheinker (GSS) syndrome.
- Creutzfeldt-Jakob disease.
- Fatal familial insomnia.

Symptoms are related to site:

- Cerebral cortex – Loss of memory and mental acuity, and visual imparement (CJD).
- Thalamus – Insomnia (FFI).
- Cerebellum – Problems to coordinate body movements and difficulties to walk (Kuru, GSS).

PRACTICE MCQ's

Hepatitis

1. Cell – fraction derived vaccine is:

(a) Hepatitis B (b) Measles

(c) Mumps (d) Rubella.

2. Chronic hepatitis is seen in:

(a) Hepatitis C (b) Hepatitis D

(c) Hepatitis A (d) Hepatitis E.

3. Which of the following does not go into chronic hepatitis stage?

(a) HBV (b) HCV

(c) HDV (d) HEV.

HIV

4. The gene coding for core of HIV is:

(a) GAG (b) ENV

(c) POL (d) TAT.

5. Gloves, syringes, needles etc., used for patients whose HIV test results is not known, should be immersed in:

(a) Providone – iodine
(b) Cresol
(c) 1% solution of sodium hypochlorite
(d) Lysol.

6. During the window period of patient with AIDS, diagnostic test is:

(a) ELISA
(b) Western Blot
(c) Line immunoassay
(d) PCR.

7. Reverse Transcriptase is:

(a) DNA polymerase
(b) DNA dependant RNA polymerase
(c) RNA dependant DNA polymerase
(d) RNA dependant RNA polymerase.

8. P24 antigen disappears from the blood after how many weeks in HIV:

(a) 2-4 weeks
(b) 4-6 weeks
(c) 6-8 weeks
(d) 8-10 weeks.

9. Sero conversion in HIV infection takes place in:

(a) 2 weeks
(b) 4 weeks
(c) 9 weeks
(d) 12 weeks.

ANSWERS TO PRACTICE MCQ's

Hepatitis

1. Ans. (a) Hepatitis B

[*Ref.:* Ananthnarayan, 8th ed., page no. 544]

- ❖ Hepatitis B is a Cell – fraction derived (sub unit) vaccine composed of non-glycosylated HbsAg component derived from Baker's yeast by recombinant DNA technique.

2. Ans. (a) Hepatitis C

[*Ref.:* Ananthnarayan, 8th ed., page no. 545, 547]

- ❖ Chronic hepatitis and carrier state is seen in Hepatitis B and C and D (more commonly in Hepatitis C).
- ❖ Chronicity and carrier state not seen in Hepatitis A and E.
- ❖ HBV – The risk of chronic infection and carrier rate is higher in those infected at birth (90%) and in patients who are immunocompromised. Only 5-10% of older children or adult progress to develop chronic infection.
- ❖ HCV – about 50-80% develops chronic infection. Carrier rate is 1-20%.

3. Ans. (d) HEV

[*Ref.:* Ananthnarayan, 8th ed., page no. 547]

- ❖ Chronicity and carrier state not seen in Hepatitis A and E.

HIV

4. Ans. (a) gag gene

[*Ref.:* Ananthnarayan, 8th ed., page no. 571]

Antigens of HIV	Gene coded
Envelope antigens Spike antigen-gp120 (principal antigen) Transmembrane pedicle protein-gp41	Coded by Env gene
Shell antigen Nucleocapsid protein-p18	Coded by Gag gene
Core antigen Principal core antigen-p24 Other core antigens-p15, p55	Coded by Gag gene
Polymerase antigens p31, p51, p66	Coded by Pol gene

5. Ans. (c) 1% solution of sodium hypochlorite

[*Ref.:* Ananthnarayan, 8th ed., page no. 572]

- ❖ The standard recommendation for gloves, syringes, needles etc., used for HIV patients is solution of sodium hypochlorite of 0.5% available chlorine (5g/l).
- ❖ The standard recommendation for treatment of contaminated medical instrument – 2% glutaraldehyde.

  Also know:

  - HIV is a thermolabile virus. It is readily inactivated at 60°C in 10 minutes.
  - The virus survives in dried blood, at room temperature (20-25°C).
  - HIV is inactivated by treatment with 50% ethanol, 35% isopropanol, 0.5% lysol, 0.5% formaldehyde, 0.3% hydrogen peroxide.
  - Bleaching powder is an effective disinfectant for use as surface decontaminants. It is effective at a concentration of 0.5%, free chlorine (5 g/L; 5000 ppm).

6. Ans. (d) PCR

[*Ref.:* Ananthnarayan, 8th ed., page no. 578-79]

The time interval before antibody appears in the serum is known as window period and it may vary for 3-4 weeks. The serum of the patient tested during this period is negative for serum antibodies but positive for viral antigens and RNA.

Window Period in HIV

- ❖ Initial period when the antibody detection methods are negative.
- ❖ It may vary for 3-4 weeks.
- ❖ Diagnosed by:
  - p24 antigen detection (30% sensitive)
  - HIV RNA – best.

7. Ans. (c) RNA dependant DNA polymerase

[*Ref.:* Ananthnarayan, 8th ed., page no. 570-71]

VIROLOGY IV

- ❖ The HIV characteristically possess an RNA-dependent DNA polymerase called reverse transcriptase which synthesizes DNA by using the genome RNA as a template.
- ❖ Three Enzymes of HIV (coded by Pol gene) – reverse transcriptase, integrase and protease.

8. Ans. (b) 4-6

[*Ref.:* Ananthnarayan, 8th ed., page no. 576; NACO, Guideline for HIV Testing, 2007, page no. 73]

- ❖ The p24 antigen often becomes undetectable after P24 antibodies develop in the blood. This is due to formation of immune complex by p24 with the antibodies.
- ❖ IgM p24 antibody appears in 4-6 weeks followed by IgG. *–Ananthnarayan*

The viral capsid core antigen (p24) antigen:

- ❖ Appears usually 1-3 week safter infection. The antibody sandwich ELISA using specific monoclonal antibodies to HIV p24 are used to detect p24 antigen.
- ❖ **The p24 antigen often becomes undetectable after p24 antibodies develop in the blood. This is due to formation of immune complex by p24 with the antibodies.**
- ❖ IgM p24 antibody appears in 4-6 weeks followed by IgG.
- ❖ However, p24 antigen may appear later in the course of infection suggesting a very poor prognosis.

P24 antigen detection is useful in:

- ❖ Monitoring HIV.
- ❖ Diagnosis of HIV in pediatric individuals.
- ❖ Diagnosis of HIV in window period.

9. Ans. (a) 2 weeks

[*Ref.:* Ananthnarayan, 8th ed., page no. 578; NACO, Guideline for HIV Testing, 2007, page no. 73]

- ❖ Sero conversion in HIV infection takes place in 2-8 weeks to several months. *–Ananthnarayan*
- ❖ Antibodies appear in blood in 2-8 weeks, but become detectable after 3 weeks to 12 weeks with the tests available currently. *–NACO*

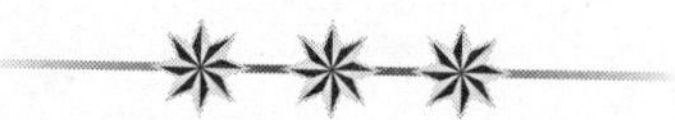

VIROLOGY IV

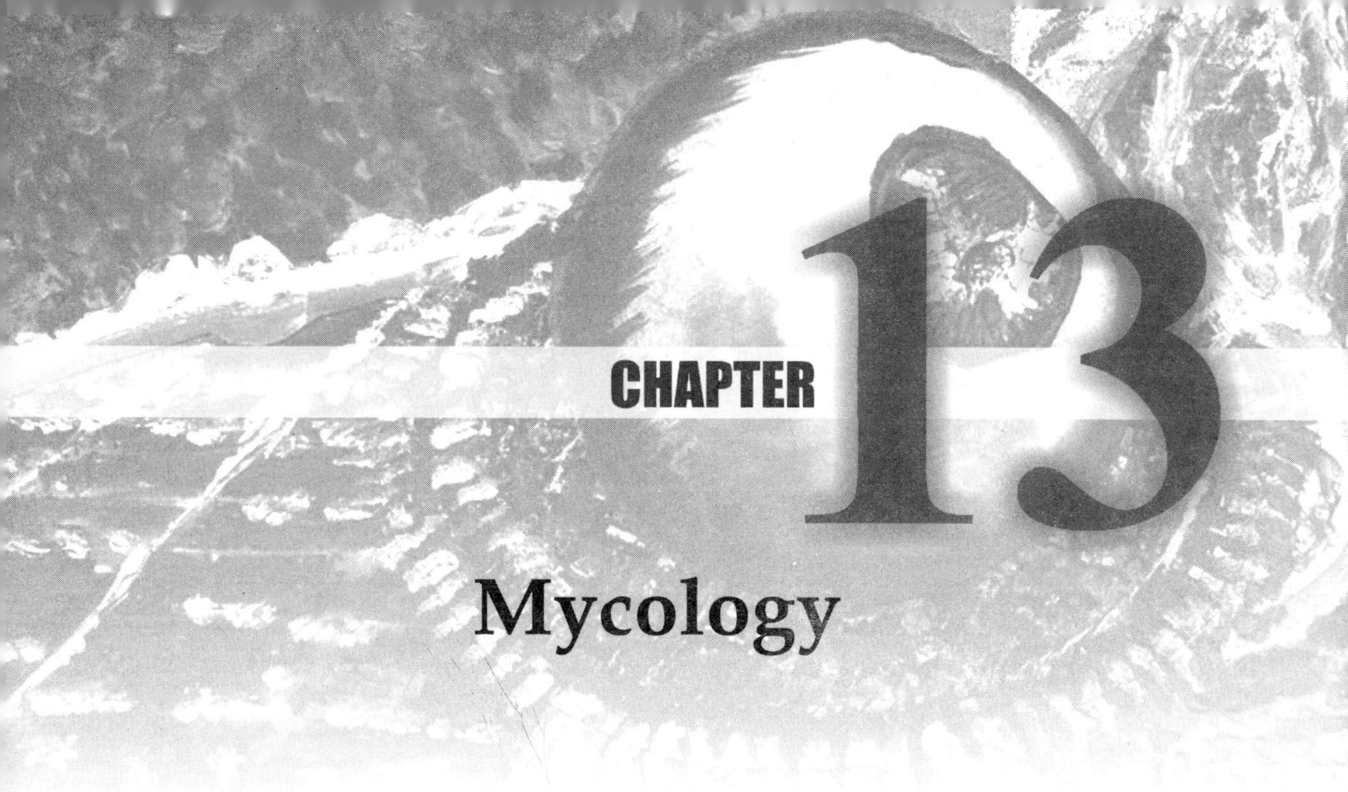

Mycology

CLASSIFICATION OF FUNGI

Morphological Classification

Yeast: Cryptococcus.

Yeast like: Produces pseudohyphae, e.g., Candida.

Mould: Dermatophyte, Aspergillus, Zygomycetes, Penicillium.

Dimorphic: Produces mould form at 25°C and environmental temperature, yeast form at 37°C and at body temperature.

Examples:

- Histoplasma
- Coccidiodes
- Sporothrix
- Blastomyces
- Paracoccidioides
- Penicillium marneffi.

Classification Based on Sexual Spore:

- *Phyco/zygomycetes*: Zygospore, broad aseptate hyphae, e.g., Rhizopus, Mucor, Absidia.
- *Ascomycetes*: Ascospores, Noarrow septate hyphae, e.g., Aspergillus.
- *Basidiomycetes*: Basidiospore, e.g., Cryptococcus.
- *Fungi imperfectii*: Deuteromycetes/hypomycetes
    - Sexual phase not found yet
    - Candida, Dermatophyte, Dimorphic group.

Classification Based on Disease:

I. *Superficial*: Tinea versicolor, Tinea nigra, Dermatophytes

II. *Subcutaneous*: Mycetoma, Chromoblastomycosis, Sporothrix, Rhinosporidium

III. *Systemic*:

(a) Histoplasma
(b) Blastomyces
(c) Coccidiodes
(d) Paracoccidioides
(e) Candida
(e) Cryptococcus.

IV. *Oppurtunistc fungi*:

(a) Aspergillus
(b) Zygomycetes
(c) Penicillium spp
(d) Penicillium marneffi
(e) Pneumocystis jerovecii
(f) Fusarium
(g) Candida
(h) Cryptococcus.

❖ **Sexual spore (ZAB)**
- Zygospore
- Ascospore
- Basidiospore

❖ **Asexual spore (ABC)**
- Arthrospore,
- Blastospore,
- Chlamydospore (Candia – Cornmeal agar).

Fungal Media:

❖ Sabaraud's Dextrose agar:
- Antibiotic – Cycloheximide, Chloramphenicol and Gentamicin
- pH – 5.6

❖ Niger seed agar – For Cryptococcus

❖ BHI broth – Histoplasma and Cryptococcus.

Fungal Stains:

❖ Lactophenol cotton blue (LPCB) – demonstrate the hyphae.

❖ PAS – Widely used histopathological fungal stain.

❖ Mucicarmine – Cryptococcus and Rhinosporidium.

❖ India Ink and Nigrosin – Cryptococcus capsule.

❖ Gomori Methinamine Silver – Pneumocystis.

Not Cultivable Fungi:

❖ Rhinosproridium

❖ Pneumocystis jerovecii

❖ Locazia.

SUPERFICIAL MYCOSES

Tinea Versicolor:

❖ Agent – Malassezia furfur

❖ Chronic recurrent, Non-inflammatory, Non-pruritic lesion

❖ Hypo to hyper pigmentation

- ***Diagnosis*:**
  - Sphagetti and meat ball appearance
  - Lipohilic (SDA with olive oil overlay is used)
  - Fried egg colony
  - Urease +ve
  - Wood's lamp examination – Scaly lesion show golden yellow fluorescens.
- ***Other Infection by Malassezia furfur:***
  - Seborrheic dermatitis (Dendroff)
  - Atopic dermatitis
  - Malassezia folliculitis
  - Systemic infections – In immunocompromised.

Tinea nigra:

- Agent – Hortaea werneckii
- Painless black non scaly, non inflammatory patch on palm and sole.

Piedra:

- *White Piedra*:
  - Agent – Trichosporon bigeli
  - White nodule on hair shaft (less firmly attached)
  - Hyaline septate hyphae and rectangular arthrospores
- *Black Piedra*:
  - Agent – Piedra hortae
  - Black nodule on hair shaft (firmly attached)
  - Dark brown septate hyphae with ascus containing ascospores.

DERMATOPHYTE (TINEA OR RING WORM)

- Trichohyton – skin, nail, hair *(Tri – Three)*
- Microsporoon – skin, hair *(M not for N)*
- Epidermophyton – skin, nail

Clinical Types:

- Tinea capitis
- Tinea cruris
- Tineapedis
- Tinea corporis
- Tinea barbae
- Tinea ungium.

Tinea capitis:

- **Endothrix:** Arthrospore formations occurs within the hair completely filling hair shaft.
  Caused by: *T. tonsurans* and *T. violaceum.*
- **Ectothrix:** Arthrospore on the surface of hair shaft.
  Caused by: *M. audounii, M. canis, T. mentagrophytes.*
- **Kerion:** Painful inflammatory reaction producing boggy lesions on scalp.
  Caused by: *T. verricosum.*

- **Favus:** Cup like crust (scutula) forms around the infected hair follicle minimal hair shaft involvement.

  Caused by: *T. schoenleinii.*

Other Dermatophyte:

- Most common agent western world – T. rubrum, M. canis.
- Most common type of dermatophytosis – T. pedis.
- Trichophyton concentricum – Causes Tinea imbricata.

Lab Diagnosis

- Culture on SDA at 25°C for 3 weeks.
- LPCB mount of culture isolate shows two types of conidiation – Macro and Micro conidia.
- Based on the conidiation the three agents can be differentiated.

Dermatophytes	Macroconidia	Microconidia
Trichophyton	Rare, thin walled, smooth, pencil shaped	Abundant
Microsporum	Numerous, thick walled, rough, spindle shaped	Rare
Epidermophyton	Numerous, smooth walled, club shaped	Absent

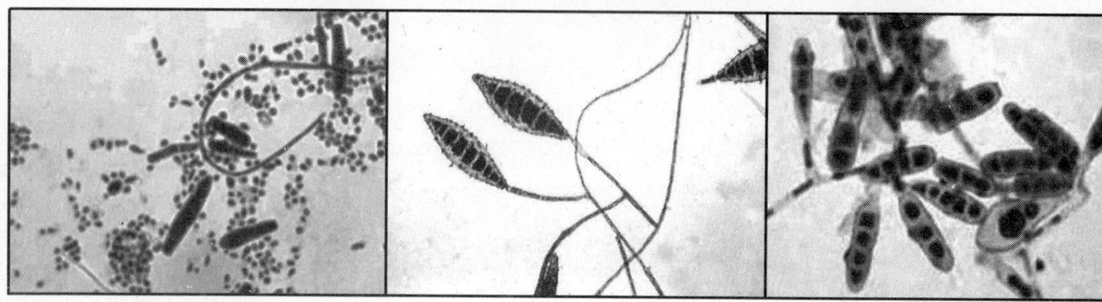

Trichophyton Microsporum (Macroconidia) Epidermophyton (Macroconidia)

Fig. 13.1

Other Tests done:

- Wood lamp – For Microsporon spp.
- Hair perforation test – T. mentagrophyte and M. canis.
- Urease – T. mentagrophyte.
- T/T – Gresiofulvin.

Wood Lamp Examination:

Fungi	Fluorescence
Micosporum audouinii, M. canis and *M. ferrugineum*	Bright green
Trichophyton schoenleinii	Dull green
All other Dermatophytes	No fluorescence
Pityriasis versicolor	**Golden yellow**
Corynebacterium minutissimum	Coral-red

MYCOLOGY

Dermatophytid or id reaction:

- Hypersensitivity to fungus antigens may lead to secondary eruption in sensitized patients because of circulation of allergenic products.
- Occurs distal to primary site and culture negative.

SUBCUTANEOUS MYCOSES

Mycetoma

- **Chronic granulomatous SC infection – Triad – swelling, discharging sinus and granules.**
- Affects extremities like hand and foot (bone), which are more prone for accidental trauma.
- Can be caused by bacteria (Actinomycetoma) or fungi (Eumycetoma).
- Overall most common – Actinomycetoma.
- Eumycetoma – More prevalent in North India, Actinomycetoma more common in South India.

Eumycetoma	Actinomycetoma (White)
(a) **Black Grain Eumycetoma**	*Actinomadura madurae*
• *Madurella mycetomatis*	*Actinomadura pelletieri (red*
• *Madurella grisea*	*Nocardia brasiliensis*
• *Exophiala jeanselmei*	*Nocardia caviae*
• *Curvularia spp.*	
(b) **White Grain Eumycetoma**	*Nocardia asteroides*
Aspergillus nidulans	*Nocardiopsis dassonvillei*
Acremonium spp.	*Streptomyces somaliensis*
Fusarium spp.	***Botryomycosis:*** Most common agent – Staphylococcus
Pseudallescheria boydii	*Others* – Streptococcus, E. coli, Proteus species, Pseudomonas

	Actinomycotic	Eumycotic
Tumor	Multiple tumour masses with ill defined margins	Single, well defined margins
Sinuses	Appear early, numerous, raised inflammed opening	Appear late, few in no.
Discharge	Purulent	Serous
Granule	White/red	Black/white
Bone	Osteolytic lesions	Osteosclerotic lesions
Filament	< 2μm (bacilli)	>2μm (hyphae)

Sporothrix:

- Also known as ***Rose Gardner disease.***
- Commonly seen in gardner, carpenter, mine worker.
- Chronic subcutaneous pyogranulomatous nodulo-ulcerative lesion.
- Lymphatic spread occurs.
- Risk – Bare foot.
- Common in Sub Himalya region.

MYCOLOGY

Lab Diagnosis

- It is a Dimorphic fungi.
- Yest form – Cigar shaped asteroid body.
- Mould form – Hyphae with Flower like sporulation.

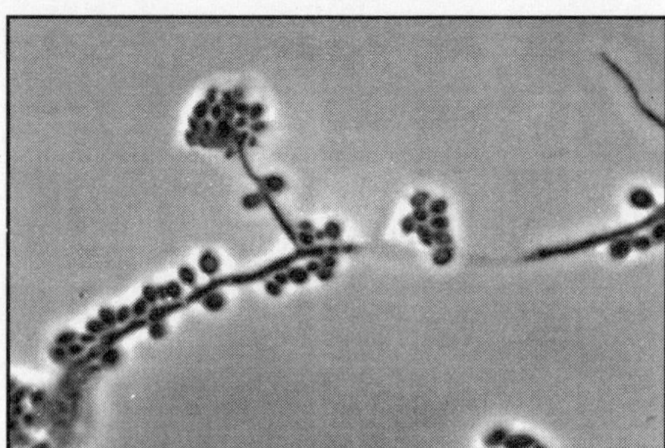

Fig. 13.2: Hyphae with Flower like sporulation

Chromoblastomycosis

- Chronic localized infection of skin and subcutaneous tissue, most often involving limb with brown walled, globose bodies 5-13 m in size, called **sclerotic bodies or muriform cells/**Medlar body.
- **Agents are Phialophora, Cladosporium, Rhinocladiella.**

Rhinospordiosis

- Chronic granulomatous disease by development of large polyps in the nose, conjunctiva and occasionally in ears, larynx, bronchus genitalia etc.
- Sri-lanka and India are endemic zones of Asia (Orissa, Kerala, Chennai).
- *Rhinosporidium seeberi* has not been cultured.
- Stagnant water is reservoir of infection.
- Spherules – Sporangia upto 350 mm contains endospores (6-9 m in size).
- Stains with mucicarmine stain.
- *Treatment* – Radical surgery, dapsone.

SYSTEMIC MYCOSES

Candida

- Commonest mycoses involving skin and its appendages, mucosa and internal organs.
- *Predisposing factors*:
  - DM
  - ↓ immunity
  - Steroid
  - Malignancy
  - Febrile neutropenia.
- Pseudo hyphae seen – constricted wall near septa.

- C. albicans – Most pathogenic species.
- *Diagnosed by*:
  - Germ tube test (Renauld Braune Phenomena) +ve.
  - Chamydospore on corn meal agar.
  - C. dublinensis also shows +ve GTT and Chamydospore.
- Most common non albican spp – C. Parapsilosis >C. glabrata
- *Disease produced by Candidia*:
  - Mucocutaneous
  - Nail fold
  - Systemic infections.
- Treatment:
  - Superficial – Nystatin, Mucocutaneous – Fluconazole.
  - Systemic – Amphotericin B.

Cryptococcus:

- True yeast.
- Sexual spore – Basidiospore.
- Also known as European Blastomycosis.
- Most common source – Feces of Pigeon.
- Mode of transmission – Inhalation > skin.
- ***Pathogenesis:*** Virulence factors
  - Polysaccharide capsule – Not immunogenic, no anti-capsular ab formed.
  - Phenyloxidase enzyme responsible for production of melanin when grown on substrate like niger seed agar.
- ***Clinical Feature:*** Pulmonary infection, Meningitis, Bone, Skin infection.

Lab Diagnosis:

- India Ink/nigrosin – Capsule (Polysaccharide).
- Mucicarmine stain.
- Latex agglutination test – Capsular Ag detection.
- *Culture*:
  - SDA – smooth, mucoid, cream coloured colonies.
  - Niger seed agar – Brown colony.
- Urease +ve.

Histoplasma capsulatum:

- Dimorphic fungi
- Intracellular
- Affects Reticuloendothelial system
- Darling Disease
- Does not have true capsule.

Clinical Features:

- Pulmonary – Acute, Chronic (Histoplasmoma).
- Fever, weight loss, hepatosplenomegaly and lymphadenopathy are the common features.
- Skin (India).
- Presence of calcification and caseation necrosis, mimics Tuberculosis.

Lab Diagnosis:

❖ It is a Dimorphic fungi
  - Yeast at 37, Mould at 25
  - Narrow based budding yeast cell 4-6 μ
  - Tuberculate macroconidia.

❖ Ag detection in serum and urine.

❖ Histoplasmin skin test.

❖ Immunodiffusion for the detection of antibody (Exoantigen test).

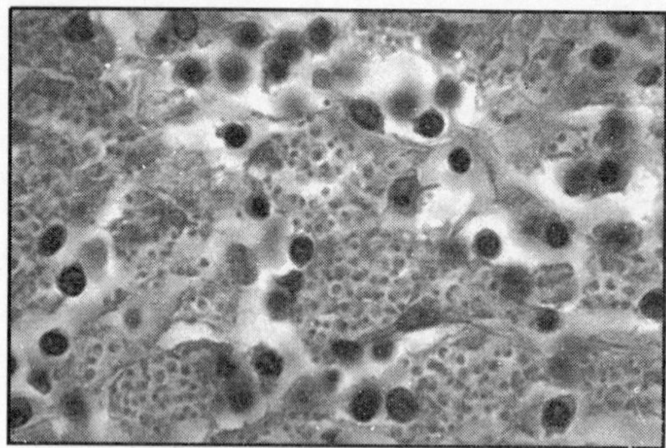

Narrow based budding yeast cell

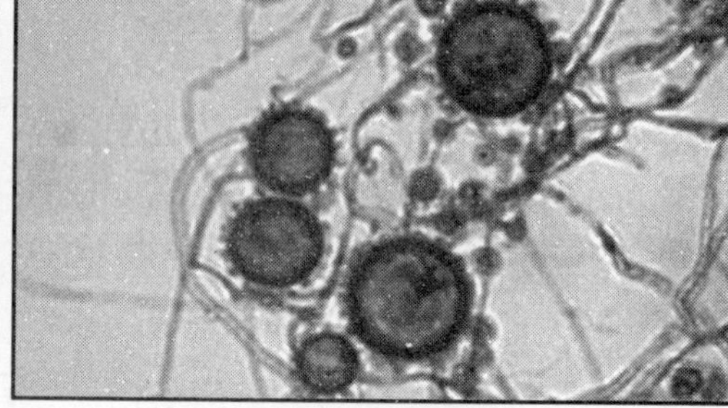

Tuberculate macroconidia

Fig. 13.3

Blastomycosis:

❖ It is a dimorphic fungi.

❖ Also known as North American Blastomycosis, Gilchrist disease.

❖ **Broad based budding yeast cell 8-15 μ.**

❖ Pulmonary, other tissue – Bone, skin.

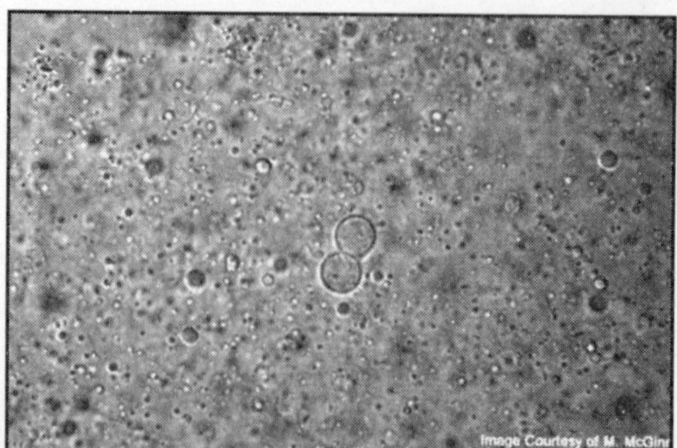

Fig. 13.4: Broad based budding Yeast Cell 8-15 μ.

Coccidiodes:

❖ It is also dimorphic fungi.

- ❖ Also known as Desert Rheumatism/Valley fever.
- ❖ Endemic in South, North and Central USA and Mexico.
- ❖ Not reported from India.
- ❖ Agent for Bioterrorism.
- ❖ *Clinical feature* – Pulmonary symptoms and bone involvement.
- ❖ Spherule filled with endospores at 37°C.
- ❖ Hyphae with arthroconidia at 25°C.

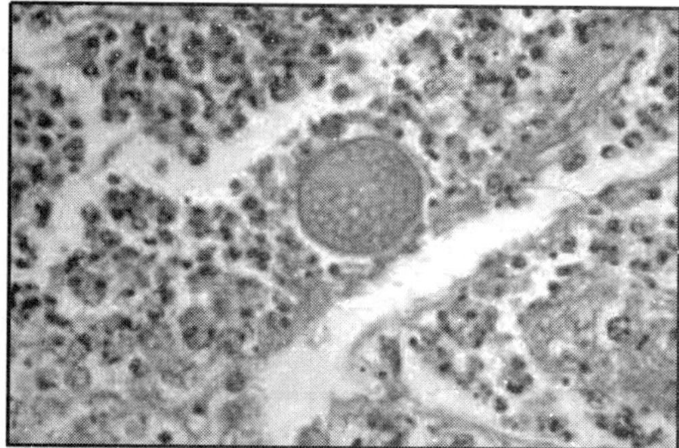

Spherule filled with endospores at 37°C

Hyphae with arthroconidia at 25°C

Fig. 13.5

Paracoccidioides:

- ❖ It is also dimorphic fungi.
- ❖ Also known as South American Blastomycosis.
- ❖ Most common symptom – Pulmonary infection
- ❖ Multiple budding yeast cell
  - Micky mouse appearance
  - Pilot wheel appearance.

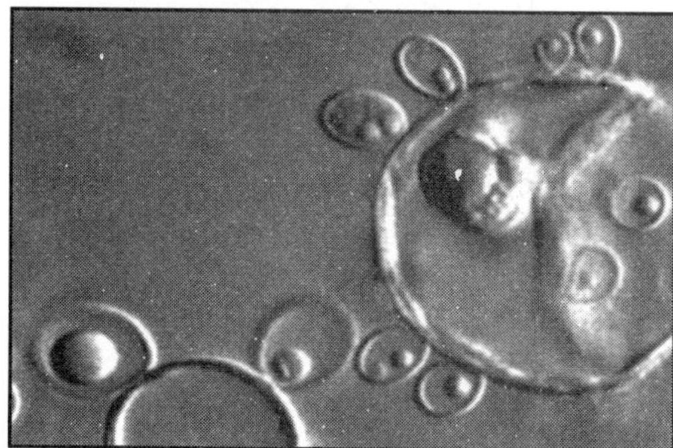

Micky mouse appearance

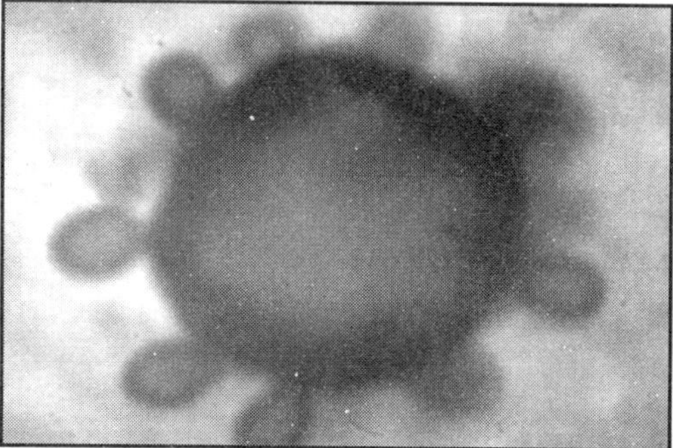

Pilot wheel appearance

Fig. 13.6

OPPORTUNISTIC MYCOSES

Zygomycosis:

- ❖ Broad aseptate wide angle hyphae

- Zygospore
- *Example:* Rhizopus, Mucor, Absidia
- Risk factor – Diabetes (DKA), dialysis, iron overload
- *Clinical feature*:
  - Rhinocerebral zygomycosis
  - Pulmonary zygomycosis
  - Orbital cellulitis
  - Skin.

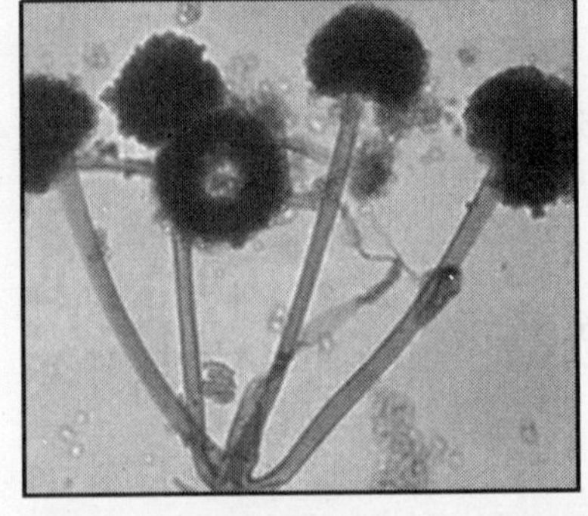

Fig. 13.7: Rhizopus with rhizoid

Aspergillus:

- Narrow septate hyphae with acute angle branching.
- ABPA
- Asthma
- Aspergilloma
- Invasive aspergillosis
- Otomycoses (most common)
- Oculomycoses
- Paranasal sinusitis
- Aspergillus flavus – produces Aflatoxin that can cause Carcinoma liver.

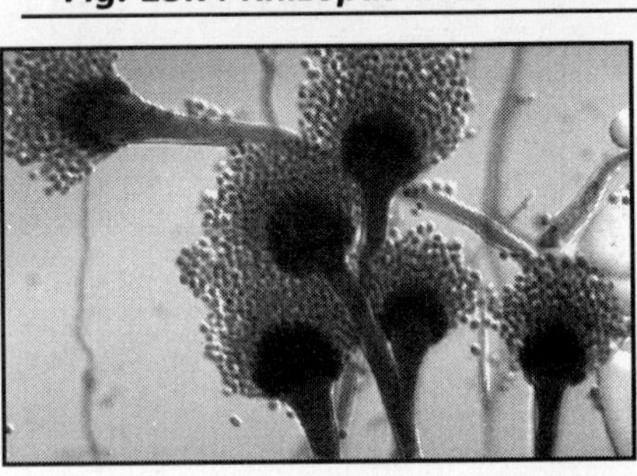

Fig. 13.8: Aspergillus fumigatus

Penicillium marneffi:

- Brick red pigment on SDA
- Isolated from Bamboo rat
- Shows thermal dimorphism
- Seen in S.E. Asia
- Produces wart like skin lesion, may spread systemically.
- Morphology – Sausage shaped cells with transverse septa which divide by ***binary fission.***

FMGE MCQ's

1. Fungus having non-septate hyphae and producing sporangiospores is: [*March 2011*]

(a) Ascomycetes (b) Basidiomycetes

(c) Phycomycetes (d) Fungi imperfectii.

2. Most common fungus causing chronic meningitis is: [*March 2009*]

(a) Blastomyces (b) Cryptococcus neoformans

(c) Histoplasma (d) Coccidioidomycosis.

3. Sclerotic bodies are seen in: [*September 2009*]

(a) Sporotrichosis (b) Histoplasmosis

(c) Chromoblastomycosis (d) Rhinosporodiosis.

4. Amongst the following, which is the rarest opportunistic fungal infection seen in AIDS patient: [*September 2008*]

(a) Cryptococcosis (b) Candidiasis
(c) Histoplasmosis (d) Pneumocystis.

5. All of the following causes subcutaneous fungal infections except: [*September 2007*]
(a) Blastomycosis (b) Sporotrichosis
(c) Maduramycosis (d) Rhinosporodiosis.

6. Which of the following is not a fungal infection? [*September 2007*]
(a) Blastomycosis (b) Cryptococcus
(c) Actinomycosis (d) Histoplasmosis.

7. All are dimorphic fungi except: [*March 2005*]
(a) Blastomycoses (b) Cryptococcus
(c) Histoplasma (d) Paracoccidia.

8. True about Cryptococcus neoformans are all except: [*September 2005*]
(a) Possess a prominent polysaccharide capsule
(b) Abundant in pigeon droppings
(c) Dimorphic fungi
(d) Causes meningitis in the immunocompromised.

9. Which is a yeast like fungi? [*March 2003*]
(a) Cryptococcus (b) Candida
(c) Blastomyces (d) Histoplasma.

ANSWERS TO FMGE QUESTIONS

1. Ans. (c) Phycomycetes

[*Ref.:* Ananthnarayan, 8th ed., page no. 601]

❖ **Phycomycetes or zygomycetes:**
- Possess sexual spore as zygospore.
- Possess broad aseptate hyphae, e.g., Rhizopus, Mucor, Absidia.

❖ **Ascomycetes:**
- Possess sexual spore Ascospores.
- *Possess* narrow septate hyphae, e.g., Aspergillus.

2. Ans. (b) Cryptococcus neoformans

[*Ref.:* Ananthnarayan, 8th ed., page no. 610]

❖ Cryptococcus neoformans is the most common fungal cause of chronic meningitis especially in immunocompromised state, i.e., in HIV patients.

3. Ans. (c) Chromoblastomycosis

[*Ref.:* Ananthnarayan, 8th ed., page no. 609]

Chromoblastomycosis:

❖ Chronic localized infection of skin and subcutaneous tissue, most often involving limb.

- Chracterized by brown walled, globose bodies 5-13 m in size, called ***sclerotic bodies or muriform cells/Medlar body.***
- Agents are – Phialophora,Cladosporium, Rhinocladiella.

4. Ans. (c) Histoplasmosis

[*Ref.:* Ananthnarayan, 8th ed., page no. 612]

- Histoplasmosis though is not rare in HIV patients (quite common) but among the options provided it is less common than others in HIV patients.
- **Oppurtunistic fungi that are commonly occur in HIV patients:**
    - Candida
    - Cryptococcus
    - Aspergillus
    - Zygomycetes
    - Penicillium spp
    - Penicillium marneffi
    - Pneumocysts jerovecii
    - Fusarium.

5. Ans. (a) Blastomycosis

[*Ref.:* Ananthnarayan, 8th ed., page no. 608; Jagdish Chander's, Mycology, 3rd ed., page no. 148]

- ***Subcutaneous mycoses (Systemic classification):***
    - Mycetoma
    - Chromoblastomycosis
    - Sporothrix
    - Rhinosporidium
    - Lobomycosis (Locazia).

6. Ans. (c) Actinomycosis

[*Ref.:* Ananthnarayan, 8th ed., page no. 608; Jagdish Chander's, Mycology, 3rd ed., page no. 149]

- ***Actinomycosis is a bacterial cause of mycetoma caused by bacteria like:***
    - *Actinomadura madurae*
    - *Actinomadura pelletieri (red)*
    - *Nocardia brasiliensis*
    - *Nocardia caviae*
    - *Nocardia asteroides*
    - *Nocardiopsis dassonvillei*
    - *Streptomyces somaliensis.*

7. Ans. (b) Cryptococcus

[*Ref.:* Ananthnarayan, 8th ed., page no. 600]

Yeast: Produces true yeast, e.g., Cryptococcus.

Yeast like fungi: Produces pseudohyphae, e.g., Candida.

Mould: Produces true hypahe, e.g., Dermatophyte, Aspergillus, Zygomycetes, Penicillium.

Dimorphic Fungi:

- Produces mould form at 25°C and environmental temperature.
- Yeast form at 37°C and at body temperature.

Examples:

- Histoplasma
- Blastomyces
- Coccidiodes
- Paracoccidides
- Sporothrix
- Penicillium marneffi.

MYCOLOGY

8. Ans. (c) Dimorphic fungi

[*Ref.:* Ananthnarayan, 8th ed., page no. 601]

- Cryptococcus is a *true* yeast and it is not a dimorphic fungi.

Cryptococcus:

- Possess a prominent polysaccharide capsule.
- Source of infection is abundant in pigeon droppings.
- Most common fungal cause of meningitis in the immunocompromised.

9. Ans. (b) Candida

***Ref.:* Ananthnarayan, 8th ed., page no. 600]**

- ***Yeast like fungi*** produces pseudohyphae.

Example: Candida.

PRACTICE MCQ's

Mycology

1. All are yeast or yeast like fungi except:

(a) Candida (b) Geotrichum

(c) Cryptococcus (d) Trichophyton.

2. Fungi which do not have sexual stage:

(a) Phycomycetes (b) Ascomycetes

(c) Basidiomycetes (d) Fungi imperfecti.

3. All are asexual spores of fungi except:

(a) Arthrospores (b) Chlamydospores

(c) Blastospores (d) Ascospores.

4. Which stain is most suitable for fungus demonstration in biopsy?

(a) PAS (b) H and E

(c) Indian Ink (d) Mason's Trichrome.

5. Which antimicrobial is added in SDA to prevent growth of contaminant moulds?

(a) Griseofulvin (b) Clotrimazole

(c) Cycloheximide (d) Gentamicin.

Superficial and Subcutaneous Mycosis

6. Hair perforation test is positive in:

(a) Trichophyton mentagrophyte (b) Microsporum gypseum

(c) Epidermophyton floccosum (d) Trichosporon bigeli.

7. Pityriasis Versicolor is caused by:

(a) E. floccosum (b) M. furfur

(c) M. gypseum (d) T. tonsurans.

8. **Tinea imbricata is caused by:**
   (a) Trichophyton verruconsum (b) Trichophyton rubrum
   (c) Trichophyton concentricum (d) Epidermophyton floccosum.
9. **Organism that does not affect nail:**
   (a) Trichophyton rubrum (b) Epidermophyton floccosum
   (c) Microsporum (d) Hortaea werneckii.
10. **The causative agent of Favus is:**
   (a) Microsporum audonii (b) Trichophyton schoenleinii
   (c) Microsporum canis (d) Trichophyton mentagrophytes.
11. **Microconidia are absent in:**
   (a) Trichophyton rubrum (b) Trichophyton mentagrophytes
   (c) Microsporum audonii (d) Epidermophyton floccosum.
12. **All are dermatophyte infections of hair except:**
   (a) Ectothrix (b) Favus
   (c) Kerion (d) Piedra.
13. **Examination of skin scraping from a patient having hypopigmented, non-itchy lesions on chest show yeast like cells and branched filaments. (Sphagetti – meat ball appearance) Probable fungus is:**
   (a) Malassezia furfur (b) Dimorphic fungus
   (c) Candida albicaus (d) Dermatophyte.
14. **Drug of choice for extensive Tinea corporis is:**
   (a) Topical clotrimazole (b) Amphotericin – B
   (c) Oral Griseo fulvin (d) Topical miconazole

MYCOLOGY

Subcutaneous Mycosis

15. **All are true about Botryomycosis except:**
   (a) Clinical features similar to mycetoma (b) Caused by staphylococcus aureus
   (c) Microscopy shows cocci (d) Amphotericin – B is effective.
16. **A patient coming from Himachal Pradesh, presents with multiple skin lesions. Microscopy reveals cigar shaped yeast cells and asteroid bodies. Microscopy of culture shows 'Flower like' pattern most likely fungus is:**
   (a) Candida (b) Sporothrix schencki
   (c) Epidermophyton floccosum (d) Rhizopus.
17. **Red coloured grains are seen in mycetoma caused by:**
   (a) Actinomadura pelletieri (b) Madurella mycetomatis
   (c) Madurella grisea (d) Actinomadura madurae.
18. **Not true about Rhinosporidiosis is:**
   (a) Cannot be cultured (b) Most common site is Vagina
   (c) Fungal Spherules in biopsy (d) Bleeds to touch.

Candidiasis

19. Most common fungal infection in febrile neutropenia:

(a) Aspergillus niger
(b) Mucormycosis
(c) Candida albicans
(d) Cryptococcus.

20. Candida infection is predisposed by all except:

(a) Menstruation
(b) Diabetes
(c) HIV
(d) OCP.

21. An HIV infected female has an ulcer over the tongue. Lab findings show growth in corn meal agar at 20°C. Microscopy shows Pseudo hyphae and growth in human serum at 37°C show budding yeast cells. The probable cause is:

(a) Candida albicans
(b) Histoplasmosis
(c) Blastomyces
(d) Cryptococcus neoformans.

22. Germ tube test is diagnostic for:

(a) Candida glabrata
(b) Candida albicans
(c) Cryptococcus neoformans
(d) Coccidiodes immitis.

Cryptococcosis

23. Capsulated fungus is:

(a) Histoplasma capsulatum
(b) Candida albicans
(c) Cryptococcus neoformans
(d) Rhinosporidium seeberi.

24. The capsule of Cryptococcus neoformans in CSF sample is best seen by:

(a) Gram stain
(b) Gemsa stain
(c) Indian Ink preparation
(d) Methanamine silver stain.

Dimorphic Fungi

25. Blastomycosis is characterized by all except:

(a) Dimorphic
(b) Narrow based budding yeast cells in tissues
(c) Commonly involves lung
(d) Common in North America.

26. What is true about Histoplasmosis?

(a) Tuberculate Macroconidia seen
(b) Pseudohypha seen
(c) Broad based budding yeast cells in tissues
(d) Hyphal forms not infectious.

27. All of the following are dimorphic fungi except:

(a) Coccidiodes immitis
(b) Penicillium griseofulvum
(c) Histoplasma capsulatum
(d) Blastomyces dermatitidis.

Opputunistic Fungi

28. Which of the following is not an opportunistic fungus:

(a) Cryptococcus
(b) Aspergillosis
(c) Dermatophyte
(d) Penicillium marneffei.

29. Which rays are used in wood's lamp?

(a) X-rays
(b) UV rays
(c) Gamma rays
(d) Infra red rays.

30. A patient presents with chronic cough, resistant to routine antibiotics; whose X-ray chest shows cavity filled with mass. Sputum microscopy shows acutely branching septate hyphae. Probable organism:

(a) Histoplasma capsulatum
(b) Aspergillus fumigatus
(c) Mycobacterium tuberculosis
(d) Actinomyces.

31. Aflatoxin is produced by:

(a) Aspergillus flavus
(b) Aspergillus fumigatus
(c) Aspergillus nidulans
(d) Aspergillus niger.

32. Example for fungus having Branching, Aseptate hyphae are all except:

(a) Rhizopus
(b) Absidia
(c) Penicillium
(d) Mucor.

33. Most common fungus causing orbital cellulitis in a patient with diabetic ketoacidosis is:

(a) Mucor
(b) Aspergillus
(c) Candida
(d) Cryptococcus.

34. Which of the following is the most common etiologic agent in paranasal sinus mycoses?

(a) Aspergillus
(b) Histoplasma
(c) Coccidioides coronatus
(d) Candida albicans.

35. Pneumocystis carini is diagnosed by:

(a) Silver nitrate staining
(b) H and E stain
(c) Gram stain
(d) Acid fast stain.

ANSWERS TO PRACTICE MCQ's

1. Ans. (d) Trichophyton

[*Ref.:* Ananthnarayan, 8th ed., page no. 604]

❖ Trichophyton is a dermatophyte (true mould).

2. Ans. (d) Fungi imperfecti

[*Ref.:* Ananthnarayan, 8th ed., page no. 601]

❖ *Fungi which do not have sexual stage know as* ***Fungi imperfecti or deuteromycetes.***

3. Ans. (d) Ascospores

[*Ref.:* Ananthnarayan, 8th ed., page no. 601-02]

❖ ***Sexual spore (ZAB):***

- Zygospore
- Ascospore
- Basidiospore.

❖ *Asexual spore (ABC):*
   - Arthrospore
   - Blastospore
   - Chlamydiospore.

4. Ans. (a) PAS

[*Ref.:* Ananthnarayan, 8th ed., page no. 601]

❖ PAS stain is most suitable for fungus demonstration in biopsy.

❖ LPCB stain is most suitable for fungus demonstration from culture isolates.

5. Ans. (c) Cycloheximide

[*Ref.:* Ananthnarayan, 8th ed., page no. 601; Jagdish Chander's, Mycology, 3rd ed., page no. 149, 508]

❖ Antimicrobial is added in SDA to prevent growth of contaminant moulds:
   - Cycloheximide (actidione) – Most commonly added.
   - Gentamicin.
   - Chloramphenicol.

❖ **Also know Sabouraud Dextrose agar:**
   - pH is 5.6 and contains dextrose 4%.
   - Low pH might inhibit some of the important fungi.

❖ Emmon's modification of Sabouraud Dextrose agar – pH is 6.8 and dextrose 2%.

6. Ans. (a) Trichophyton mentagrophyte

[*Ref.:* Ananthnarayan, 8th ed., page no. 606; Jagdish Chander's, Mycology, 3rd ed., page no. 522]

❖ **Hair perforation test is positive in:**
   - Trichophyton mentagrophyte
   - Microsporum canis.

7. Ans. (b) M. furfur

[*Ref.:* Ananthnarayan, 8th ed., page no. 603]

❖ Pityriasis Versicolor is caused by – Malassezia furfur.

8. Ans. (c) Trichophyton concentricum

[*Ref.*: Jagdish Chander's, Mycology, 3rd ed., page no. 129]

❖ **Tinea imbricata is caused by:**
   - Trichophyton concentricum
   - Concentric rings of scaling which spreads out to periphery.

❖ Tinea incognito – occurs after topical corticosteroid application.

9. Ans. (c) Microsporum

[*Ref.:* Ananthnarayan, 8th ed., page no. 604]

❖ Trichohyton – skin, nail, hair *(Tri – Three)*

- ❖ Microsporoon – skin, hair *(M not for N)*
- ❖ Epidermophyton – skin, nail.

10. Ans. (b) Trichophyton schoenleinii

[*Ref.:* Jagdish Chander's, Mycology, 3rd ed., page no. 127]

- ❖ Favus is characterized by Cup like crust (scutula) forms around the infected hair follicle minimal hair shaft involvement, caused by – T. schoenleinii

11. Ans. (d) Epidermophyton floccosum

[*Ref.:* Jadish Chander's, Mycology, 3rd ed., page no. 129-30]

Dermatophytes	Macroconidia	Microconidia
Trichophyton	Rare, thin walled, smooth, Pencil shaped	Abundant
Microsporum	Numerous, thick walled, rough, Spindle shaped	Rare
Epidermophyton	Numerous, smooth walled, Club shaped	Absent

12. Ans. (d) Piedra

[*Ref.:* Ananthnarayan, 8th ed., page no. 606]

- ❖ Ectothrix, Favus and Kerion are variants of Tenia capitis (infection of scalp hair).
- ❖ Piedra is not dermatophyte.

13. Ans. (a) Malassezia furfur

[*Ref.:* Ananthnarayan, 8th ed., page no. 603; Jagdish Chander's, Mycology, 3rd ed., page no. 96-99]

- ❖ Laboratory diagnosis of the Tinea Versicolor is usually made by demonstration of both budding yeast cell and hyphae in KOH preparation of skin scrapings giving rise to characteristic "Sphagetti and meatball appearance of fungus."
- ❖ **Tinea Versicolor**
- ❖ Agent are Malassezia furfur.
- ❖ Chronic recurrent, non inflammatory, non pruritic lesion
- ❖ Hypo to hyper pigmentation
- ❖ *Diagnosis*:
  - ***Sphagetti and meat ball appearance***
  - Lipophilic (SDA with olive oil overlay is used)
  - Fried egg colony
  - Urease +ve
  - Wood's lamp examination – Scaly lesion show golden yellow fluorescens.

14. Ans. (c) Oral Griseo fulvin

[*Ref.:* Ananthnarayan, 8th ed., page no. 607; Jagdish Chander's, Mycology, 3rd ed., page no. 141]

- ❖ Drug of choice for extensive Tinea corporis is **Oral Griseofulvin.**

15. Ans. (d) Amphotericin – B is effective

[*Ref.:* Jagdish Chander's, Mycology, 3rd ed., page no. 159]

- ❖ Amphotericin – B is an antifungal, but Botryomycosis is caused by staphylococcus aureus.

16. Ans. (b) Sporothrix schencki

[*Ref.:* Ananthnarayan, 8th ed., page no. 609; Jagdish Chander's, Mycology, 3rd ed., page no. 163-98]

Clue to the Diagnosis:

- ❖ Himachal Pradesh, presents with multiple skin lesions – Endemic area of Sporothrix.
- ❖ Microscopy reveals cigar shaped yeast cells and asteroid bodies.
- ❖ Microscopy of culture shows 'Flower like' pattern most likely fungus is:
- ❖ **Sporothrix –** Also as ***Rose Gardner disease***
  - Commonly seen in gardner, carpenter, mine worker
  - Chronic subcutaneous pyogranulomatous nodulo ulcerative lesion
  - Lymphatic spread occurs
  - Risk – Bare foot
  - ***Endemic area – Sub Himalya***
  - ***Lab diagnosis:***
    - It is a dimorphic fungi
    - Yest form – ***Cigar shaped asteroid body***
    - Mould form – ***Hyphae with Flower like sporulation.***

17. Ans. (a) Actinomadura pelletieri

[*Ref.:* Jagdish Chander's, Mycology, 3rd ed., page no. 150]

- ❖ Red coloured grains are seen in mycetoma caused by – Actinomadura pelletieri.

18. Ans. (b) Most common site is Vagina

[*Ref.:* Ananthnarayan, 8th ed., page no. 609]

- ❖ Most common site of Rhinosporidiosis is Nose (inferior turbinate).

19. Ans. (c) Candida albicans

[*Ref.:* Ananthnarayan, 8th ed., page no. 607; Jagdish Chander's, Mycology, 3rd ed., page no. 272]

Predisposing factors for Candida infection:

- ❖ Natural receptive stages – old age, pregnancy, infants
- ❖ DM
- ❖ ↓ immunity
- ❖ HIV
- ❖ Steroid
- ❖ Malignancy
- ❖ Febrile neutropenia
- ❖ Zn or iron deficiency.

20. Ans. (a) Menstruation

[*Ref.:* Ananthnarayan, 8th ed., page no. 607; Jagdish Chander's, Mycology, 3rd ed., page no. 272]

- Menstruation is not a predisposing factors for Candida infection.

21. Ans. (a) Candida albicans

[*Ref.:* Ananthnarayan, 8th ed., page no. 607]

Clue to the Diagnosis:

- ❖ Ulcer over the tongue.
- ❖ Microscopy shows Pseudo hyphae.
- ❖ Growth in human serum at 37°C show budding yeast cells – Positive germ tube test.

22. Ans. (b) Candida albicans

[*Ref.:* Ananthnarayan, 8th ed., page no. 608]

- ❖ Germ tube test is diagnostic for Candida albicans and Candida dublinensis.

23. Ans. (c) Cryptococcus neoformans

[*Ref.:* Ananthnarayan, 8th ed., page no. 610]

- ❖ Cryptococcus neoformans is the only fungus that has a capsule (polysaccharide capsule).
- ❖ Histoplasma capsulatum is non-capsulated (name is misnomer).

24. Ans. (c) Indian Ink preparation

[*Ref.:* Ananthnarayan, 8th ed., page no. 610; Jagdish Chander's, Mycology, 3rd ed., page no. 303]

Cryptococcus Neoformans is Diagnosed by:

Demonstration of Capsule (Polysaccharide) by India Ink/nigrosin stain

- ❖ Mucicarmine stain
- ❖ Latex agglutination test – Capsular Ag detection from CSF
- ❖ *Culture*
  - SDA – smooth, mucoid, cream coloured colonies
  - Niger seed agar – Brown colony
- ❖ Urease +ve.

25. Ans. (b) Narrow based budding yeast cells in tissues

[*Ref.:* Ananthnarayan, 8th ed., page no. 611, Jagdish Chander's; Mycology 3rd ed., page no. 216]

- ❖ Broad based budding yeast cells in tissues- characteristic of blastomycosis.
- ❖ Narrow based budding yeast cells in tissues- characteristic of histoplasmosis.

26. Ans. (a) Tuberculate Macroconidia seen

[*Ref.:* Ananthnarayan, 8th ed., page no. 610; Jagdish Chander's, Mycology, 3rd ed., page no. 216]

- ❖ Tuberculate Macroconidia and Narrow based budding yeast cells in tissues – characteristic of histoplasmosis.

27. Ans. (b) Penicillium griseofulvum

[*Ref.:* Jagdish Chander's, Mycology 3rd ed., page no. 28]

- ❖ Only Penicillium marneffi is dimorphic fungi whereas other Penicillium spp are true moulds.

28. Ans. (c) Dermatophyte

[*Ref.:* Ananthnarayan, 8th ed., page no. 133-35]

29. Ans. (b) UV rays

[*Ref.:* Jagdish Chander's, Mycology, 3rd ed., page no. 135]

- Wood's lamp emits UV rays.

Table: Wood's Lamp Examination

Fungi	Fluorescence
Micosporum audouinii, M. canis and M. ferrugineum	Bright green
Trichophyton schoenleinii	Dull green
All other Dermatophytes	No fluorescence
Pityriasis versicolor	Golden yellow
Corynebacterium minutissimum	Coral-red

30. Ans. (b) Aspergillus fumigatus

[*Ref.:* Ananthnarayan, 8th ed., page no. 613]

Clue to the Diagnosis:

- Chest shows cavity filled with mass may be Aspergilloma.
- Sputum microscopy shows acutely branching septate hyphae.

31. Ans. (a) Aspergillus flavus

[*Ref.:* Ananthnarayan, 8th ed., page no. 615]

- Aflatoxin is produced by Aspergillus flavus.
- Ergotoxin is produced by Claviceps pupura.

32. Ans. (c) Penicillium

[*Ref.:* Ananthnarayan, 8th ed., page no. 613]

- Penicillium and Aspergillus– Possess septate hyphae.

33. Ans. (a) Mucor

[*Ref.:* Ananthnarayan, 8th ed., page no. 613, Jagdish Chander's, Mycology, 3rd ed., page no. 365]

Clue to the Diagnosis:

- Fungus causing orbital cellulitis mainly caused by zygomycetes.
- Patient with diabetic ketoacidosis – Risk factor for zygomycetes.

34. Ans. (a) Aspergillus

[*Ref.:* Jagdish Chander's, Mycology, 3rd ed., page no. 348, 481]

- Most common etiologic agent in paranasal sinus mycoses – Aspergillus.

35. Ans. (a) Silver nitrate staining

[*Ref.:* Jagdish Chander's, Mycology, 3rd ed., page no. 322]

- Silver nitrate staining is used for the diagnosis of Pneumocystis carini.

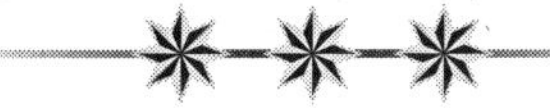

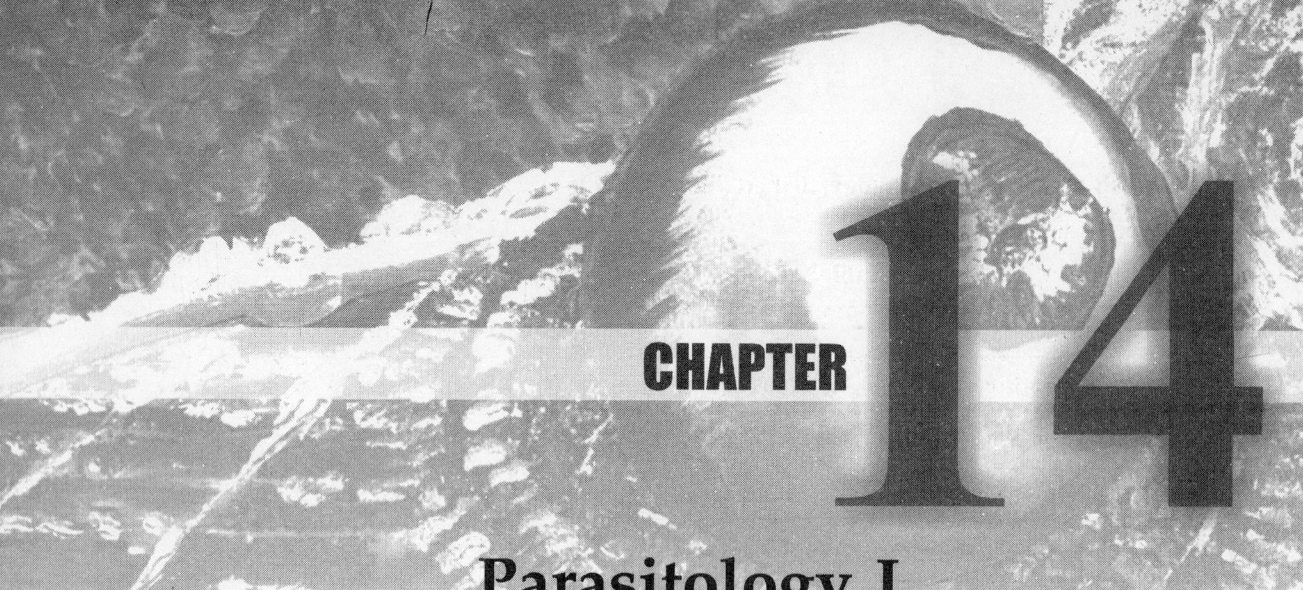

CHAPTER 14

Parasitology I

Protozoa (Amoeba, Flagellates, Malaria, Coccidian Parasites and Miscellaneous Protozoa)

ENTAMOEBA

Life Cycle

- ❖ Definitive host – Man.
- ❖ Infective form – Mature quadrinucleate cyst.
- ❖ Mode of infection – Food or water contaminated with cyst (resistant to chlorination).
- ❖ Mode of transmission – **Faeco-oral route** and Sexual transmission (20-30% in homosexuals).
- ❖ Reservoir of infection – Asymptomatic carriers.

Culture Media:

- ❖ *Polyaxenic* – Bacterial supplement (for diagnosis)
  - Boeck and Drbohlav's Media
  - Locke's egg serum/egg albumin
  - Balamuth, Nelson's Medium
- ❖ *Axenic Medium* – Diamond medium.
- ❖ For study of pathogenesis, anti amoebic susceptibility, preparation of antigen.

Virulence Factors

- ❖ Lectin antigen (galactose inhibitable adherence lectin)
- ❖ Cysteine proteinase.

Clinical Picture:

- ❖ *Amoebic dysentery*:
  - Flask shaped ulcer
  - Most common site – Caecum

- *Amoebic liver abscess*:
  - 10% of amoebic dysentery
  - Ancovy sauce pus (chocolate syrup)
- *Extra intestinal* – Brain, lung etc.

Diagnosis

- Stool examination – Done to differentiate E. histolytica from E. coli
- Lectin antigen in stool.
- Serology – Important for Amoebic Liver Abscess
- PCR.

Characteristics	E. histolytica/E. dispar	E. coli
Trophozoites	Actively motile with finger shaped pseudopodia cytoplasm is presence of RBCs	Sluggishly motile, Blunt pseudopodia
Cysts	10-20 µm nucleus – Four nuclei Fine uniform granules, evenly distributed	20–25 µm, Nucleus – Eight nuclei Coarsely granular – unevenly arranged

E. Histolytica and E. dispar

- **Differences**
  - Only *E. histolytica* – Causes invasive disease
  - Both can be differentiated by:
    - Lectin antigen present only in E. histolytica
    - PCR
    - Distinct surface antigens and isoenzyme markers.

Free Living Amoebae

	Naegleria fowleri	Acanthamoeba
Disease	Primary amoebic meningoencephalitis	Granulomatous amoebic Meningoencephalitis Ulcerative keratitis
Portal of entry	Nose – Olfactory N route	Upper respiratory tract – hematogenous route
Predisposing factor	Swimming in contaminated water	Immunodeficiency
Clinical course	Acute	Subacute – Chronic
Pathology	Acute suppurative changes	Granulomatous inflammation
Morphological form	Trophozoite, cyst, flagellated form	Cyst and trophozoites
Culture	Frequently positive	Negative
Trophozoites	Single pseudopodium	**Thorn like Pseudopodium**
Leukocytes in CSF	Neutrophils	Lymphocytes

- **Other free living amoeba:**
  - Balamuthia
  - Sappinia.

GIARDIA LAMBLIA

- **Habitat:** Mucosa of duodenum and upper ileum.
- **Morphology:** Two forms:
  - **Trophozoites**
    - Tear-drop shaped with **two nuclei**
    - Four pairs of flagella
    - Axostyles, parabasal body and Ventral sucking disk.
  - **Cyst** – Mature cyst consists of **four nuclei** and cysts.
- **Life Cycle**
  - Infective stage – Cyst
  - Route of infection – Faeco-oral route
  - Trophozoite has ***falling – Leaf like motility.***
- **Susceptibility to Infection**
  - Children and immunocompromised individual
  - Individuals with Achlorhydria
  - Antigenic variation.
- **Clinical disease**
  - Chronic diarrhea with malabsorption
  - Steatorrhoea – malabsorption of fats.
- **Lab Diagnosis**
  - Stool Microscopy – for cyst and trophozoites
  - Demonstrates either trophozoites or cyst
  - **String test/Entero test:** Duodenal contents
  - Serology.

TRICHOMONAS VAGINALIS

- Twitching motility
- Only Trophozoites – Pear shaped, 5 flagella
- Most common Parasitic cause of STD
- *Foul smelling discharge, strawberry appearance.*

HAEMOFLAGELLATES

Parasite	Epidemiology	Location	Mode	Symptoms
Leishmania tropica	Mediterranean area, Asia	Skin	Sandfly (Phlebotomus)	Skin lesion *(Oriental sore)*

PARASITOLOGY I

Leishmania brasiliensis	Central and South America	Skin and muco-cutaneous	Sandfly (Lutzomyia)	Skin lesions, espundia
Leishmania donovani	Asia, Africa	Skin and somatic organs	Sandfly Phlebotomus	Skin lesions, liver and spleen
L. mexicana	America	muco-cutaneous		Chiclero ulcer

- **Leishmania**
  - Amastigote form – human (LD body) – diagnostic from.
  - Promastigote – infective form (by bite of sandfly).
- **Trypanosoma**
  - Human – Non-multiplying Trypomastigote (Infective form and Diagnostic from).
  - Released with faeces while insect is taking blood meal and then faeces is rubbed into the bite wound site.
  - Insect – Epimastigote and Multiplying Trypomastigote.
- **Kala Azar**
  - Anemia, leucopenia, thrombocytopenia.
  - Hyper gammaglobulinemia.
  - Spleen ↑, Liver ↑.
  - Fever.
  - Hyper pigmentation (Indian).
  - LN↑ (African but not in Indian cases).
- **Kala Azar with HIV**
  - Absence of hepatosplenomegaly.
  - GIT and resp. symptoms.
- **PKDL**
  - Two year after treatment.
  - 3% (African), 10% (Indian).
  - Non-ulcerative hypopigmented lesions.

Laboratory Diagnosis

- Microscopy – Stained peripheral blood smear examination.
- Sample – Spleen (most Sn)/Bone marrow aspiration (most common preferred).
- Lymphnode aspirate (Not useful in Indian cases).
- Blood culture – NNN medium (Promastigotes grown).
- *Serological tests*:
  - Napier's aldehyde test – +ve after three months and also false +ve seen.
  - Chopra's antimony test.
  - ICT – Ab to K39 antigen.
  - CFT – Using WKK antigen.
- Leishmanin (Montenegro) skin test – Negative in acute case of Kala azar.
- Molecular diagnosis – Kinetoplast DNA.
- Animal inoculation – Chinese and Golden Hamsters.

TRYPANOSOMA CRUZI

Parasite	Epidemiology	Location in Host	Mode	Symptoms of Infection
T. cruzi *(Chagas'disease)*	South America	Cardiac muscle, blood and other tissues	Reduviid bugs	Chagoma Muscle pain, LN, Myocarditis, Megacolon Meningoencephalitis, Romana's sign (eye edema)

T. brucei

Comparison	West African	East African sleeping sickness
Organism	*T. b. gambiense*	*T. b. rhodesiense*
Vectors	Tsetse flies (palpalis group)	Tsetse flies (Morsitans group)
Primary reservoir	Humans	Antelope and cattle
Human illness	Chronic CNS disease	Acute (early CNS disease) < 9 m
Lymphadenopathy	Prominent Cervical LN (Winter bottom sign)	Minimal Axially and Inguinal lymphadenopathy
Parasitemia	Low	High

COCCIDIAN PARASITES

Property	Cryptosporidium	Cyclospora	Isospora
Size	4-6 μ size	8-10 μ	10-20 μ
Shape	Round	Round	Oval
Cyst contains	Four sporozoites	Two sporoblast, each having two sporozoites	Two sporoblast, each having four sporozoites
Acid fast	Uniformly acid fast	Variable acid fast	Uniformly acid fast
Autoflouroscence	No, but can be stained with fluorescent dye	Autoflouroscence ++	Autoflouroscence +/–
Treatment	Co-trimoxazole	Co-trimoxazole	Spiramycin, Nitazoxanide

Toxoplasmosis

- Cat – Definite host – producing oocyst.
- Man – Intermediate host.
- All three morphological forms are infective – Oocyst, tissue cyst, tachyzoites.
- *Congenital toxoplasmosis*:
    - 1st Trimester – More sever infection.
    - 3rd Trimester – More chance of infection.

- If mother is previously infected – Asymptomatic.
- IgM detection, IgA can also be used (experimental but better sensitivity).

❖ Sabin Feldman test.

❖ Most common manifestation of congenital toxoplasmosis – chorioretinitis.

❖ Most common manifestation of toxplasmosis in HIV – encephalitis.

❖ Most common manifestation of Acquired Toxoplasmosis – Asympt. and if Sympt. – Cervical LN↑.

❖ ***Treatment***

- Immunocompetent hosts – No treatment is typically indicated.
- Congenital toxoplasmosis – Cotrimoxazole.
- Toxoplasmosis during pregnancy – Spiramycin is typically used.
- Prophylaxis in HIV patients – Cotrimoxazole.

Balantidium coli

❖ Largest protozoa.

❖ *Habitat* – Large intestine of man.

❖ *Morphology* – Trophozoite and cyst.

❖ *Trophozoite*:

- Revolving motility.
- Contains two nuclei – Macronucleus and Micronucleus.

❖ *Cyst*:

- Infective form
- Contains two nuclei.

❖ *Diagnosis* – Dysentery.

❖ In large intestine – Ulcers mimic amoebic ulcers but never invade muscular layer.

❖ *Treatment* – Tetracycline – DOC.

PLASMODIUM

Species	Disease	Periodicity (hours)
Plasmodium vivax	Beningn tertian	48
Plasmodium falciparum	Malignant tertian	24-48
Plasmodium ovale	Ovale tertian	48
Plasmodium malariae	Quartan	72
Plasmodium knowlesi	Quartan	24-48

Life-cycle

❖ Man – Intermediate host.

❖ Mosquito – Definitive host.

❖ Sporozoites are infective forms.

❖ Present in the salivary gland of female anopheles mosquito.

- After bite of infected mosquito sporozoites are introduced into blood circulation.
- Other modes of transmission include blood transfusion and transplacentally. (Infective stage–Merozoites and No EE cycle).
- Africa (Sub Saharan).
- India (Orissa and North East).

Recrudescence Vs Relapse

- Recrudescence due to treatment failure.
- Occurs after 2-3 weeks of treatment.
- Occurs in all spp (Most common P. falciparum).
- Relapse – due to hypnozoites.
- Seen in P. vivax and ovale.

Pathogenesis of P. falciparum

- Sequestration (binding of RBC to endothelium).
- Rossetting – Unparasitized RBC clump together with parasitized RBC.
- Antigenic diversity.

Immunity

- *Nature of Haemoglobin*:
  - Sickle cell anemia trait protective.
  - Thalassemia trait protective.
  - Fetal Hb – protective.
- *Nature of RBC*:
  - Pf – All RBC.
  - P. malariae – old RBC.
  - P. ovale/vivax – Young RBC.
- *Nature of Enzyme* – G6PD deficiency – protection.

Clinical Features – Triad

- Malarial paroxysm – fever, chill and rigor.
- Anemia.
- Hepatosplenomegaly.

Complications of Severe Falciparum Malaria

- Recrudescence and relapse.
- Black water fever.
- Cerebral malaria.
- Tropical splenomegaly syndrome.
- Pulmonary edema.
- Renal failure.
- Hypoglycaemia with lactic acidosis.

Laboratory Diagnosis:

- Microscopy – For demonstration of parasites and for speciation.
- Stained peripheral blood smear examination.

- Thick and thin smears – Gold standard method.
- Thick smear – For identification, quantification.
- Thin smears – For speciation.
- Quantitative Buffy Coat examination – Rapid method for detection of parasites.

Ring form of P. vivax:

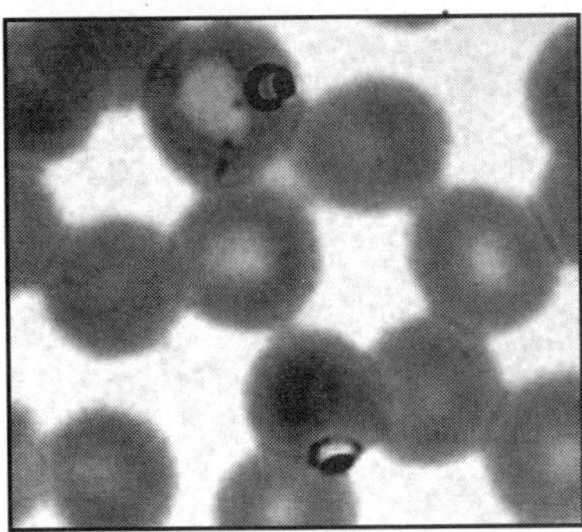

Fig. 14.1: Ring form of P. vivax

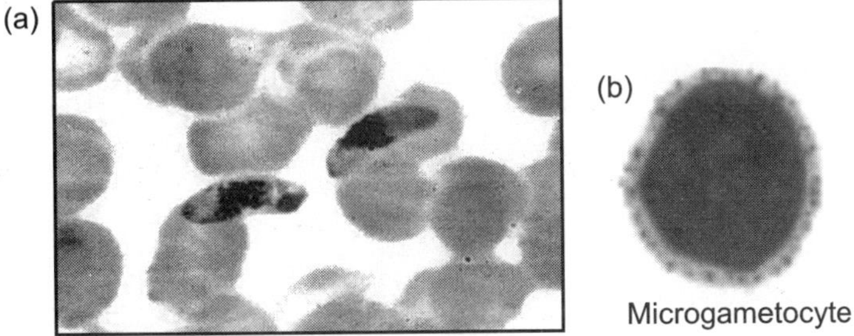

Fig. 14.2: (a) Gametocyte of P. Falciparum and (b) Gametocyte of other Plasmodium spp.

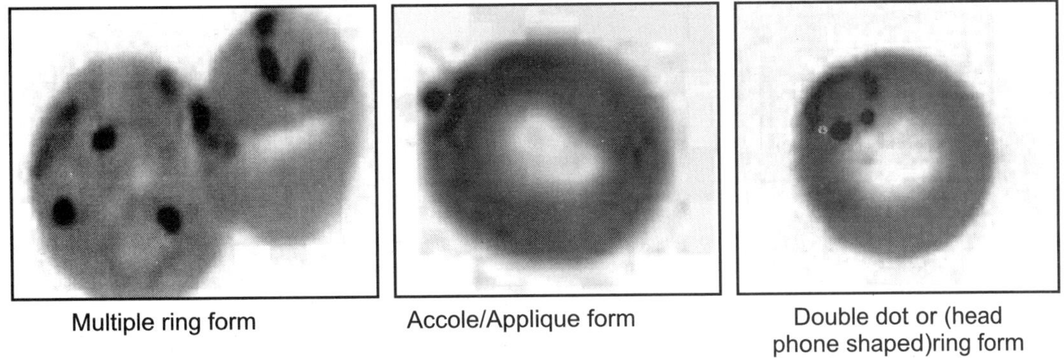

Fig. 14.3: Ring form of P. Falciparum

Band form – P. malariae

Enlarged RBC and fimbrianated – P. ovale

Other test:

- Antigen Detection – Immunochromatographic tests
- Rapid and simple
- pLDH – Pan malarial
- HRP-2 Ag detection – for P.f

- Serology – antibodies against malaria parasites
- Molecular Diagnosis – PCR.

Characteristic	P. falciparum	P. vivax	P. ovale	P. malariae
Red cell preference	All age RBC	Reticulocytes and young RBC	Reticulocytes and young RBC	Older cells
Morphology	**Ring forms** • Multiple • Double dot • Accolle form **Banana-shaped** gametocytes	Irregularly shaped large rings and trophozoites; Schizont and late trophozoites also seen	Erythrocytes enlarged and fimbrinated Schizont and late trophozoites also seen	Band form Schizont and late trophozoites also seen
Relapses	No	Yes	Yes	No
Recrudescence	Yes	No	No	Yes

Babesia

- ❖ Intra erythrocytic protozoa
- ❖ Not found in India
- ❖ Tick borne malaria like illness in animal
- ❖ Zoonotic – Opportunistic to human
- ❖ Treatment – Clindamycin with oral quinine
- ❖ Differ from Plasmodium:
  - Hemozoin absent
  - Gametocyte absent
  - *Maltese cross form* seen – Ring in tetrad in merozoites
  - Vermicule in Tick.

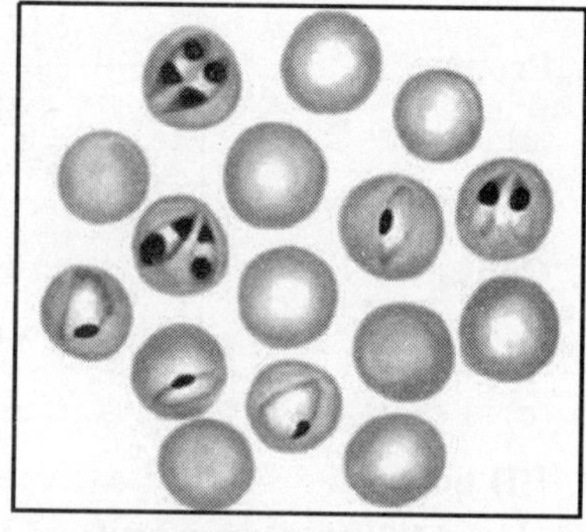

Fig. 14.4: Maltese cross form

Species	B. microti	B. bovis/divergens
Distribution	North America	Europe
Host	Rodent	Cattle
Immunity of host	Spleen is usually normal	Seen in splenectomised and immunocompromised patient
Clinical feature	Asymptomatic/mild fever	Severe, but no cerebral involvement
Clinical course	Self-limiting	Severe, fulminant

FMGE MCQ's

Amoeba and Intestinal/Genital Flagellates

1. Which of the following infestations lead to malabsorption? [*March 2011*]

(a) Giardia lamblia
(b) Ascaris lumbricoides
(c) Necator americana
(d) Ancylostoma duodenale.

Leishmania

2. Highly specific and sensitive test for diagnosing kala-azar: [*March 2010*]

(a) Complement fixation test with WKK antigen

(b) Napier's aldehyde test

(c) Chopra's antimony test

(d) Immunofluorescent antibody test.

3. Novy-McNeal-Nicolle [NNN] medium is used for: [*September 2008*]

(a) Giardia lamblia
(b) Leishmania donovani
(c) Echinococus
(d) Toxoplasma gondii.

4. Rk39 antigen is used in diagnosis of: [*September 2007*]

(a) Kala azar
(b) Tuberculosis
(c) Leprosy
(d) Diphtheria.

5. Kala azar is transmitted by: [*March 2007, September 2007*]

(a) Sand fly
(b) Tsetse fly
(c) Flea
(d) Hard tick.

6. Promastigote form of Leishmania is found in which part of sandfly: [*March 2005*]

(a) Lymph node
(b) GIT
(c) Spleen
(d) Bone marrow.

7. Causative agent for oriental sore is: [*September 2007, March 2003*]

(a) Onchocerca volvulus
(b) Leishmania donovani
(c) Leishmania tropica
(d) Brugya malayi.

8. LD bodies are associated with: [*September 2009*]

(a) Larva migrans
(b) Kala azar
(c) Malaria
(d) Loa loa.

Malaria

9. Infective stage of Malaria to man is: [*September 2011*]

(a) Sporozoite
(b) Trophozoite
(c) Merozoites
(d) Male and female gametocytes.

10. Stage of Plasmodium falciparum NOT seen in peripheral blood smear is: [*March 2011*]

(a) Schizonts
(b) Male gametocyte
(c) Female gametocyte
(d) Ring forms.

11. True about plasmodium falciparum is: [*September 2005*]

(a) Preferentially infects old erythrocytes only
(b) Schuffner's dots is characteristic
(c) Crescentic macrogametocyte
(d) Large schizonts.

12. Drug of choice for benign tertian malaria: [*March 2008*]

(a) Primaquine
(b) Mefloquine
(c) Chloroquine
(d) Azithromycin.

13. Drug of choice for cerebral malaria in pregnancy: [*September 2006*]

(a) Primaquine
(b) Mefloquine

(c) Chloroquine
(d) Quinine.

14. Black malarial pigment is seen in all except: [*September 2010*]

(a) P. vivax
(b) P. falciparum
(c) P. malariae
(d) P. ovlae.

15. Babesiosis is most commonly transmitted by: [*March 2005*]

(a) Pigs
(b) Rats
(c) Sand fly
(d) Ticks.

Coccidian Parasite

16. Which of the following infection, if occurs in the first trimester, leads to maximum incidence of congenital malformations: [*March 2010*]

(a) Rubella
(b) Toxoplasmosis
(c) CMV
(d) All of the above.

17. Investigation for definitive identification of Cryptosporidium: [*March 2010*]

(a) ELISA
(b) Immunofluorescence test
(c) Demonstration of oocyte in feces
(d) Fluoroscent staining with auramine.

18. Sabin-Feldman dye test is used for diagnosis of: [*March 2005, 2009 and September 2007*]

(a) Cryptosporidium
(b) Babesia
(c) Pneumocystis
(d) Toxoplasma.

ANSWERS TO FMGE MCQ's

Amoeba and Intestinal/Genital Flagellates

1. Ans. (a) Giardia lamblia

[*Ref.:* Parija's, Parasitology, 3rd ed., page no. 67; Mandell's Principles of Infectious Diseases, 6th ed., page no. 3201]

- Infection with G. lamblia includes asymptomatic cyst passage, acute self-limited diarrhea, and a chronic syndrome of diarrhea, malabsorption, and weight loss.
- Steatorrhea and malabsorption of vitamins A and B_{12}, protein, D-xylose, and iron have been documented.
- The most common disaccharidase deficiency has been that of lactase with post-Giardia lactose intolerance sometimes persisting for several weeks after treatment.

Leishmania

2. Ans. (d) Immunofluorescent antibody test

[*Ref.:* Parija's, Parasitology, 3rd ed., page no. 91-92; Mandell's, Principles of Infectious Diseases, 6th ed., page no. 3149]

- Several serologic techniques are currently used to detect specific antibodies to Leishmania like ELISA, indirect hemagglutination test (IHA) and the indirect immunofluorescent antibody test (IFAT) which are more sensitive and specific.

–Harrison

About Other Options:

- Both Napier's aldehyde test and Chopra's antimony test are no specific tests and they detect hypergammaglobulinemia.
- Complement fixation test detects antibody by using WKK antigen (Witebsky, Klingenstein and Kuhn antigen derived from Mycobacterium tuberculosis), hence shows false +ve results may occur due to cross-reacting antibodies in patients with leprosy, Chagas' disease, cutaneous leishmaniasis, and other infections.

Also Remember:

The diagnosis of kalazar can be confirmed by:

- Demonstrating amastigotes (LD body) in tissue. ***Splenic aspiration*** for Wright-Giemsa stained smears and for culture is the most sensitive method for parasite identification.
- Isolating promastigotes in culture.
- Best – Antileishmanial antibodies against recombinant k39 (sensitivity is 98% and its specificity is 90%). *–Harrison*

3. Ans. (b) Leishmania donovani

[*Ref.:* Parija's, Parasitology, 3rd ed., page no. 86]

- **Novy-McNeal-Nicolle [NNN] medium is the recommended medium used for the isolation of Leishmania & Trypanosoma.**
- NNN medium consists of salt agar and defrinated rabbit blood.
- Leishmania donovani Promastigote form is isolated in culture (sensitivity 75%).

4. Ans. (a) Kala azar

[*Ref.:* Parija's, Parasitology, 3rd ed., page no. 92; Mandell's, Principles of Infectious Diseases, 6th ed., page no. 3149]

- **Rk39 antibody:** Antileishmanial antibodies against recombinant k39, a kinesin-like antigen, by ELISA or are dipstick tests have **good sensitivity and specificity** for the diagnosis of visceral leishmaniasis.

Laboratory Diagnosis of Kala azar

- Microscopy – Stained smear to demonstrate LD bodies (amastigote form).
- **Sample:**
  - Spleen (most Sensitive).
  - Bone marrow aspiration (most common preferred sample).
  - Lymphnode aspirate (not useful in Indian cases).
  - Peripheral blood smear examination.
- Blood culture – NNN medium (Promastigotes grown).
- *Serological tests:*
  - Napier's aldehyde test – +ve after 3 months and also false +ve seen.
  - Chopra's antimony test.
  - CFT – detecting antibody using WKK antigen.
  - ICT or ELISA – detecting antibody to Rk 39 antigen.
- Leishmanin (Montenegro) skin test – Negative in acute case of Kala azar.

- Molecular diagnosis – Kinetoplast DNA.
- Animal inoculation – Chinese and Golden Hamsters.

5. Ans. (a) Sand fly

[*Ref.:* Parija's, Parasitology, 3rd ed., page no. 84; Mandell's, Principles of Infectious Diseases 6th ed., page no. 3147]

- **Kala azar is transmitted by Sandfly of Genus Phlebotomus argentipes.**
- Visceral leishmaniasis (also known as kala azar, a Hindi term meaning "black fever") is caused by the L. donovani complex, which includes L. donovani and L. infantum/chagasi.
- These species are responsible for anthroponotic and zoonotic transmission, respectively.
- India and neighbouring Nepal, Bangladesh, Sudan, and Brazil are the four largest foci of VL and account for 90% of the world's VL burden, ***with India the worst affected.***

6. Ans. (b) GIT

[*Ref.:* Parija's, Parasitology, 3rd ed., page no. 85]

- Amastigote form of Leishmania are ingested by the female Sandfly during the blood meal.
- In the midgut of sandfly, the amstigote forms transform to promastigote form and migrate to buccal cavity of sandfly.

In Leishmania

- ***Amastigote form:***
  - Found in humans.
  - They are the diagnostic from (LD body).
- ***Promastigote:***
  - Infective form (by bite of sandfly).
  - Found inside midgut of sandfly.
  - Seen in culture.

PARASITOLOGY I

7. Ans. (c) Leishmania tropica

[*Ref.:* Parija's, Parasitology, 3rd ed., page no. 94; Mandell's, Principles of Infectious Diseases, 6th ed., page no. 3149]

- The classic form of Old World cutaneous leishmaniasis is the **"oriental sore."**
- **It is most frequently caused by L. tropica complex** (includes L. major, L. tropica, or Leishmania aethiopica).
- It has also been termed bouton D'Orient, bouton de Crete, Bouton D'Alep, Bouton de Biskra, Aleppo evil, Baghdad boil, and Dehli boil in various regions.
- **Forms of Old World cutaneous leishmaniasis:**
  - Anthroponotic cutaneous leishmaniasis – by L. tropica.
  - Zoonotic cutaneous leishmaniasis – by L. major.
  - Leishmaniasis Recidivans – by L. aethiopica.

8. Ans. (b) Kala azar

[*Ref.:* Parija's, Parasitology, 3rd ed., page no. 91]

- **Leishmania donovani bodies (LD bodies)** are the amastigote form of the parasite found in various organs in patients suffering from Kala azar (Visceral leishmaniasis).
- LD body is demonstrated in smears of spleenic aspirate (most sensitive), bone marrow aspirate (most common preferred sample, but less sensitive), LN aspirate (African patients) and peripheral blood smear.

Malaria

9. Ans. (a) Sporozoite

[*Ref.:* Parija's, Parasitology, 3rd ed., page no. 123]

- **Infective stage of Malaria to man is Sporozoite.**
- **Infective stage of Malaria to man when transmitted by blood transfusion – Merozoite.**
- **Infective stage of Malaria to mosquito is- Gametocyte.**

10. Ans. (a) Schizonts

[*Ref.:* Parija's, Parasitology, 3rd ed., page no. 126]

- In Plasmodium falciparum, the later half of erythrocytic cycle (i.e. eythrocytic schizogony) occurs in the blood vessels of deep viscera. Therefore, late trophozoites, schizonts and merozoites are not demonstrated in peripheral blood smear examination in a case of Plasmodium falciparum infection. *–Parija's*
- However, the early of half of erythrocytic cycle occurs in peripheral blood, so stages of early half of erythrocytic cycle like the early trophozoite (i.e., ring form) and also gametocyte.

Peripheral blood smear examination in Plasmodium falciparum

- ***Demonstrated:***
  - Ring form (and variants of ring forms like accolle form, double dot/headphone shaped ring form and multiform ring form).
  - Gametocyte.
- ***Not demonstrated:***
  - Late trophozoites.
  - Schizonts.
  - Merozoites.

11. Ans. (c) Crescentic macrogametocyte

[*Ref.:* Parija's, Parasitology, 3rd ed., page no. 124]

Plasmodium falciparum

- Infects erythrocytes of all ages. (P. malariae infects old RBCs).
- Maurer's dots is characteristically found (Schuffner's dots is found in P. vivax and P. ovale).
- Schizont is small and compact – Never seen in peripheral blood (Schizont is large P. vivax).

12. Ans. (c) Chloroquine

[*Ref.:* Park, 21st ed., page no. 239]

- Drug of choice for benign tertian malaria – Chloroquine (1st line drug).

13. Ans. (d) Quinine

[*Ref.:* Park, 21st ed., page no. 239]

- Drug of choice for cerebral malaria in pregnancy – Quinine.

14. Ans. (a) P.vivax

[*Ref.:* Parija's, Parasitology, 3rd ed., page no. 124]

- All Plasmodium spp produces black and coarse pigment except P. vivax where golden yellow and fine pigments are seen.

Species	Colour of pigment	Merozoites per Schizont	Dots seen
P. falciparum	Dark brown	18-24 no.	Maurer's dots
P. vivax	Yellowish-brown	12-24 no.	Schuffner's dots
P. ovale	Dark Yellowish-brown	8 no.	Schuffner's dots(larger and darker)
P. malariae	Dark-brown	8 no.	Ziemann's dot

15. Ans. (d) Ticks

[*Ref.:* Parija's, Parasitology, 3rd ed., page no. 153]

- Babesisosis is an **Tick borne malaria like illness** (zoonotic disease) caused by mainly B.microti (and other spp also) and seen in North America and Europe.

Babesia

- Not found in India.
- Tick borne malaria like illness in animal.
- Zoonotic – Opportunistic to human.
- *Treatment* – Clindamycin with oral quinine.
- Differ from Plasmodium:
  - Hemozoin absent.
  - Gametocyte absent.
  - ***Maltese cross form*** seen – Ring in tetrad in merozoites.
  - Vermicule in Tick.

Species	B. microti	B. bovis/divergens
Distribution	North America	Europe
Host	Rodent	Cattle
Immunity of host	Spleen is usually normal	Seen in splenectomised and immunocompromised patient
Clinical feature	Asymptomatic/mild fever	Severe, but no cerebral involvement
Clinical course	Self-limiting	Severe, fulminant

Coccidian Parasite

16. Ans. (d) All of the above

[*Ref.*: Ananthnarayan, 8th ed., page no. 551; Field's Virology, 5th ed., page no. 2741; Parija's, Parasitology, 3rd ed., page no. 175]

- **CMV:** Although the association between time of maternal infection and outcome of congenital infection is not as strong for CMV as it is for rubella, still then evidence have shown that primary maternal infection early in gestation is more likely to lead to sequelae than later maternal infection. *–Field's*
- **Rubella:** The fetal risk is maximum if transmitted in 1st trimester. *–Ananthnarayan*
- **Toxoplasma:** The severity of fetal anomaly is maximum if transmitted in 1st trimester. But the transmission risk is maximum if mother gets infected in 3rd trimester. *–Parija's*
- **Congenital infection where maximum incidence of congenital malformations occurs in** 3rd trimester – Varicella infection.

17. Ans. (a) ELISA

[*Ref.*: Parija's, Parasitology, 3rd ed., page no. 163; Mandell's, Principles of Infectious Diseases, 6th ed., page no. 3149]

- Antigen-detection assays are being increasingly used for diagnosis of cryptosporidiosis from stool. The ELISA kits for Cryptosporidium antigen detection from stool have generally performed well for diagnosis of cryptosporidiosis with sensitivities ranging from 66% to 100% with excellent specificity.

About Other Options:

- **Demonstration of oocyte in feces (by wet mount examination):** Least sensitive, useful only if the feces has moderate to high number of oocyst.
- **Fluoroscent staining with auramine:** More sensitive than acid fast staining. However, these assays are plagued by false-positive results. All of the acid-fast stains detect other parasites that may cause similar illnesses (e.g., Isospora and Cyclospora).
- **Immunofluorescent assays (IFA):** Employing oocysts specific monoclonal antibodies are now commonly used to test for cryptosporidiosis. IFA has been reported to be as sensitive as acid fast staining.

18. Ans. (d) Toxoplasma

[*Ref.*: Parija's, Parasitology, 3rd ed., page no. 178]

- **Sabin-Feldman dye test is the GOLD STANDARD method for diagnosis of Toxoplasmosis.**

Sabin-Feldman Dye Test:

- Is the reference serologic test against which other methods have been evaluated.
- Highly sensitive and specific test.
- **Positive test indicates:** Immobilization of live Tachyzoites of T. gondii when incubated with patients's serum (containing antibody) and complement and alkaline methylene blue dye.
- It measures primarily IgG antibodies, does not indicate recent or old infection.
- The titer does not correlate with the severity of illness.
- A negative Sabin-Feldman dye test practically rules out prior exposure to *T. gondii.*

PRACTICE MCQ's

1. E. histocytica, true is:

(a) E. histolytica sub spp dispar is pathogenic
(b) Cyst contains eight nuclei
(c) Flask-shaped ulcers are present
(d) Premalignant condition.

2. E. histocytica, true are:

(a) Mostly symptomatic
(b) E. histocytica can be differentiated morphologically from E. dispar
(c) E. histocytica can be differentiated antigenically from E. dispar
(d) Most common site – Liver.

3. Acute Primary Amoebic meningoencephalitis true is:

(a) Meningitis caused by Naegleria
(b) Diagnosis is by demonstration of trophozoite in CSF or sometimes cyst
(c) Caused by feco-oral transmission
(d) More common in India.

4. The Pathogenecity of Entamoeba histolytica is indicated by:

(a) Zymodeme pattern
(b) Size
(c) Nuclear pattern
(d) Shape.

5. Chronic amoebic keratitis is seen in:

(a) E. histolytica
(b) Acanthamoeba
(c) Naegleria
(d) Haemoflagellates.

6. Winter bottoms sign in sleeping sickness refers to:

(a) Posterior cervical lymphadenopathy
(b) Conjunctivitis
(c) Skin rashes
(d) Eye edema.

7. RBC's are enlarged in infection with:

(a) P. vivax
(b) P. malariae
(c) P. ovale
(d) P. falciparum.

8. All RBCs are mainly attacked in:

(a) Vivax malaria
(b) Ovale malaria
(c) Falciparum malaria
(d) Quartan malaria.

9. Which antigen detection test is used for the diagnosis of P. falciparum malaria?

(a) Histidine-Rich-Protein I (HRP-I)
(b) Histidine-Rich-Protein II (HRP-II)
(c) Histidine-Rich-Protein III (HRP-III)
(d) Merozoite surface antigen.

10. Infectious stage of Plasmodium when transmitted by blood transfusion is:

(a) Schizont
(b) Cryptozoite
(c) Sporozoite
(d) Merozoite.

ANSWERS TO PRACTICE MCQ's

1. Ans. (c) Flask-shaped ulcers are present

[*Ref.*: Parija's, Parasitology, 3rd ed., page no. 46]

- ❖ E. histolytica sub spp histolytica is pathogenic where as E. histolytica sub spp dispar is non-pathogenic.
- ❖ Cyst of E. histolytica contains four nuclei, E. coli has eight nuceli.
- ❖ E. histolytica – intestinal ulcers are Flask-shaped.
- ❖ It is not a premalignant condition.

2. Ans. (c) E. histocytica can be differentiated antigenically from E. dispar

[*Ref.:* Parija's, Parasitology, 3rd ed., page no. 46]

- ❖ Amoebiasis is mostly asymptomatic.
- ❖ Most common site – Intestine (most common *site of extraintestinal amoebiasis* – Liver).
- ❖ **E. histocytica& E. dispar are morphologically similar and can only can be differentiated by:**
  - Antigenically from E. dispar (Lectin antigen is present only in E. histocytica).
  - Zymodeme pattern (Isoezyme study).
  - PCR.

3. Ans. (a) Meningitis caused by Naegleria

[Ref.: Parija's, Parasitology, 3rd ed., page no. 51-55]

- ❖ Acute Primary Amoebic meningoencephalitis caused by Naegleria.
- ❖ Diagnosis is by demonstration of only trophozoite in CSF (cysts are not seen).
- ❖ Caused by nasal route.
- ❖ Not common in India.

4. Ans. (a) Zymodeme pattern

[*Ref.:* Parija's, Parasitology, 3rd ed., page no. 46]

- ❖ Refer Text.

5. Ans. (b) Acanthamoeba

[*Ref.:* Parija's, Parasitology, 3rd ed., page no. 58]

Acanthamoeba causes:

- ❖ Chronic amoebic keratitis.
- ❖ Granulomatous amoebic encephalitis.

6. Ans. (a) Posterior cervical lymphadenopathy

[*Ref.:* Parija's, Parasitology, 3rd ed., page no. 116]

- ❖ **Winter bottoms sign:** Enlarged non-tender mobile posterior cervical lymphadenopathy is classically seen in African trypanosomiasis.
- ❖ **Romana sign:** Unilateral painless periorbital swelling seen in Chaga's disease.

7. Ans. (c) P. ovale

[*Ref.:* Parija's, Parasitology, 3rd ed., page no. 148]

- ❖ RBC's are enlarged in infection with P. ovale > P. vivax.

8. Ans. (c) Falciparum malaria

[*Ref.*: Parija's, Parasitology, 3rd ed., page no. 129]

- ❖ All RBCs are mainly attacked in – Plasmodium falciparum.
- ❖ Young RBCs R reticulocytes are mainly attacked in – Plasmodium vivax and P. ovale.
- ❖ Old RBCs are mainly attacked in – Plasmodium malariae.

9. Ans. (b) Histidine-Rich-Protein II (HRP-II)

[*Ref.*: Parija's, Parasitology, 3rd ed., page no. 137]

- ❖ Histidine-Rich-Protein II (HRP-II) is specific to Plasmodium falciparum.
- ❖ LDH (Lactate dehydrogenase) is present in all species of Plasmodium.

10. Ans. (d) Merozoite

[*Ref.*: Parija's, Parasitology, 3rd ed., page no. 134]

- ❖ Infectious stage of Plasmodium to man is *Sporozoites.*
- ❖ Infectious stage of Plasmodium when transmitted by blood transfusion is *Merozoites.*
- ❖ Infectious stage of Plasmodium to mosquito is *Gametocyte.*

***

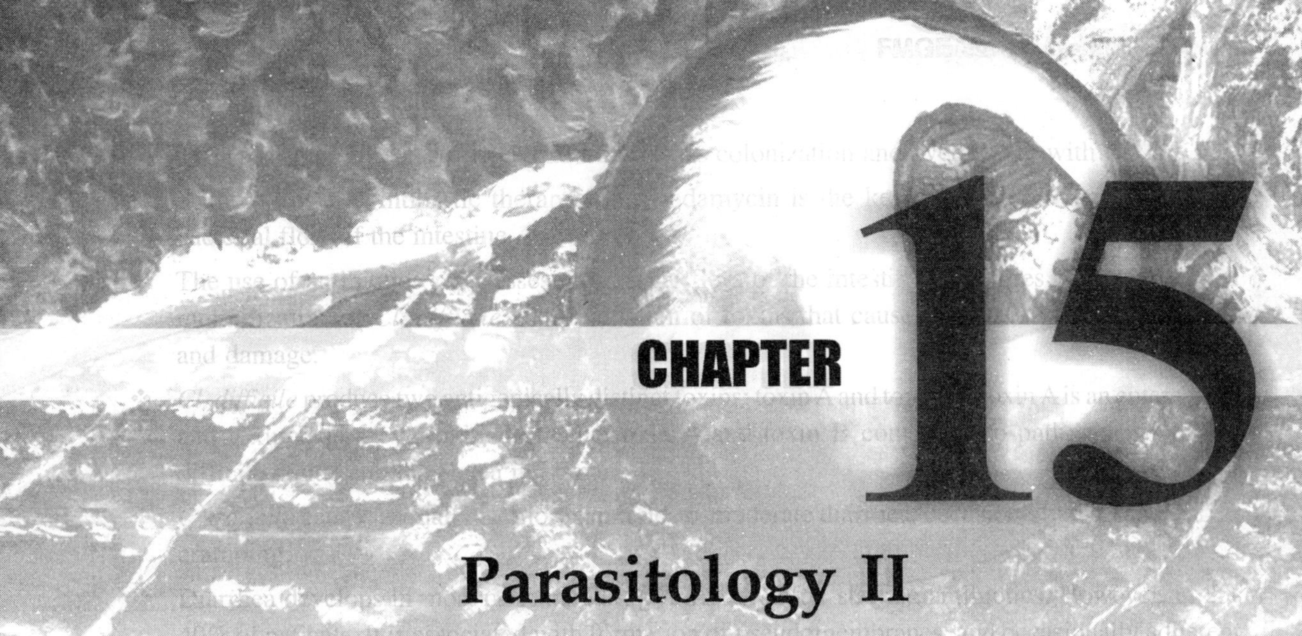

CHAPTER 15

Parasitology II

Helminthes (Cestodes, Trematodes and Nematodes)

CESTODES

- Cestodes, or tapeworms, are segmented worms.
- Habitat – adults reside in the GIT and larvae can be found in any organ.

Intestinal Cestodes – Humans are definitive host

- *Taenia saginata* and *T. solium*
- *Diphyllobothrium*
- *Hymenolepis*
- *Dipylidium caninum.*

Tissue Cestodes (Larval stage) – Humans are intermediate host

- Echinococcus granulosus.
- Sparganum.
- Multiceps spp.
- *Taenia solium* – causing cysticercoisis.

Taenia

Characters	Taenia saginata	Taenia solium
Length	5-10 metres	2-3 metres
Scolex	Large and quadrate	Small and globular
Neck	Short	Long
Proglottid	1000-2000	Less than 1000
Larva	Cysticercus bovis	Cysticercus cellulosae

❖ Both *Taenia saginata and T. solium* causes intestinal Taeniasis.

❖ T. solium in addition causes Cysticercosis in humans, when they act as intermediate hosts.

Characters	Intestinal taeniasis	Cysticercosis
Infective stage	Cysticercus cellulosae	Taenia solium egg
Clinical symptoms	Intestinal symptoms only	Depending on the location of the cyst
Diagnosis	Demonstration of eggs in the faeces	Demonstration of larvae in tissues. Serological tests are of great value.

Cysticercosis

❖ Potentially dangerous systemic disease.

❖ Most commonly found in subcutaneous and intermuscular tissues followed by the **eye and then the brain.**

Man acquires cysticercosis by:

❖ Ingestion of food and water contaminated with eggs.

❖ **Auto infection** through anus-hand-mouth transfer of eggs.

❖ Reverse peristalsis of eggs throwing back the eggs to duodenum where they hatch and cause tissue infection.

Neurocysticercosis

❖ Most serious form of cysticercosis.

❖ Two types:
- Parenchymal
- Extra-parenchymal.

❖ Convulsions, intracranial hypertension and psychiatric disturbances are the three important manifestations.

Echinococcus

❖ **Echinococcus granulosus – hydatid tape worm or dog tape worm.**

❖ Hydatid cyst is the larval stage.

❖ Causes cystic echinococcosis or hydatid disease in man and other herbivorous animals.

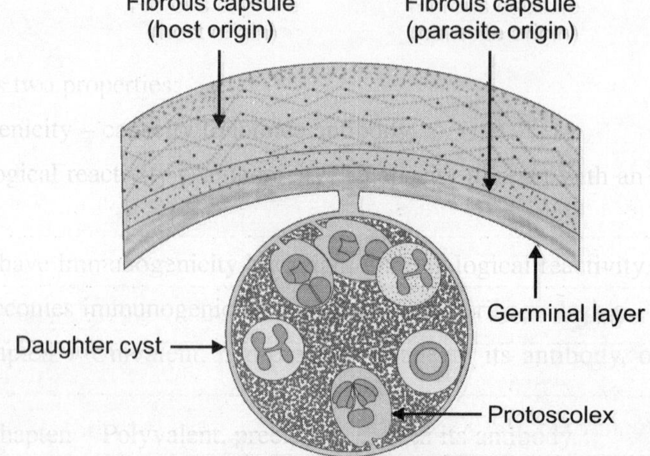

Fig. 15.1: Hydatid cyst

Life Cycle

- Definitive host – Dog and wild carnivores.
- Intermediate hosts – Man and other herbivorous animals.
- Man is an accidental host.
- Eggs – Infective stage of the parasite.

Clinical Features

- Hepatomegaly with or without palpable abdominal mass.
- Bone – Rapid erosion leading to fractures.
- Other sites – Tumor like condition or an abscess.

Parasitic Diagnosis

- Hydatid fluid microscopy – on wet mount examination protoscolices appear as colourless white **structures.**
- **Acid fast staining of centrifuged deposit – acid fast scolices and protoscolices seen.**
- **Casoni's skin test – Immediate hypersensitivity reaction.**
- IHA, CIEP, ELISA and Western Blot used for the detection of antibodies.
- *Detection of antigen:*
  - In serum by ELISA, CIEP, latex agglutination test etc.
  - Recently, in urine by CoA or CIEP.
- Imaging methods like USG, MRI and X-ray are of immense importance to show the size and condition and to pinpoint the exact location of the cysts.

Treatment

- Surgery is the mainstay of this condition.
- Albendazole and mebendazole are the only antihelminthics useful in cystic Echinococcosis.
- Percutaneous Aspiration Injection Reaspiration (PAIR) of the cyst is the latest alternative to surgery.

Hymenolepis nana – dwarf tapeworm

- Infection – fecal/oral contamination.
- Common among institutionalized children.
- **H. nana is the only cestode of humans that does not require an intermediate host. Both the larval and adult phases of the life cycle take place in the human.**
- **Autoinfection** cycle perpetuates the infection.

Clinical Manifestations

- *H. nana* infection – asymptomatic.
- When infection is intense, anorexia, abdominal pain, and diarrhea develop.

Diagnosis

- Infection is diagnosed by the finding of eggs in the stool.

Hymenolepiasis Diminuta

- Cestode of rodents.
- Occasionally infects small children, who ingest the larvae in uncooked cereal foods contaminated *by **fleas.***

- Diagnosed by the detection of eggs in the stool.
- Treatment – praziquantel.

TREMATODES

Trematodes or flatworms – belong to the phylum Platyhelminthes.

Major Human Trematode Infections

Blood Flukes	Mode of Transmission
➢ *Schistosoma haematobium* ➢ *Schistosoma mansoni* ➢ *S. japonicum*	Skin penetration by **cercariae** released from snails.
Biliary Flukes ➢ *Clonorchis sinensis* ➢ *Opisthorchis viverrini* ➢ *O. felineus*	Ingestion of metacercariae in freshwater fish.
Hepatic Flukes ➢ *Fasciola hepatica* ➢ *F. gigantica*	Ingestion of metacercariae in freshwater fish.
Intestinal Flukes ➢ *Fasciolopsis buski* ➢ *Heterophyes heterophyes*	➢ Ingestion of metacercariae on aquatic plants. ➢ Ingestion of metacercariae in freshwater or brackish-water fish.
Lung Flukes ➢ *Paragonimus westermani*	Ingestion of metacercariae in crayfish or crabs.

- All human parasitic trematodes are hermaphroditic (except for schistosomes).

Life Cycle

- Definitive host – mammal/human.
- Intermediate host – Snails or for some trematodes more than one intermediate host may be

Metacercariae – infective stage.

Blood Fluke (Schistosomiasis)

Five species infecting humans:

- **Eggs with a terminal spine** – *Schistosoma haematobium, Schistosoma intercalatum.*
- **Eggs with a lateral spine** – *Schistosoma mansoni.*
- **Eggs with a rudimentary knob** – *Schistosoma japonicum.*

Habitat

- *S. hematobium* – vesicle plexus.
- *S. mansoni* – inferior mesentric plexus.
- *S. japonicum* – superior mesentric plexus.

Clinical Spectrum of Disease:

Acute schistosomiasis

- Most cases are asymptomatic.
- **Schistosomal dermatitis – swimmer's itches.**
- Migration of schistosomule may be associated with inflammatory and mechanical effects in liver and lung.
- **Katayama fever – serum sickness like illness.**

Intestinal Schistosomiasis

- *S. mansoni, S. japonicum, S. mekongi.*
- Intermittent diarrhea with constipation.

Hepatosplenic Schistosomiasis

- *S. haematobium, S. japonicum.*
- *Massive splenomegaly.*
- *Hyper splenism* – anemia.

Genito Urinary Disease

- Intermittent hematuria, dysuria, urinary frequency.
- Hydronephrosis, pyelonephritis, UTI – due to persistant obstruction.

Malignancy

- *S. haematobium* – Squamous cell carcinoma of bladder.
- Drug Therapy for Human Trematode Infections – Praziquantel.

Laboratory Diagnosis

Urine Diagnosis

- *S. haematobium* eggs are passed with diurnal frequency.
- Sedimentation or filtration methods – concentration techniques.

Stool Diagnosis

- Useful for *S. mansoni, S. japonicum, S. intercalatum.*
- Concentration techniques should be used.
- Formol ether sedimentation technique.
- Kato Katz thick smear preparation.

Biopsy

- Rectal biopsy is much more sensitive than Kato Katz thick smear.
- Liver biopsy may be useful in ruling out comorbid conditions like Hepatitis B and C.

Serology

- Antibody detection systems.
- Antigen detection
  - Detects antigen in blood and other body fluids.
  - Circulating anodic antigen (CAA) and Circulating cathodic antigen (CCA).

NEMATODES

General Features of Nematodes:

- Unsegmented, elongated and cylindrical.
- Separate sexes.
- Buccal capsule present.
- GIT is complete.
- Body cavity is present.
- *Size:*
  - Smallest <5 mm: *Trichinella spiralis, Strongyloides stercoralis.*
  - Largest > 1 metre: *Dracunculus medinensis.*
- Body is covered with a tough cuticle.

Nematodes according to egg/larva producing capacity:

Name	Birth to	Example
Viviparous	Larva	*D. medinensis* *W. bancrofti* *B. malayi* *T. spiralis*
Oviparous	Laying eggs	*A. lumbricoides* *T. trichiuria* *A. duodenale* *N. americanus* *E. vermicularis*
Ovo-viviparous	Egg containing larva which immediately hatchout	*S. stercoralis*

Nematodes according to mode of infection:

Mode	Forms	Examples
Ingestion	Eggs contaminated food Growing embryo in intermediate host Encysted embryo in flesh	Ascaris Enterobius Trichuris Trichinella
Penetration through skin	Filariform larva	Hook worm Strongyloides
Bite	Blood sucking insects	Filarial worm

Classification of Nematodes according to Habitat:

(A) Intestinal Nematodes

Small Intestine

- Ascaris lumbricoides/round worm.
- Ancylostoma duodenale/hook worm.

- Necator americanus/American hook worm.
- Strongyloides stercoralis.
- Trichinella spiralis.
- Capillaria philippinensis.

Large Intestine (vermiform appendix and caecum)

- Enterobius vermicularis/pin worm.
- Trichuris trichuira/whip worm.

B. Tissue or Somatic Nematode

Lymphatic system

- Wuchereria bancrofti.
- Brugia malayi.

Subcutaneous tissues

- Loa loa/African eye worm.
- Onchocerca volvulus.
- Mansonella.
- Dracunculus medinensis/Guinea worm.

Conjunctiva

- Loa loa.

Table: Human Intestinal Parasitic Nematodes

Parasitic Nematode					
Feature	**Ascaris lumbricoides (Roundworm)**	**Necator americanus, Ancylostoma duodenale (Hookworm)**	**Strongyloides stercoralis**	**Trichuris trichiura (Whipworm)**	**Enterobius vermicularis (Pinworm)**
Infective stage	Egg	Filariform larva	Filariform larva	Egg	Egg
Route of infection	Oral	Percutaneous	Percutaneous or autoinfection	Oral	Oral
Gastrointestinal location of worms	Jejunal lumen	Jejunal mucosa	Small-bowel mucosa	Cecum, colonic mucosa	Cecum, appendix
Pulmonary passage of larvae	Yes	Yes	Yes	No	No
Principal symptoms	Rarely gastrointestinal or biliary obstruction	Iron-deficiency anemia in heavy infection	Gastrointestinal symptoms; malabsorption or sepsis in hyperinfection	Gastro-intestinal symptoms, anemia	Perianal pruritus

PARASITOLOGY II

Diagnostic stage	Eggs in stool	Eggs in fresh stool, larvae in old stool	Larvae in stool or duodenal aspirate; sputum in hyperinfection	Eggs in stool	Eggs from perianal skin on cellulose acetate tape
Treatment	Mebendazole Albendazole	Mebendazole Albendazole	1. Ivermectin 2. Albendazole	Mebendazole Albendazole	Mebendazole Albendazole

1. Trichinella spiralis

❖ ***Habitat:*** Encysts in striated muscles of the animal.

❖ ***Morphology:***

- Adult worm – Male and female – ***smallest nematode infecting man.***
- Encysted larvae

❖ ***Life cycle:***

- Definitive host – Pig.
- Intermediate – Rat or man.
- Infection passes from pig to pig/rat. And rat to rat.
- Mode of infection – Ingestion of the raw flesh containing viable encysted larvae.

❖ ***Laboratory diagnosis:***

- Demonstration of larvae:
  - In muscle biopsy/autopsy specimen.
  - Site – Tendinous insertion of deltoid/gastrocnenius muscle.
- Stool examination – For adult worm/larvae.
- Blood – Eosinophilia.
- Serology:
  - CFT
  - Precipitation.
  - Bentonite flocculation test/latex agglutination test with Trichinella antigen.
- Skin test – intradermal injection of Bachman's antigen cause an immediate erythematous reaction. Positive test persist for 10-20 years.
- X-ray: If cyst is calcified.

❖ ***Treatment:*** Thiabendazole.

2. Trichuris trichiura (whip worm)

❖ ***Habitat*** Male adult worm live in large intestine – caecum, appendix.

❖ ***Morphology:***

- Adult worm – shape of whip-anterior 3/4th is very thin and hair like, posterior 2/5th is thick and stout.
- Oviparous.

❖ ***Eggs:***

- ***Brown, bile stained egg***
- Barrel shaped with a mucus plug at each pole.
- Contains an unsegmented ovum.

- Floats in saturated solution of common salt.
- Embryonated egg is infectious.

❖ ***Pathogenesis and clinical disease – Trichuriasis:***

- Acute appendicitis – when the worm inhabits in appendix.
- C/o abdominal pain, mucus diarrhoea, blood streaked stool and loss of weight.
- Prolapse of rectum in massive trichuriasis.

❖ ***Laboratory diagnosis:***

- Stool examination – characteristic egg.
- Adult worm occasionally found in stool.

❖ ***Treatment*** – Thiabendazole and mebendazole.

3. Ascaris lumbricoides

❖ Largest intestinal nematode parasite of humans – 40 cm in length.

❖ Most infected individuals have low worm burdens and are asymptomatic

❖ ***Life Cycle:***

- Adult worms live in the lumen of the small intestine.
- Transmission typically occurs through fecally contaminated soil and is due either to a lack of sanitary facilities.
- Younger children are most affected.

❖ ***Clinical Features:***

- Non-productive cough.
- Burning substernal discomfort.
- Dyspnea.
- Blood-tinged sputum are less common.
- Chest X-ray evidence of **eosinophilic pneumonitis (Löffler's syndrome).**
- In heavy infections – Pain and small-bowel obstruction, perforation, intussusception, or volvulus, biliary colic, cholecystitis, cholangitis, pancreatitis, intrahepatic abscesses.
- In highly endemic areas, intestinal and biliary ascariasis can mimic **acute appendicitis and gallstones** as causes of surgical acute abdomen.

❖ ***Laboratory Findings:***

- Microscopic detection of characteristic *Ascaris* eggs – stool/bile.
- *Treatment* – Albendazole, mebendazole effective.

4. Hookworm: A. duodenale and N. americanus

❖ Infective stage and mode of infection – Filariform larvae, penetrate the skin.

❖ ***Clinical Features:***

- Most hookworm infections are asymptomatic.
- Infective larvae may provoke pruritic maculopapular dermatitis **(ground itch)** at the site of skin penetration as well as serpiginous tracks of subcutaneous migration in previously sensitized hosts.
- Chronic hookworm infection leads – iron deficiency.
- **Hypochromic microcytic anemia, occasionally with eosinophilia or hypoalbuminemia, is characteristic of hookworm disease.**

❖ ***Laboratory Diagnosis:***
- Oval non bile stained eggs, that floats in saturated salt solution – in the feces.
- Stool-concentration procedures – to detect light infections.
- Eggs of the two species are indistinguishable by light microscopy.
- If stool sample that is not fresh, the eggs may have hatched to release rhabditiform larvae, which need to be differentiated from those of *S. stercoralis*.

❖ ***Treatment:*** Albendazole, mebendazole.

5. Strongyloides stercoralis:

❖ *Dwarf thread worm* – **Smallest pathogenic nematode causing human infection.**

❖ Has both parasitic and free living stages.

❖ ***Life Cycle:***
- Completed in a single host, man is the principle host.
- Dog and other animals can act as reservoir hosts.
- Has potential for autoinfection and multiplication within infected host.

❖ **Clinical Spectrum:**
- Acute strongyloidosis – Presents as acute watery or mucoid diarrhoea.
- Chronic strongyloidosis – Diffuse abdominal pain, nausea, vomiting, diarrhoea.
- Hyper-infection syndrome – Affecting CNS (in HTLV1 or HIV infected people). therapy etc.

❖ ***Laboratory Diagnosis:***
- Specimens to be collected:
  - Stool.
  - Duodenal aspirate.
  - Sputum.
  - Urine, etc.
- Larval demonstration in stool – low sensitivity ~ 20%.
- At least three specimens to be examined.
- Formalin ethyl acetate concentration technique preferred.
- For isolation of larvae:
  - Baermann method.
  - Harada Mori filter paper method – not very sensitive.
  - Agar plate method – 96% sensitive but laborious and time consuming.
- Skin test.
- Serology – IgG ELISA – about 85-95% sensitivity.

❖ ***Treatment:*** Ivermectin is drug of choice (Alternate thiabendazole and albendazole).

PARASITOLOGY II

FILARIAL WORMS

Characteristics of the Filarial worms:

Organism	Periodicity	Vector	Location of Adult	Microfilarial Location	Sheath
Wuchereria bancrofti	Nocturnal subperiodic	*Culex Anopheles Aedes*	Lymphatic tissue	Blood	+
Brugia malayi	Nocturnal subperiodic	*Anopheles Mansonia*	Lymphatic tissue	Blood	+
Loa loa	Diurnal	*Chrysops* (deerflies)	Subcutaneous tissue	Skin, eye	+
Onchocerca volvulus	None	*Simulium* (blackflies)	Subcutaneous tissue	Skin, eye	–
Mansonella	None	*Culicoides* (midges)	Subcutaneous tissue	Skin	–

FMGE MCQ's

Cestodes

1. **Hydatid cyst is commonly seen in:** [*September 2011*]
   (a) Liver (b) Spleen
   (c) Lungs (d) Bones.
2. **Intermediate host for hydatid disease is:** [*March 2010*]
   (a) Cow (b) Man
   (c) Dog (d) Pig.
3. **Most common site of Hydatid cyst in human:** [*September 2007*]
   (a) Spleen (b) Right posterior superior of liver
   (c) Left lobe of liver (d) Right anterior inferior of liver.
4. **Most common site of Hydatid cyst in human:** [*September 2007*]
   (a) Spleen (b) Liver
   (c) Lung (d) Brain.
5. **Megaloblastic anemia caused by:** [*March 2005*]
   (a) Taenia saginata (b) Diphylobothrium latum
   (c) Taenia solium (d) Echinococcus granulosus.

Trematodes

6. **Paragonismus westermanii is commonly called:** [*March 2005*]
   (a) Lung fluke (b) Tapeworms
   (c) Intestinal flukes (d) Liver flukes.

Nematodes

7. **Iron deficiency anemia is commonly caused by:** [*March 2009, September 2005*]
   (a) Enterobius vermicularis
   (b) Taenia solium
   (c) Ancylostoma duodenale
   (d) All of the above.
8. **Non bile stained eggs is found in:** [*March 2009*]
   (a) Ancylostoma duodenale
   (b) Trichuris trichura
   (c) Ascaris lumbricoides
   (d) All of the above.
9. **Microfilaria is not seen in:** [*September 2009*]
   (a) Lymphatics
   (b) Hydrocoele fluid
   (c) Chylous urine
   (d) Blood.
10. **Two nuclei at the tail tip is seen in:** [*September 2009*]
   (a) Brugia malayi
   (b) Wucheria bancrofti
   (c) Onchocerca volvulus
   (d) Mansonella ozzardi.
11. **Most common parasitic infection in AIDS:** [*Septemberr 2008*]
   (a) Ancylostoma duodenale
   (b) Echinococcus granulosus
   (c) Strongyloides stercoralis
   (d) Enterobius vermicularis
12. **Cyclops is a part of life cycle of:** [*September 2007*]
   (a) Toxoplasmosis
   (b) Echinococcus
   (c) Leishmaniasis
   (d) Dracunculosis.
13. **All of the following are arthropod borne diseases except:** [*September 2007*]
   (a) Malaria
   (b) Filariasis
   (c) Dengue
   (d) Dracunculosis.
14. **Chandler's index is associated with:** [*September 2006*]
   (a) Round worm
   (b) Hook worm
   (c) Pin worm
   (d) Tape worm.

ANSWERS TO FMGE MCQ's

1. **Ans. (a) Liver**

[*Ref.:* Park, 21st ed., page no. 278]

- ❖ The liver is involved in about two-thirds of hydatid disease due to E. granulosus infections and in nearly all E. multilocularis infections.
- ❖ In humans, hydatid disease involves the liver in approximately 75% of cases, the lung in 15%, and other anatomic locations in 10%.
- ❖ The right lobe is the most frequently involved portion of the liver.

2. **Ans. (b) Man**

[*Ref.:* Parija's, Parasitology, 3rd ed., page no. 222]

- ❖ Definitive host – Dog and wild carnivores.
- ❖ Intermediate hosts – Herbivorous animals like sheep and man.

- Man is an accidental host.
- Eggs – Infective stage of the parasite.

3. Ans. (b) Right posterior superior of liver

[*Ref.:* Park, 21st ed., page no. 278; Journal – Hydatid Disease: Radiologic and Pathologic Features and Complications Iván Pedrosa et al., *Radio Graphics*, May 2000, 20, 795-817]

- The right lobe is the most frequently involved portion of the liver *–Park*
- Trans diaphragmatic migration of hydatid disease from the posterior segments of the right hepatic lobe has been reported to be a common complication and is probably related to their proximity to the diaphragm.

4. Ans. (b) Liver

[*Ref.:* Park, 21st ed., page no. 278]

- See Q. No. 1.

5. Ans. (b) Diphylobothrium latum

[*Ref.:* Parija's, Parasitology, 3rd ed., page no. 201]

- The adult worm Diphylobothrium latum has extraordinary affinity for vitamin B_{12} and it absorbs most of the vitamin B_{12} from stomach hence can cause megaloblastic anemia.

Diphylobothrium latum (fish tape worm)

- Longest parasite found in intestine.
- Definitive host – man.
- Intermediate host:
  - 1st intermediate host – Cyclops/diaptomus.
  - 2nd intermediate host – Fresh water fish.
- Infective form – Plerocercoid(L3).
- Mode – Ingestion of raw fish.
- *Causes Megaloblastic anemia.*
- *More prevalent in Baltic country.*
- *In India – only one case from Vellore.*

6. Ans. (a) Lung fluke

[*Ref.:* Parija's, Parasitology, 3rd ed., page no. 239]

- Paragonimus westermani is also commonly called as Lung fluke.

A. Intestinal Flukes

- Fasciolopsis buski
- Gastrodiscoides hominis
- Heterophyes heterphyes
- Metagonimus Yokogawai.

B. Liver Flukes

- Fasciola hepatica
- Clonorchis sinensis
- Opisthorchis felineus.
- Fasciola gigantica
- Opisthorchis viverrini

C. **Lung Flukes**
   - Paragonimus westermani.

D. **Blood Flukes**
   - Schistosoma haematobium
   - Schistosoma mansoni
   - Schistosoma japonicum.

Paragonimus westemani (Lung fluke):

- ❖ Definite host man.
- ❖ Intermediate host:
  - 1st – Snail
  - 2nd – Crey/crab fish
- ❖ Infective form – Metacercariae.
- ❖ Mode of transmission – Ingesting of metacercariae encysted in the muscles and viscera of crayfish and freshwater crabs.
- ❖ Cyst in Right lung – Most common.
- ❖ Golden brown sputum.
- ❖ Causes endemic hemoptysis.
- ❖ Diagnostic – Operculated eggs.
- ❖ Most common place in India – Manipur.

7. Ans. (c) Ancylostoma duodenale

[*Ref.:* Parija's, Parasitology, 3rd ed., page no. 305]

Parasite	Type of anemia
Ancylostoma duodenale	Iron deficiency
Necator americanus	Iron deficiency
Babesia	Hemolytic
Plasmodium spp.	Autoimmune hemolytic
Trichuris trichiura	Iron deficiency
Leishmania donovani	Autoimmune hemolytic
Diphyllobothrium latum	Vit. B_{12} Deficiency/Megaloblastic

8. Ans. (a) Ancylostoma duodenale

[*Ref.:* Parija's, Parasitology, 3rd ed., page no. 303]

- ❖ **Non-bile stained eggs *(NEHA)***
  - *Necator*
  - *Enterobius vermicularis*
  - *Ancylostoma*
  - *Hymenolepis nana*

- *Also know,* Saline Mount is recommended to demonstrate bile staining property. Iodine mount cannot differentiate bile stained and non bile stained eggs.

9. Ans. None

[*Ref.:* Parija's, Parasitology, 3rd ed., page no. 336]

- Microfilaria is usually demonstrated in peripheral blood but can also be demonstrated from urine micrscopy and microscopy of hydrocele fluid and lymphnode aspiration. *–Parija's*

Also know: Microfilaria is not seen in peripheral blood:

- Occult Filariasis (Tropical pulmonary syndrome).
- Chronic Filarisis (rarely seen).
- Collection in Wrong time.

10. Ans. (a) Brugia malayi

[*Ref.:* Parija's, Parasitology, 3rd ed., page no. 328]

- **Microfilaria that has no nuclei at the tail tip:**
  - Wucheria bancrofti.
  - Onchocerca volvulus.
  - Mansonella ozzardi.
- **Microfilaria that has nuclei at the tail tip:**
  - Brugia malayi.
  - Loa loa.
  - Mansonella perstans.
  - Mansonella streptocerca.

Table: Differences between microfilaria of Wucheria bancrofti and Brugia malayi

Wucheria bancrofti	Brugia malayi
Sheathed	Sheathed
Large cephalic space	Large cephalic space
Nuclei overlapping	Nuclei overlapping
No nuclei at the tail tip	Two nuclei at tail tip
Pointed tail tip	Pointed tail tip

PARASITOLOGY II

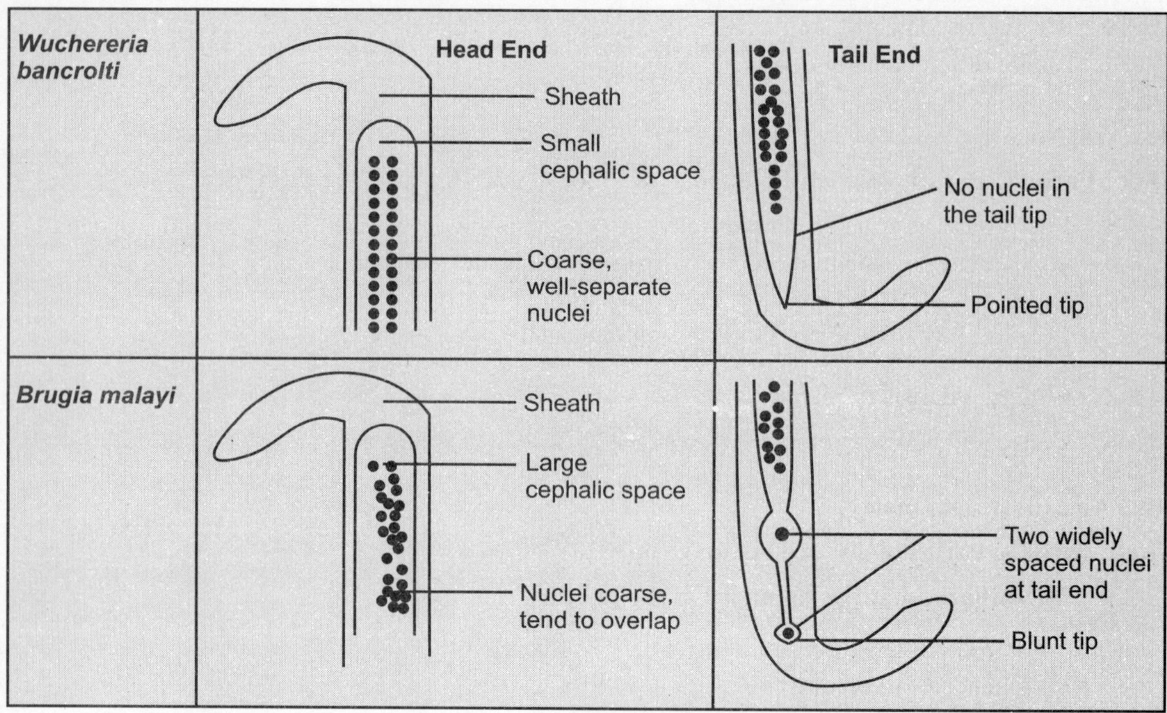

Fig 15.2: Differences between microfilaria of Wucheria bancrofti and Brugia malayi

Also know:

Sheathed Microfilaria:

- Wucheria bancrofti
- Brugia malayi
- Loa loa.

Habitat of Microfilaria:

- *Nocturnal:* Wucheria and Brugia
- *Diurnal:* Loa loa
- *Non periodic:* Onchocerca and Mansonella.

11. Ans. (c) Strongyloides stercoralis

[*Ref.:* Parija's, Parasitology, 3rd ed., page no. 296]

- Among the options, Strongyloides stercoralis is a common oppurtinistic parasite in HIV patients.
- HIV patients, strongyloides causes hyperinfection syndrome and disseminated strongyloidiasis.

Most common parasitic infection in AIDS:

- Cryptospordium (MC)
- Isospora
- Cyclospora
- Toxoplasma
- Strongyloides
- Leishmania.

12. Ans. (d) Dracunculosis

[*Ref.:* Parija's, Parasitology, 3rd ed., page no. 355]

- **Cyclops is a part of life cycle of (2D):**
  - Dracunculosis
  - Diphyllobothrium latum.

13. Ans (d) Dracunculosis

[*Ref.:* Parija's, Parasitology, 3rd ed., page no. 355]

- ❖ Dracunculosis is caused drinking unfiltered water containing Cyclops infected with 3rd stage larva of Dracunculus medinensis.

14. Ans. (b) Hook worm

[*Ref.:* Park 21st ed., page no. 221, 20th ed., page no. 215]

- ❖ Chandler's index is indicator of morbidity mortality from hookworm infection.
- ❖ Average number of stool per gram of stool in the entire community.
  - *Below 200: Suggestive of hook worm infection is not of much significance*
  - *200-500: May be regarded as potential dangerous*
  - *250-300: Minor public health problem*
  - *>300: Important public health problem*

PRACTICE MCQ's

1. Cysticercosis is caused by:

(a) T. solium (b) T. saginata

(c) T. asciatica (d) E. granulosus.

2. The following regarding cysticercosis are true except:

(a) Calcification is usually seen (b) Commonest sites is eyes

(c) The main d/d is tuberculoma (d) Found in subcutaneous tissues.

3. Neurocysticerosis, following are true except:

(a) Acquired by eating contaminated vegetables

(b) Acquired by feco-oral route

(c) Caused by larva (d) Acquired by eating pork.

4. Commonest parasite of CNS in India is:

(a) Hook worm (b) Hydatid cyst

(c) Schistosomiasis (d) Cysticercosis.

5. The egg which of the following parasites consist of polar filaments arising from either end of the embrophore:

(a) Taenia saginata (b) Hymenolepis nana

(c) Echinococcus (d) Diphyllobothrium latum.

6. Cholangiocarcinoma is caused by:

(a) Fasciola infestation (b) Clonorchis infestation

(c) Paragonimus infestation (d) Ascaris infestation.

7. In which stage of filariasis are microfilaria seen in peripheral blood:

(a) Occult filariasis (b) Acute stage

(c) Chronic stage (d) Elephantiasis.

8. Abdominal pain, bloody diarrhea and rectal prolapse in children is caused by:

(a) Trichuris trichura (b) Hook worm

(c) Ascariasis (d) Trichinella spiralis.

9. Which of the following is viviparous:

(a) Strongyloidis stercoralis (b) Hookworm

(c) Trichinella spiralis (d) Ascaris.

10. Eosinophilic meningoencephalitis is caused by:

(a) Angiostrongylus cantonensis (b) Capillaria

(c) Naegleria (d) Toxocara canis.

ANSWERS TO PRACTICE MCQ's

1. Ans. (a) T. solium

[*Ref.:* Parija's, Parasitology, 3rd ed., page no. 216]

- ❖ Cysticercosis is caused by only by T. solium whereas intestinal taeniasis is caused by both T. solium and T. saginata.

2. Ans. (b) Commonest sites are meninges

[*Ref.:* Parija's, Parasitology, 3rd ed., page no. 216]

- ❖ Calcification is usually seen detected by CT scan.
- ❖ Commonest sites are subarachnoid space followed by brain parenchyma.
- ❖ The main differential diagnosis of Neurocysticerosis, is the space occupying lesions like Tuberculoma.
- ❖ Cysts are found in subcutaneous tissues, muscle, eye and CNS.

3. Ans. (d) Acquired by eating pork

[*Ref.:* Parija's, Parasitology, 3rd ed., page no. 217]

- ❖ Intestinal teniasis is acquired by eating pork contaminated with larva of T. solium or T. saginata.
- ❖ **Neurocysticerosis:**
  - Acquired by eating contaminated vegetables with T. solium eggs.
  - Autoinfection of T. solium eggs (Faeco-oral route).
  - Main pathogenesis of Neurocysticerosis is due to larva.

4. Ans. (d) Cysticercosis

[*Ref.:* Parija's, Parasitology, 3rd ed., page no. 217]

- ❖ Commonest parasite of CNS in India is – Toxoplasma and Cysticercosis.
- ❖ Neurocysticerosis is a common cause of neurological disease in India.
- ❖ It is one of the common cause of epilepsy.
- ❖ Next to tuberculosis, it is the 2nd most common space occupying lesion of brain.

5. Ans. (b) Hymenolepis nana

[*Ref.:* Parija's, Parasitology, 3rd ed., page no. 230]

- ❖ Hymenolepis nana egg contains three pairs of hooklets and polar filaments arising from either end of the Embryophore.

6. Ans. (b) Clonorchis infestation

[*Ref.:* Parija's, Parasitology, 3rd ed., page no. 275]

PARASITOLOGY II

❖ **Cholangiocarcinoma is caused by Clonorchis and Opisthorchis infestation.**

Table: Parasites associated with Malignancy

Parasites	Malignancy
Schistosoma haematobium	Squamous cell carcinoma of urinary bladder
Clonorchis sinensis	Cholangiocarcinoma of liver, bile duct and adenocarcinoma of pancreas
Opisthorchis viverrini	Cholangiocarcinoma of bile duct

7. Ans. (b) Acute stage

[*Ref.:* Parija's, Parasitology, 3rd ed., page no. 336]

Microfilaria is not seen in peripheral blood:

❖ Occult Filariasis (Tropical pulmonary syndrome).

❖ Chronic Filarisis (rarely seen).

❖ Collection in wrong time.

8. Ans. (a) Trichuris trichura

[*Ref.:* Harrison 18th ed., page no. 1743]

❖ Most infections with Trichuris trichiura are asymptomatic, but heavy infections may cause gastrointestinal symptoms like ***abdominal pain***, anorexia, and ***bloody or mucoid diarrhea*** resembling inflammatory bowel disease.

❖ ***Rectal prolapse*** can result from massive infections in children, who often suffer from malnourishment and other diarrheal illnesses.

❖ Trichuris trichura is a large intestinal nematode.

9. Ans. (c) Trichinella spiralis

[*Ref.:* Parija's, Parasitology, 3rd ed., page no. 282]

Nematodes according to egg/larva producing capacity:

Name	Birth to	Example
Viviparous	Larva	*D. medinensis* *W. bancrofti* *B. malayi* *T. spiralis*
Oviparous	Laying eggs	*Asciairs* *Trichuris* *Hook worm* *E. vermicularis*
Ovo-viviparous	Egg containing larva which immediately hatchout	*S. stercoralis*

10. Ans. (a) Angiostrongylus cantonensis

[*Ref.:* Parija's, Parasitology, 3rd ed., page no. 312]

❖ Angiostrongylus cantonensis is the agent of Eosinophilic meningoencephalitis.

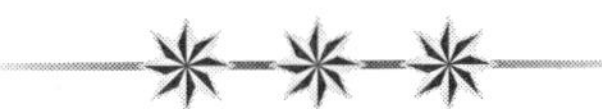

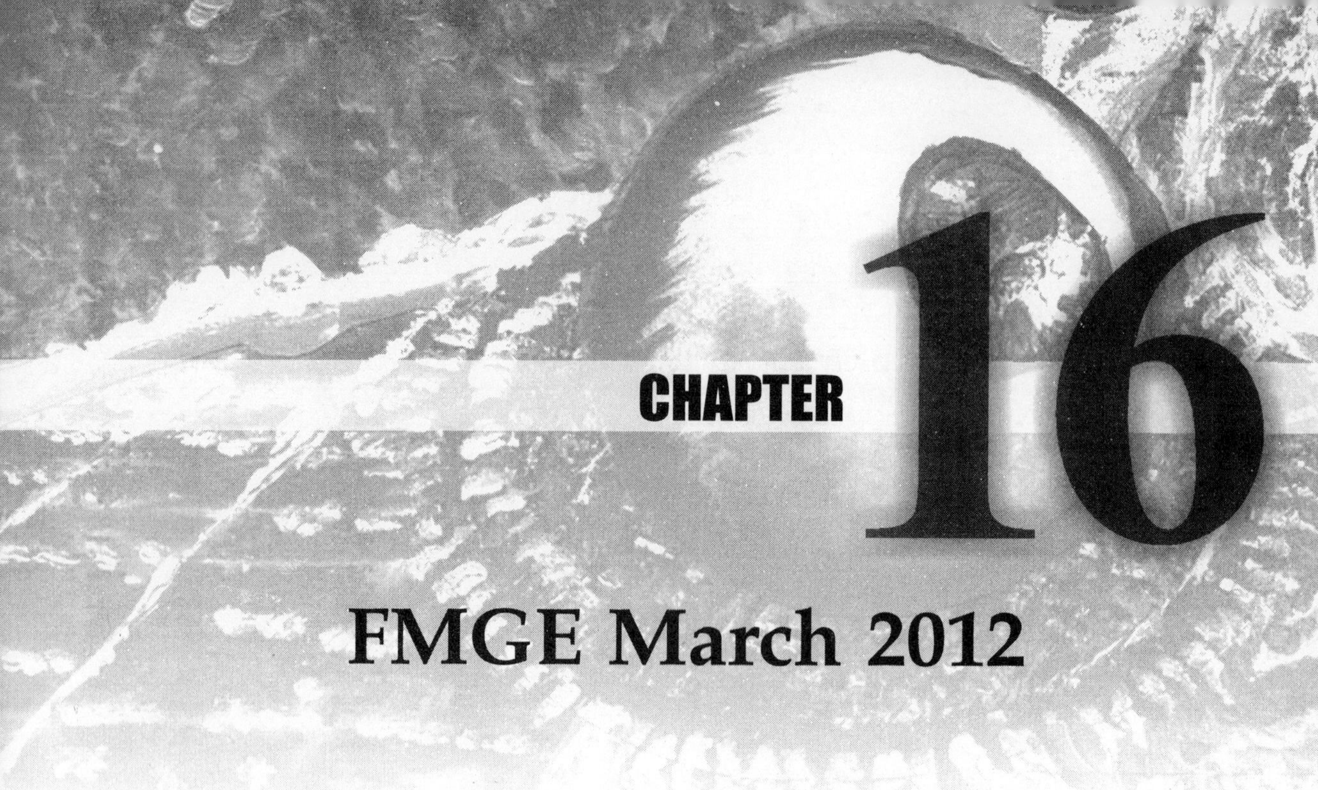

CHAPTER 16

FMGE March 2012

1. The role of adjuvant in a D.P.T. vaccine is:

(a) Decrease hypersensitivity
(b) Decrease absorption of vaccine
(c) Increase antigenicity
(d) Increase the shelf life of a vaccine.

2. Herd immunity in human population plays a role in all of the following except:

(a) Pertussis
(b) Rabies
(c) Measles
(d) Diphtheria.

3. Paul Bunnell test is used for diagnosis for diagnosis of:

(a) Yellow fever
(b) Genital Herpes
(c) Infectious mononucleosis
(d) Chicken pox.

4. Which of the following is an example of precipitation reaction:

(a) WidalTest
(b) Coomb's Test
(c) Counter current immunoelectrophoresis
(d) Weil-Felix Test.

5. All of the following are strategies of polio eradication in India except:

(a) Mass immunization campaign against Polio
(b) Good personal hygiene
(c) AFP surveillance
(d) Strengthening complete routine immunization.

6. All of the following are the components of DOTS plus in India except:

(a) Register & uninterrupted supply of drugs
(b) Political will
(c) Case detection with the help of X-Ray chest
(d) Systemic evaluation and monitoring.

7. **Reverse cold chain is used for:**
   (a) Transportation of vaccines to Lab to check its potency
   (b) Carrying stool samples of Polio patients from Primary Health Centre (PHC) to lab.
   (c) Transportation of outdated vaccines from PHC to district hospital
   (d) Transportation of vaccines from camps to sub centre.
8. **T cells are derived from:**
   (a) Tonsils (b) Thymus
   (c) Thalamus (d) Thyroid.
9. **Diagnosis of rabies may be made postmortem by demonstration of which of the following inclusion bodies in the brain:**
   (a) HP bodies (b) Negri bodies
   (c) Paschen bodies (d) Lipschutz inclusions.
10. **During epidemic of Hepatitis E fatality is maximum in:**
   (a) Adolescents (b) Infants
   (c) Pregnant women (d) Malnourished male.
11. **Which of the following is transmitted by mites:**
   (a) Epidemic typhus (b) Trench fever
   (c) Scrub typhus (d) Endemic typhus.
12. **XDR tuberculosis is defined by:**
   (a) Resistance to all first and second line anti-tubercular agents
   (b) Resistance to any three first line anti-tubercular agents
   (c) Resistance to isoniazid & rifampicin and any three classes of second line anti-tubercular agents
   (d) Resistance to isoniazid & rifampicin.
13. **Which of the following pneumonia is common in AIDS cases:**
   (a) Staphylococcal (b) Pneumocystis carinii
   (c) Viral (d) Pneumococcal.
14. **Pathogenesis of rheumatic fever is due to immunological injury caused by:**
   (a) Forbidden clones (b) Neo antigens
   (c) Hidden antigens (d) Cross reacting antigens.
15. **Re-infection tuberculosis affects which of the following region of the lung:**
   (a) Lower part of the upper lobe (b) Hilar region
   (c) Apical region (d) Upper part of the lower lob.
16. **Which one of the following microbe, found in ear discharge, has a high predilection for meningitis**
   (a) Staphylococcus aureus (b) Streptococcus pneumoniae
   (c) Pseudomonas aeruginosa (d) Proteus mirabilis.
17. **Human herpes virus 8 infection is associated with**
   (a) Hairy cell leukemia (b) Kaposi sarcoma
   (c) Oral hairy leucoplakia (d) Molluscum contagiosum.

ANSWER TO FMGE MACH 2012

1. Ans. (c) Increase antigenicity.

[*Ref.:* Ananthnarayan, 8th ed., page no 143; Park, 21st ed., page no. 152, 20th ed., page no. 142]

- ❖ Alum is a repository adjuvant which is used for increase the immunogenicity of the vaccine antigen.
- ❖ Aluminium hydroxide or phosphate antigens in the water phase of a water-in-oil emulsion (Freund's incomplete adjuvant) delay the release of antigen from the site of injection and prolong the antigenic stimulus.
- ❖ Aluminum phosphate is more immunogenic than hydroxide.

2. Ans. (b) Rabies

[*Ref.:* Ananthnarayan, 8th ed., page no. 89; Park, 21st ed., page no. 97]

- ❖ Herd immunity refers to an overall level of immunity in a community.
- ❖ Eradication of an infectious disease depends on development of a high level of herd immunity against the pathogen.
- ❖ Epidemics of a disease is likely to occur when herd immunity against that disease is very low, indicating the presence of a large number of susceptible people in the community.
- ❖ **Elements that contributes to Herd immunity are:**
  - Occurrence of Clinical and sub clinical cases in herd.
  - Ongoing immunization programme.
  - Herd structure – includes Population.
- ❖ **Herd immunity occurs with the following vaccines:**
  - Diphtheria
  - Pertussis
  - Measles, Mumps, Rubella
  - OPV
  - Small Pox.

3. Ans. (c) Infectious mononucleosis.

[*Ref.:* Ananthnarayan, 8th ed., page no. 476]

- ❖ The standard diagnostic procedure for infectious mononucleosis is Paul-Bunnell test.

Paul-Bunnell test

- ❖ During infectious mononucleosis heterophile antibodies agglutinate sheep erythrocytes:
- ❖ However, such antibodies may also occur after injections of sera and sometimes even in normal individuals.
- ❖ Infectious mononucleosis antibodies may be differentiated by absorption tests. Inactivated serum (56°C for 30 minutes) in doubling dilutions is mixed with equal volumes of a 1% suspension of sheep erythrocytes.
- ❖ After incubation at 37°C for four hours the tubes are examined for agglutination.
- ❖ An agglutination titre of 100 or above is suggestive of infectious mononucleosis.
- ❖ For confirmation, differential absorption of agglutinins with guinea pig kidney and ox red cells or by a slide agglutination test (monospot test) employing sensitized horse erythrocytes, with the same sensitivity and specificity.
- ❖ The Paul-Bunnell antibody develops early during the course of infectious mononucleosis and disappears within about two months.

4. Ans. (c) Counter current immunoelectrophoresis.

[*Ref.:* Ananthnarayan, 8th ed., page no. 107]

- Counter current immunoelectrophoresis is an example of precipitation test, whereas all the other options are example of agglutination test.

Counterimmunoelectrophoresis (CIE,counter-current immunoelectrophoresis):

- This involves simultaneous electrophoresis of the antigen and the antibody in gel in opposite directions resulting in precipitation at a point between them (Fig).
- This method produces visible precipitation lines within thirty minutes and is ten times more sensitive than the standard double diffusion technique.
- Used for - alfa FetoProtein, Antigen of Cryptococcus and Meningococcus

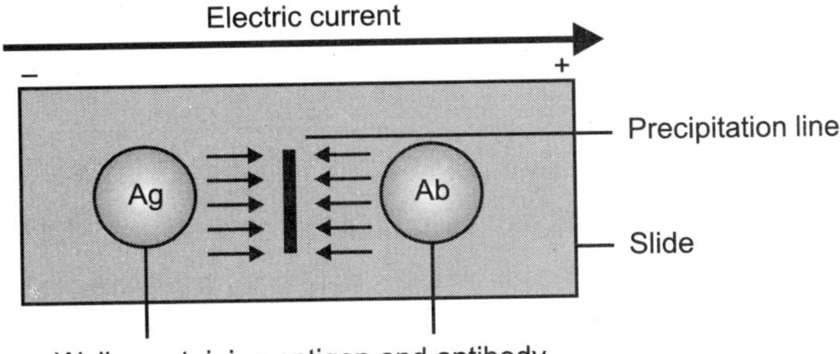

Example of Precipitation reaction

Ring test

- Ascoli thermo precipitation test (anthrax)
- Lancefield grouping (*Streptococcus)*

Slide flocculation test – VDRL, RPR

Tube flocculation test – Kahn test, standardization of toxin

Immuno-diffusion (In gel):

- Produces visible band, so interpretation is easy
- Can be preserved
- Differentiate between antigens

Example

- Elek gel precipitation (*C diphtheriae* toxigenicity testing)
- Eiken test (E.coli)

Immunoelectrophoresis

Counter current immunoelectrophoresis (CIEP)

Rocket electrophoresis

5. Ans. (b) Good personal hygiene

[*Ref.:* Park, 21st ed., page no. 188]

Strategies of polio eradication in India

- Conduct pulse polio immunization days every year until poliomyelitis is eradicated.
- Sustain high levels of routine immunization coverage.

- ❖ Monitor OPV coverage at district level and below.
- ❖ Improve surveillance capable of detecting all cases of AFP due to polio or non polio etiology.
- ❖ Ensure rapid case investigation including the collection of stool sample for virus isolation.
- ❖ Arrange follow up of all cases of AFP at 60 days to check for residual paralysis.
- ❖ Conduct outbreak control for cases confirmed or suspected to be poliomyelitis to stop transmission.

6. Ans. (c) Case detection with the help of X-Ray chest.

[*Ref.:* Revised National Tuberculosis Control Programme/DOTS-Plus Guidelines/February 2009/ p10, Park, 21st ed., page no. 179]

Five Components of DOTS-Plus

DOTS-Plus refers to DOTS programmes that add components for MDR-TB diagnosis,management and treatment.

1. **Sustained political and administrative commitment**
   - A well functioning DOTS programme
   - Long term investment of staff and resources
   - Coordination efforts between community, local governments, and internationalagencies
   - Addressing the factors leading to the emergence of MDR-TB.
2. **Diagnosis of MDR-TB through quality-assured culture and drugsusceptibility testing**
   - Proper triage of patients for Culture & DST testing and management under DOTS-Plus
   - Co-ordination with National and Supra-National Reference Laboratories
3. **Appropriate treatment strategies that utilize second-line drugs underproper management conditions**
   - Rational standardized treatment design (evidence-based)
   - Directly observed therapy (DOT) ensuring long-term adherence
   - Monitoring and management of adverse drug reactions
   - Adequate human resources.
4. **Uninterrupted supply of quality assured anti-TB drugs.**
5. **Recording and reporting system designed for DOTS-Plus programmes that enable performance monitoring and evaluation of treatment outcome.**

7. Ans. (b) Carrying stool samples of Polio patients from Primary Health Centre (PHC) to lab.

[*Ref.:* Internet source, Park, 21st ed., page no. 188-89]

- ❖ **Reverse cold chain means:** The process of maintaining the cold chain when heat sensitive items are stored and transported in the reverse direction, i.e., upwards from the clinic to a depot or laboratory.
- ❖ This process is also used for transporting specimen samples, i.e., used for Carrying stool samples of Polio patients from Primary Health Centre (PHC) to lab.

8. Ans. (b) Thymus.

[*Ref.:* Ananthnarayan, 8th ed., page no.127]

- ❖ T cells are derived from thymus.
- ❖ B cells are derived from bone marrow.

9. Ans. (b)Negri bodies.

[*Ref.:* Ananthnarayan, 8th ed., page no. 530]

Demonstration of Negri body *(inclusion bodies) is* still the method most commonly used for the post mortem diagnosis of rabies.

Negri body

- Impression smears of the brain are stained by Seller's technique (basic fuchsin and methylene blue in methanol), which has the advantage that fixation and staining are done simultaneously.
- Negri bodies are seen as intra cytoplasmic; round or oval, purplish pink structures with characteristic basophilic inner granules.
- Negri bodies vary in size,3-27μ.
- Other types of inclusion bodies sometimes may be seen in the brain in diseases such as canine distemper but the presence of inner structures in the Negri bodies makes differentiation easy.
- Most common site for Negri body – Hippocampus (next-cerebellum).
- Negri body may be absent in 20% cases.
- So, failure to find Negri bodies does not exclude the diagnosis of rabies.

10. Ans. (c) Pregnant women

[*Ref.:* Ananthnarayan, 8th ed., page no. 546]

- A unique feature of Hepatitis E infection is the clinical severity and high case fatality rate of 20-40 per cent in pregnant women, especially in the last trimester of pregnancy.

Hepatitis E:

- Belongs to Caliciviruses.
- Spherical non enveloped virus.
- Single-stranded RNA genome.
- *Causes enterically transmitted non A non B hepatitis.*
- Incubation period ranges 2 to 9 weeks.
- Affect-Young to middle aged adults (15-40 years old).
- Faeco-oral transmission.
- No carriers seen.
- ***More severe in pregnancy.***
- In India, HEV is responsible for the. Majority of epidemic and sporadic hepatitis in adults.
- Diagnosed by:
  - IgM antibody detection
  - Electron microscopy of stool
  - Viral RNA detection.

11. Ans. (c) Scrub typhus

[*Ref.:* Ananthnarayan, 8th ed., page no. 406]

- Epidemic typhus – transmitted by Louse.
- Trench fever – transmitted by Louse.
- Scrub typhus – transmitted by trombiculid mite.
- Endemic typhus – transmitted by rat flea.

12. Ans. (c) Resistance to isoniazid & rifampicin and any three classes of second line anti-tubercular agents

[*Ref.:* Park, 21st ed., page no. 178-79]

Drug Resistance in Tuberculosis:

MDRTB: (Multi drug resistance **Tuberculosis**) – Resistant to INH and Rifampicin +/ Resistant to other 1st line drug like Ethambutol, Streptomycin and Pyrazinamide.

XDRTB: (Extended drug resistance **Tuberculosis**) – MDRTB + Resistant to quinolone + Resistant to aminoglycoside (amikacin/capreomycin/ kanamycin).

13. Ans. (b)Pneumocystis carinii

[*Ref.:* Ananthnarayan, 8th ed., page no. 574]

- Pneumocystis pneumonia (PCP) or pneumocystosis is a form of pneumonia, caused by the yeast-like fungus (which had previously been wrongly classified as a protozoan) Pneumocystis jirovecii.
- Pneumocystis is commonly found in the lungs of healthy people, but, being a source of opportunistic infection, it can cause a lung infection in people with a weak immune system.
- Pneumocystis pneumonia is especially seen in people with cancer, HIV/AIDS especially when *CD4 T cell count falls below 200/cmm.*

14. Ans. (d) Cross reacting antigens

[*Ref.:* Ananthnarayan, 8th ed., page no. 210]

- Pathogenesis of rheumatic fever is due to immunological injury caused due to the cross reacting streptococcal antigens cross reacts with mammalian antigen.

Structural components of Strept pyogenes cross reacts with human tissue:

Strept pyogenes	Human tissue	Disease
Capsular hyaluronic acid	Synovial fluid	Reactive arthritis
Cell wall protein **M**	**M**yocardium	**ARF**
Cell wall **c**arbohydrate	**C**ardiac valves	ARF
Cytoplasmic membrane	Vascular intima	AGN

- Due to antigenic cross reactivity, antibody produced against Streptococcal antigens, cross reacts with human tissue to produces lesions. This accounts for non-suppurative complications (like acute rheumatic fever and glomerulonephritis).

15. Ans. (c) Apical region

[*Ref.:* Ananthnarayan, 8th ed., page no.351]

Primary Pulmonary tuberculosis	Post primary Pulmonary tuberculosis
Occurs due to 1st time exposure to Tb bacilli	Due to endogenous reactivation or exogenous reinfection
Affect children,	Affect Adult,

FMGE MARCH 2012

Affects the Lower lobe of lungs or Lower part of the upper lobe. (Ghon focus)	Upper lobe focus (Simons focus)- Apical region
Ghon focus + hilar lymphadenopathy = k/a Primary complex	LN spread rare
Necrosis, cavitations never seen	Necrosis, cavitations seen
Ghon focus + associated fibrosis and calcification- k/a Ranke complex	Infra clavicular lesion- k/a *Assman focus*

16. Ans. (b)Streptococcus pneumoniae

[*Ref.:* Ananthnarayan, 8th ed., page no.222]

- Meningitis is the most serious complication of pneumococcal infections.
- It is usually secondary to other pneumococcal infections like pneumonia, otitis media, sinusitis or conjunctivitis

Pathogenicity of Peumococcus

- Can be commensal in nasopharynx and throat
- Most common cause of lobar pneumonia.
- *Most virulent type-3(also produces mucoid colonies).*
- In adults, types 1-8 are responsible for about 75 per cent of cases of pneumococcal pneumonia.
- In children, types 6, 14, 19 and 23 are frequent causes.
- Bronchopneumonia is almost always a secondary infection.
- This may be caused by any serotype of Pneumococcus.
- Associated with acute exacerbations in chronic bronchitis.
- Most common cause of pyogenic meningitis.
- Also causes
    - Otitis media
    - Sinusitis
    - Conjunctivitis
    - Bacterial peritonitis.

17. Ans. (b) Kaposi sarcoma

[*Ref.:* Ananthnarayan, 8th ed., page no. 477]

- In 1994, a new herpes virus was identified from tissues of Kaposi's sarcoma from AIDS patients. This has been named ***Human Herpes Virus (HHV) 8.***
- This has subsequently been identified also in Kaposi's sarcoma in persons not infected with HIV:
- It has been therefore referred to sometimes as *Kaposi's sarcoma-associated herpes virus* (KSHV), but a causative relationship is yet to be proved.

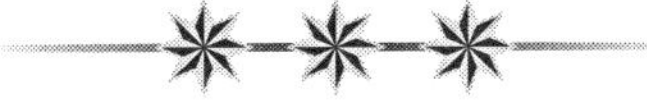

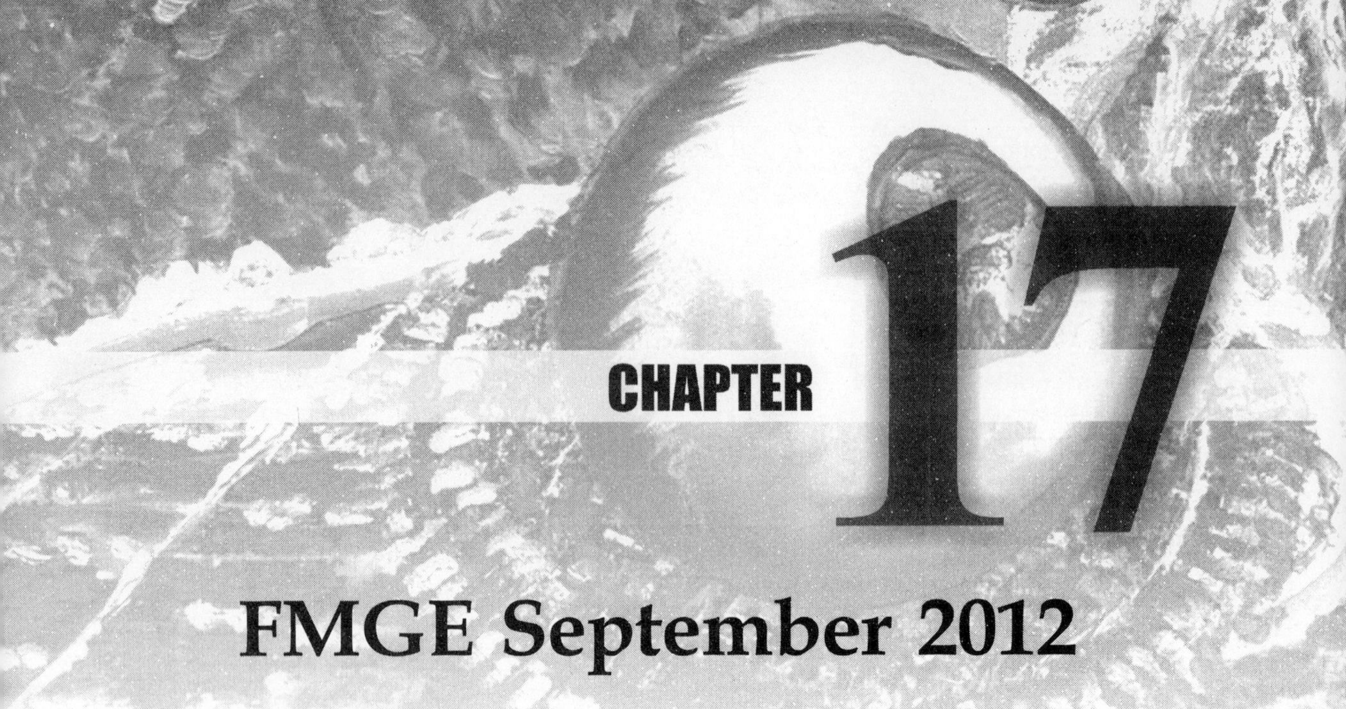

FMGE September 2012

General Microbiology

1. **Phenol coefficient indicates:** *[FMGE, March 2011]*
   (a) Efficiency of a disinfectant (b) Dilution of a disinfectant
   (c) Quantity of a disinfectant (d) Purity of a disinfectant.

Immunology

2. **Which of the following is an example of Type II hypersensitivity reaction?**
   (a) Good Pasteur syndrome (b) SLE
   (c) Arthus reaction.
3. **Delayed type hypersensitivity is:**
   (a) NK cell mediated (b) T cell mediated
   (c) B cell mediated (d) All of the above.
4. **Which of the following Cytokines are released by T Helper 1 cells?**
   (a) IL2 (b) IL4
   (c) IL5 (d) IL6.
5. **All of the following are function of CD4 T cells except?**
   (a) Macrophage activation (b) NK cell activation
   (c) Induction of fever (d) CD8 T cell activation.
6. **Which of the following condition is associated with Antibody against acetyl choline receptor:**
   (a) Grave's disease (b) Myasthenia gravis

(a) Tuberculoid leprosy (b) Lepromatous leprosy
(c) Borderline leprosy (d) Indeterminate type leprosy.

8. Male presented with urethral discharge following exposure to a prostitute. Which of the following drug should be given?
(a) Penicillin (b) Tetracycline
(c) Azithromycin (d) Doxycycline.

9. Which of the following drug shou'd be given for the treatment of a male presented with painless indurated ulcer on glans and painless inguinal lymphadenopathy?
(a) Penicillin (b) Tetracycline
(c) Azithromycin (d) Doxycycline.

10. Which of the following condition is associated with neurosyphilis?
(a) Tabes dorsalis (b) Condyloma lata
(c) Condyloma acuminate
(d) Painless indurated ulcer on glans and painless inguinal lymphadenopathy.

11. Best diagnosis of Typhoid in 2nd week.
(a) Blood culture (b) Blood culture and widal test
(c) Widal test (d) Widal test and stool culture.

12. A hospitalized patient who is on longer courses of clindamycin suddenly developed mucus diarrhea without blood. Examination revealed presence of a membrane over the colon. What is the probable diagnosis?
(a) Antibiotic associated diarrhea (b) Cholera.

13. DOC of Trachoma?
(a) Azithromycin (b) Tetracycline
(c) Penicillin (d) Doxycycline.

14. Dead end host of syphilis?
(a) Pig (b) Monkey (c) Man.

15. Significant count of E. coli in mid stream urine: *[Repeat FMGE, March 2011]*
(a) 10^4/ml (b) 10^2/ml (c) 10^3/ml (d) 10^5/ml.

16. MC cause of acute pyogenic meningitis?
(a) Meningococcus (b) Haemophilus influenzae
(c) E. coli (d) Streptococcus pneumoniae.

17. Not a commensal of conjunctival sac:
(a) Chlamydia trachomatis (b) *Streptococcus* species
(c) Diphtheriodes (d) Coagulase negative *Staphylococcus.*

18. Bacterial vaginosis is associated with all except:
(a) Abundant doderline bacillus (b) pH > 4.5
(c) Clue cell (d) Offensive smell.

19. Patient with enteric fever shows all of the following except:
(a) Leucocytopenia (b) Rose spot
(c) Intense headache (d) Bradycardia.

Virology

20. EBV is associated with all except?

(a) Nasopharyngeal carcinoma (b) Duncan syndrome
(c) Hairy cell leucoplakia (d) Mononucleosis like syndrome.

21. Kaposi sarcoma is associated with all except?
(a) Human Herpes Virus 6 (b) Human Herpes Virus 7
(c) Human Herpes Virus 8 (d) Human Herpes Virus 5.

22. Chicken pox rash lasts for?
(a) 4 day before to 5 days after rash (b) 5 day before to 2 days after rash
(c) Till the scab heals (d) 2 day before to 5 days after rash.

23. All are true about the wound management of dog bite except?
(a) Debridement of the wound (b) Stitching of the wound
(c) Clean the wound with soap and water
(d) Inject Human Rabies Immunoglobulin locally.

24. Serotypes of HPV implicated for Cervix ca.
(a) 6,11 (b) 16, 18 (c) 1, 2, 3, 4 (d) 6, 16.

25. SSPE is associated with which of the following virus?
(a) Varicella (b) Mumps (c) Rubella (d) Measles.

26. True about Yellow fever all except:
(a) Not found in India
(b) 17 D Live attenuated vaccine is given as single dose subcutaneously
(c) Vaccination last for 10 years
(d) Person can travel after 4-5 days of vaccine.

27. Which of the following test for HIV is not done in a 2 yr old child?
(a) PCR (b) Culture
(c) ELISA (d) p24 antigen detection.

28. All are RNA viruses except:
(a) Poliovirus (b) Rabies (c) Adenovirus (d) Rotavirus.

Parasitology

29. A HIV positive patient is presented with profuse diarrhea. Cryptosporidiosis is suspected. Which stain do you prefer to use?
(a) Leishman stain (b) Acid fast stain (c) LPCB (d) Silver stain.

30. Treatment of choice of malaria relapse of P. vivax:
(a) Choloquine (b) Primaquine
(c) Quinine (d) Mefloquine.

31. Which of the following can cause visceral larva migrans?
(a) Toxocara (b) Necator
(c) Ancylostoma (d) Strongyloides.

ANSWER TO FMGE SEPTEMBER 2012

1. Ans. (a) Efficiency of a disinfectant

[*Ref.:* Ananthnarayan, 8th ed., page no. 38]

Testing the efficiency of disinfectant:

Phenol coefficient (Rideal Walker) test: Compare the performance of a phelonic disinfectant with that of phenol for the ability to kill *Salmonella Typhi*. The test, however, does not show the action of disinfectant in natural condition, in the presence of organic contaminants.

Chick Martin test: It is a modification of Rideal and Walker test, in which, disinfectants acts in the presence of organic contaminants (e.g., dried yeast, faeces, etc.) to simulate the natural conditions.

Capacity (Kelsey-Sykes) test: Measures the capacity of a disinfectant to retain its activity when repeatedly used in the presence of organic material.

In-use (Kelsey and Maurer) test: Determines whether the chosen disinfectant is effective inactual use in hospital practice.

2. Ans. (a) Good Pasteur syndrome

[*Ref.:* Ananthnarayan, 8th ed., page no. 166]

Goodpasture's syndrome:

- Also known as anti-glomerular basement antibody disease.
- It is a rare autoimmune disease in which antibodies attack the lungs and kidneys, leading to bleeding from the lungs and to kidney failure.
- First reported by the American Pathologist Ernest Goodpasture.
- Goodpasture's syndrome is a type II hypersensitivity reaction.
- The specific target of the immune attack is the GBM antigen, which is found in the lungs and kidneys. The antigen is a component of the non-collagenous 1 (NCl) domain of the alpha-3 chain of type IV collagen in the glomerular basement membrane. It is treated with immunosuppressant drugs such as corticosteroids and cyclophosphamide.
- **Other examples of Type II Hypersensitivity Reaction: Refer Text of chapter 2.**

3. Ans. (b) T cell mediated

[*Ref.:* Ananthnarayan, 8th ed., page no. 168-69]

Type IV delayed (cell-mediated) hypersensitivity:

- Mediated through cell mediated immunity (i.e., due to the activation of specifically sensitized T lymphocytes).
- It is called delayed type hypersensitivity (DTH), because the response is delayed.
- Sensitization phase of 1-2 weeks after primary contact with an antigen that is uptaken by a variety of antigen-presenting cells (APCs) including Langerhans cells and macrophages and presented to T helper cells. T helper cells are activated and differentiated to TH1 subtypes.
- Effector phase – stimulated on subsequent exposure. The TH1 cells are responsible in secreting a variety of cytokines that recruit and activate macrophages and other non-specific inflammatory cells. The response is marked only after 2-3 days of the second exposure.
- Formation of granuloma is the hallmark of this hypersensitivity reaction.

Types of DTH reactions

- *Contact hypersensitivity* – occurring after sensitization with certain substances like
  - Drug – sulphonamides and neomycin
  - Plant products such as poison ivy and poison oako
  - Chemicals such as formaldehyde and nickel.
- *Tuberculin* – type hypersensitivity reaction
  - *Lepromin test*
  - Positive skin tests in coccidiomycosis, paracoccidiomycosis and other fungal infections
  - Montenegro test for Leishmaniasis.

4. Ans. (a) IL2

[*Ref.:* Ananthnarayan, 8th ed., page no. 130]

TH1 – secrete IL2, IFN - γ and TGFβ

- IFN γ – Activate macrophage, stimulate B cell and class switch to IgG2b
- IL2 – T cell growth factor, activate DTH T cell, convert NK cell → LAK cell.

TH2 – secrete IL4, 5, 6, 10

- IL4 – Inhibit Th1, class switch to **IgE, IgG**
- IL5 – Class switch to **IgA**

5. Ans. (c) Induction of fever

[*Ref.:* Ananthnarayan, 8th ed., page no. 130-31]

Function of CD4 T cells:

- Activate macrophage
- Stimulate B cell and class switch to IgG2b
- Activate DTH T cell
- Autocrine effect – Activate T helper cell
- Activate Tc cell Activate NK cell → LAK cell.

6. Ans. (b) Myasthenia gravis

[*Ref.:* Ananthnarayan, 8th ed., page no. 174]

Myasthenia gravis

- An autoimmune neuromuscular disease leading to fluctuating muscle weakness and fatiguability.
- Weakness is caused by circulating antibodies that block acetylcholine receptors at the postsynaptic neuromuscular junction, inhibiting the excitatory effects of the neurotransmitter acetylcholine on nicotinic receptors throughout neuromuscular junctions.
- Myasthenia is treated medically with:
  - Acetylcholinesterase inhibitors
  - Immunosuppressants
  - In selected cases, thymectomy.

7. Ans. (a) Tuberculoid leprosy

[*Ref.:* Ananthnarayan, 8th ed., page no. 368]

This Mitsuda reaction is positive in tuberculoid leprosy. Negative lepromin test is observed in lepromatous leprosy.

Lepromin test:

- Used to study host immunity to *M. leprae*.
- First described by Mitsuda in 1919.
- **Test** – intradermal injection of lepromin antigen into the forearm.
- ***Early or Fernandez reaction***:
  - ***Seen*** after 48 hours of injection for induration.
  - Positive reaction suggests – patient has been infected by leprae bacilli in the past.
- ***Late or Mitsuda reaction*** is characterized by – nodule at the site of inoculation after 3-4 weeks of injection, undergo necrosis followed by ulceration.
- Lepromin test is a measure of CMI induced by injected Lepromin (does not say about the past exposure not used in diagnosis).

- ***Lepromin Test is Used:***
  - Classify lesions of leprosy
    - Negative lepromin test is observed in lepromatous leprosy
    - *This Mitsuda reaction is positive in tuberculoid leprosy*
  - Assess prognosis – Negative lepromin test suggests lack of resistance to the disease and bad prognosis.
  - Assess resistance to leprosy in individuals.

8. Ans. (c) Azithromycin

[*Ref.:* Harrison, 18th ed., page no. 1427-29; Ananthnarayan, 8th ed., page no. 418-19]

- This is a case of STD induced urethritis (Male presented with urethral discharge following exposure to a prostitute).
- *Chlamydia trachomatis* is the MC cause of Nongonococcal urethritis.
- Hence the treatment should be directed against *Chlamydia trachomatis*.
- DOC of *Chlamydia trachomatis* is Azithromycin.

Causes of non gonococcal urethritis (NGU):

- Chlamydia trachomatis (MC)
- Mycoplasma genitalium and hominis
- Ureoplasma urealyticum
- Herpes simplex
- Cytomegalovirus
- Trichomonas vaginalis
- Candida albicans.

9. Ans. (a) Penicillin

[*Ref.:* Ananthnarayan, 8th ed., page no. 377; Harrison, 18th ed., page no. 1108]

- This is a case of primary syphilis – male presented with painless indurated ulcer on glans and painless inguinal lymphadenopathy.
- DOC for primary syphilis – **Penicillin.**

	Syphilis	Herpes	Chancroid	LGV	Donovanosis
Ulcer	Painless, indurated single	Multiple painful, erythematous, vesicle	Painful non-indurated irregular	Painless	Painless
LN	Painless, indurated bilateral	Painful, indurated, bilateral	Painful, non-indurated, unilateral	Painful, non-indurated, unilateral	No
Incubation period	9-90 days	2-7 days	1-14 days	3 days–6 weeks	1-4 weeks (up to 6 months)

10. Ans. (a) Tabes dorsalis

[*Ref.:* Ananthnarayan, 8th ed., page no. 377]

Tabes dorsalis, general paralysis of insane are the other manifestations of neurosyphilis which occur several decades after the infection.

Stages of Syphilis

- ***Primary Syphilis:***
  - This condition occurs within 3 weeks of sexual contact with an infected host.
  - Characterized by hard/hunterian chancre (painless LN↑) + painless ulcer
  - MC site of chancre – genitalia > mouth, nipple.
- ***Secondary Syphilis:***
  - Secondary syphilis occurs 2-10 weeks after the primary chancre and is most florid 3-4 months after infection.
  - Characterized by:
    - Skin rashes
    - Condyloma lata at mc junction
    - Mucosal patches
  - Highly infectious
  - Serology – All antibody detection tests are 100% sensitive.
- ***Latent Syphilis:*** Diagnosis by serology only.
- ***Tertiary Syphilis:***
  - CVS – aneurysm + Aortic Regurgitation.
  - Gummata – typical pathological lesion found on the skin, in the mouth and in the upper respiratory tract. Gummatous lesions may be multiple or diffuse, but are usually single lesions which measure between 1 cm to several centimeters in diameter. This tertiary lesion contains few spirochetes and represents manifestations of delayed hypersensitivity.
  - CNS – Tabes dorsalis, general paralysis of insane.
- ***Non-venereal Syphilis:***
  - Blood transfusion – primary stage is absent or lesions are extra genital.
  - Congenital syphilis.

11. Ans. (b) Blood culture and widal test

[*Ref.:* Ananthnarayan, 8th ed., page no. 295; Harrioson, 18th ed., page no. 1279]

Though widal test is the investigation of choice in second week of typhoid fever but a combination of blood culture and widal test will be more sensitive than doing widal test alone.

Week wise diagnosis of choice:

- 1st week:
  - Gold standard – Duodenal content culture > BM culture > blood culture
  - Best – combination of all three methods
  - Blood culture sensitivity – 90% in 1st week, 75% in 2nd week, 60% in 3rd week
  - Clot culture – higher sensitive than blood culture.
- End of 1st week – widal test starts positive.
- 2nd and 3rd week – widal test should be done.
- 4th week – stool and urine culture can be positive.
- Stool culture – +ve in both case/carrier, +ve even if after antibiotic start.

12. Ans. (a) Antibiotic associated diarrhea

[*Ref.:* Ananthnarayan, 8th ed., page no. 263, Harrison, 18th ed., page no.1191]

This is a case of antibiotic-associated diarrhea caused by Cl. difficile.

Antibiotic-associated diarrhea:

- Normal flora of the gastrointestinal tract resists colonization and overgrowth with *Cl. difficile.*
- Broad spectrum Antibiotic therapy like clindamycin is the key factor that alters the normal bacterial flora of the intestine.
- The use of antibiotics suppresses the normal flora of the intestine, facilitates colonization and multiplication of *Cl. difficile* and production of toxins that cause inflammation of the mucosa and damage.
- *Cl. difficile* produce two antigenically distinct toxins: toxin A and toxin B. Toxin A is an enterotoxin and toxin B is a cytotoxin. Both the toxin A and toxin B contribute to pathogenesis of Cl. difficile colitis and diarrhoea in humans.
- *C. difficile* causes as malaise, anorexia, mild-to-moderate diarrhea, occasionally with abdominal cramping.
- Diarrhea develops in most patients during or shortly after starting antibiotics. However, in 25-40% of patients. It is associated with formation of pseudomembranes, and occasionally adherent yellowish-white plaques on the intestinal mucosa.
- The condition in rare cases present with an acute abdomen and fulminant life-threatening colitis.
- *Cl. difficile* colitis is currently one of the most common nosocomial infections. Approximately, 20% of individuals who are hospitalized acquire *C. difficile* during hospitalization and of these, more than 30% patients develop diarrhea.

13. Ans. (a) Azithromycin

[*Ref.:* Harrison, 18th ed., page no. 1429]

- **Treatment of Trachoma:**
  - Azithromycin (a 1-g single oral dose) or doxycycline (100 mg twice daily for 7 days).
  - Simultaneous treatment of all sexual partners is necessary to prevent ocular reinfection and chlamydial genital disease.
  - Topical antibiotic treatment is not required for patients who receive systemic antibiotics.

14. Ans. (c) Man

[*Ref.:* Ananthnarayan, 8th ed., page no. 376-79]

Humans are the only host for syphilis and act as a dead end host for Lyme's disease.

15. Ans. (d) 10^5/ml

[*Ref.:* Ananthnarayan, 8th ed., page no. 275]

Kass' concept of significant Bacteriuria

- Significant bacteriuria concept is based on the fact that a colony count of bacteria exceeding 100,000 (10^5) bacterial per ml of urine denotes significant bacteriuria and is suggestive of active UTI.
- Counts of 10,000 bacteria or less per ml are of no significance and is due to contamination of urine during voiding.
- Bacterial counts between 10,000 (10^3) and 100,000 (10^5) are infrequent when the sample is collected properly and processed promptly. Such results are considered equivocal and the culture is repeated.
- Significant bacteria is applicable only to *E. coli* and other Gram negative bacteria and for mid-stream urine.

- It is not applicable:
  - When urine is collected directly from urinary bladder by cystoscopy.
  - For Gram positive bacteria such as *S. aureus,* any counts is significant.
  - If antibiotic already started.
- Interpretation of bacteriuria, however, requires caution and should always be with reference to clinical condition of the patient.

16. Ans. (d) Streptococcus pneumoniae

[*Ref.:* Harrison, 18th ed., page no. 3410-11]

S. pneumoniae is the most common cause of meningitis in adults >20 years of age, accounting for nearly half the reported cases (1.1 per 100,000 persons per year).

Age	Common causes
Neonates or Infants of 0-2 months	Group B streptococcus (S. agalactiae) Escherichia coli Other Gram negative bacilli (like Klebsiella pneumoniae) Listeria monocytogenes
2-20 years	Neisseria meningitides Haemophilus influenzae Streptococcus pneumoniae
> 20 years (adults)	Streptococcus pneumoniae (MC) Haemophilus influenzae Neisseria meningitides
Overall	Streptococcus pneumoniae (MC)

17. Ans. (a) Chlamydia trachomatis

[*Ref.:* Ananthnarayan, 8th ed., page no. 419]

Chlamydia trachomatis is an ocular pathogen, can cause inclusion conjunctivitis and swimming pool conjunctivitis.

18. Ans. (a) Abundant doderline bacillus

[*Ref.:* Harrison, 18th ed., page no. 1101; Ananthnarayan, 8th ed., page no. 401]

Bacterial Vaginosis is characterized by an absence of hydrogen peroxide–producing Lactobacillus spp. **(doderline bacillus),** that constitute most of the normal vaginal microbiota and help protect against certain cervical and vaginal infections.

Bacterial vaginosis (nonspecific anaerobic vaginitis) is characterized by:

- **Agent:**
  - *G. vaginalis*
  - *Mycoplasma hominis*
  - Several anaerobic bacteria (*Mobiluncus*, *Prevotella* and *Peptostreptococcus* species)
  - Absence of hydrogen peroxide–producing *Lactobacillus* spp., that constitute most of the normal vaginal microbiota and help protect against certain cervical and vaginal infections.
- **Diagnosis:** Diagnosed clinically with the ***Amsel criteria*** that include any three of the following four clinical abnormalities:

- Increased white homogeneous vaginal discharge.
- Vaginal discharge pH of >4.5.
- Distinct fishy odor (due to volatile amines detected by whiff test with 10% KOH).
- Microscopic demonstration of "clue cells" (vaginal epithelial cells coated with coccobacillary organisms).

❖ **Treatment:** Oral metronidazole 500 mg twice daily for 7 days.

19. Ans. (a) Leucocytopenia

[*Ref.:* Ananthnarayan, 8th ed., page no. 293; Harrison, 18th ed., page no. 1275-76]

❖ Leukocytosis is more common among children, during the first 10 days of illness and in cases complicated by intestinal perforation or secondary infection.

❖ However, in 15-25% of cases, leukopenia and neutropenia are detectable.

Clinical feature of Enteric fever

❖ The incubation period – ranges from 3-21 days.

❖ Fever is documented at presentation in >75% of cases.

❖ Abdominal pain (30-40%).

❖ Intense headache (80%).

❖ Relative bradycardia at the peak of high fever (50%).

❖ Other features – chills, cough, sweating, arthralgia, coated tongue, splenomegaly.

❖ Gastrointestinal symptoms included anorexia abdominal pain nausea, vomiting and diarrhea more commonly than constipation.

❖ S. paratyphi A – milder disease than S. typhi, with predominantly gastrointestinal symptoms.

20. Ans. (d) Mononucleosis like syndrome

[*Ref.:* Ananthnarayan, 8th ed., page no. 474-75]

Mononucleosis like syndrome:

❖ Caused by CMV in adult.

❖ Following blood transfusion.

❖ Atypical lymphocytosis seen.

❖ Paul bunnel test (heterophile antibody) is negative.

Infectious Mononucleosis:

❖ Caused by EBV in young adolescence.

❖ Atypical lymphocytosis seen.

❖ Paul bunnel test (heterophile antibody) positive.

Disease associated with EBV:

❖ Hodgkin lymphoma.

❖ Burkit lymphoma.

❖ Nasopharyngeal Ca– Risk factor– genetic, salted fish (nitrosamine), herbal snuff (phorbolester).

❖ Duncan syndrome– X linked lymphoproliferative disorder.

❖ Infectious mononucleosis.

21. Ans. (c) Human Herpes Virus 8

[*Ref.:* Ananthnarayan, 8th ed., page no. 477]

- In 1994, a new herpesvirus was identified from tissues of Kaposi's sarcoma from AIDS patients.
- This has been named as HHV 8.
- This has subsequently been identified also in Kaposi's sarcoma in persons not infected with HIV.
- HHV-8 has been therefore referred to sometimes as *Kaposi's sarcoma-associated herpesvirus* (KSHV), but an causative relationship is yet to be proved.

22. Ans. (d) 2 day before to 5 days after rash

[*Ref.:* Ananthnarayan, 8th ed., page no. 472]

Described earlier, refer Chapter No. 9

23. Ans. (b) Stitching of the wound

[*Ref.:* Ananthnarayan, 8th ed., page no. 530]

Post: Exposure prophylaxis

(a) Local treatment:
- Prompt cleaning of the wound.
- The wound is immediately scrubbed with soap and water.
- Followed by treatment with antiseptics.
- Bite wounds are not sutured immediately.

(b) Confirmation whether or not the animal is rabid (for 10 days).

(c) Administration of human rabies immune globulin (HRIG):

The recommended dose of HRIG is 20 IU/kg body weight 50% of the dose is given into the wound and 50% intramuscularly.

(d) Antirabies vaccine (ARV).

24. Ans. (b) 16, 18

[*Ref.:* Ananthnarayan, 8th ed., page no. 549]

Human Papillomavirus can cause

- Ca cervix:
  - Low risk – type 6,11 -- causes CIN (cervical intraepithelial neoplasia).
  - High risk – HPV 16 and less frequently, HPV 18, HPV 33, HPV 35 – causes Ca Cx.
- Benign tumours of head and neck– oral papilloma, laryngeal papilloma and conjunctival papilloma by HPV 6,11.
- Condyloma acuminata/genital wart – by Type 6,11.
- Common wart/verruca vulgaris – by HPV 2, HPV 4 and HPV 7.
- Epidermodysplasia verrucoplasia.

25. Ans. (d) Measles

[*Ref.:* Ananthnarayan, 8th ed., page no. 510]

Subacute sclerosing panencephalitis (SSPE) *are the rare complication of measles* occurs in about 7 in every 1 million patients.

SSPE

- The SSPE is a degenerating disease of the central nervous system caused by persistent measles infection.

- The disease is characterized by the development of behavioural and intellectual deterioration and seizures after many years (mean incubation period is 10.8 years) of infection by measles.
- This is a serious and late neurological sequelae of measles that affect the central nervous system.
- The condition occurs most commonly in children who were initially affected when they were below 2 years old.
- **Diagnosis:** High measles antibody titre in the blood and CSF.

26. Ans. (d) Person can travel after 4-5 days of vaccine

[*Ref.:* Ananthnarayan, 8th ed., page no. 518]

17D Live attenuated yellow fever vaccine is given single dose given sc. It is 95% effective within 10 days of inoculation. Hence the certificate for yellow fever is given after 10 days and the people can travel after 10 days of vaccine.

17D Live attenuated vaccine:

- Prepared in India (CRI, Kasuli)
- Chick embryo, no risk of encephalitis
- Single dose given sc
- 95% effective within 10 days of inoculation
- Reimmunization required every 10 years for travelers
- Cholera and YF vaccine should not be given together.

27. Ans. (c) ELISA

[*Ref.:* NACO guideline]

- Maternal antibodies persist in the baby till 18 months. Hence the antibody detection methods like ELISA or westerblot should not be done in children to diagnose neonatal HIV as they cannot differentiate the true infection with maternal transfer.
- **Diagnosis of Pediatric HIV:**
  - HIV DNA – Most recommended
  - Viral isolation
  - p24 antigen detection
  - IgG ELISA after 18 months only.

28. Ans. (c) Adenovirus

[*Ref.:* Ananthnarayan, 8th ed., page no. 439]

Adenovirus is a DNA virus

List of DNA viruses:

- Pox virus – Variola, Vaccinia, Cowpox, Monkey pox, Molluscum contagiosum
- Papova virus – HPV, Polyoma, BK, JC viruses, SV-40 virus
- Parvo virus
- Herpes virus – HSV, CMV, EBV
- Hepatitis B virus
- Adeno virus
- Bacteriophage.

29. Ans. (b) Acid fast stain

[*Ref.:* Parija's, Textbook of Parasitology, 3rd ed., page no. 163]

- **Modified Acid fast staining for Cryptosporidiosis:**
  - The oocysts of *C. parvum* are acid fast to 1% sulfuric acid or acid alcohol.
  - Appear as round, 4-6 μm red colour oocyst against blue back ground.
  - The sensitivity of acid fast staining is low.
  - It requires an oocyst concentration of greater than 500,00/μL in stool.
- **Commonly used modified acid fast staining methods are:**
  - Kinyoun's method (cold acid fast staining)
  - Rapid safranin methylene blue method
  - Carbol fuchin negative staining

Property	Cryptosporidium
Size	4-6 μ size
Shape	Round
Cyst contains	4 sporozoites
Acid fast	Uniformly acid fast
Autoflouroscence	No, but can be stained with fluorescent dye
Treatment	Co-trimoxazole

30. Ans. (b) Primaquine

[*Ref.:* Park, 21st ed., page no. 239]

Relapse rate of vivax malaria is 30% in India. To prevent this, Primaquine is given as 0.25 mg/kg daily for 14 days.

Treatment for malaria:

- Treatment of choice of P. vivax malaria – *Chlroquine*
- Treatment of choice of relapse of P. vivax malaria – *Primaquine*
- Treatment of choice of drug resistant of P. falciparum malaria – *Artemisinin combination therapy* (ACT) is given.
- Artemisinin combination therapy consists of a combination of artemisinin derivative (Artemisinin or artemether or arte-ether) and a long acting antimalarial drug like mefloquine, lumifantrine or sulfadoxine-pyrimethamine.
- In pregnancy – quinine is recommended in first trimester where as Artemisinin combination therapy (ACT) is given in second and third trimester.
- Treatment of mixed infection with P. falciparum – should be treated as falciparum malaria plus primaquine is given for radical cure.

31. Ans. (a) Toxocara

[*Ref.:* Parija's, Textbook of Parasitology, 3rd ed., page no. 323]

Larva migrans

Agents causing Visceral larva migrans	Agents causing Cutaneous larva migrans
Angiostrongylus cantonensis	Ancylostoma braziliensis
Angiostrongylus costaricensis	Ancylostoma caninum
Toxocara canis	Strongyloides stercoralis (Larva currens)
Toxocara catis	Necator americanus
Aisakine spp.	Acylostoma duodenale
Gnathostoma spinigerum	Gnathostoma spinigerum

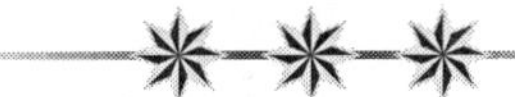

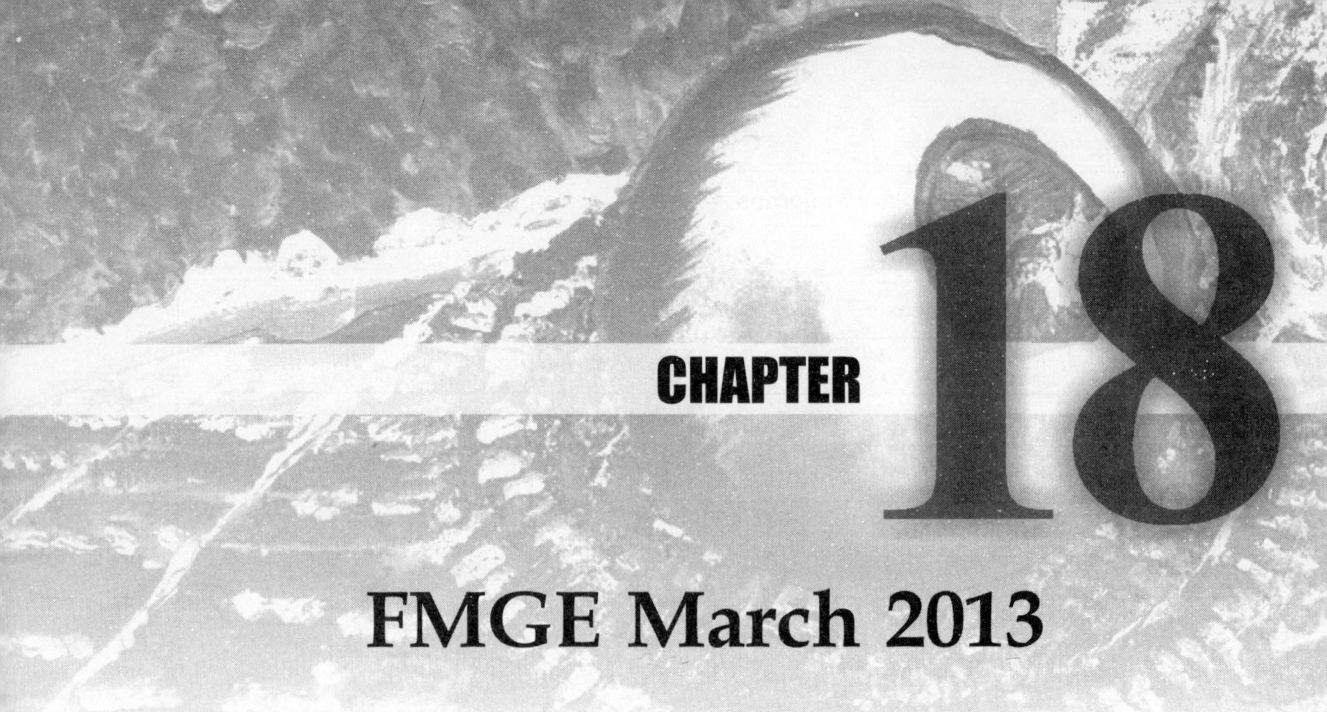

CHAPTER 18

FMGE March 2013

Immunology

1. **Delayed hypersensitivity can be passively transferred by:**
   (a) Immunoglobulins (b) Interferon
   (c) T-cells (d) Tumor necrosis factor.
2. **The central component of complement system is:**
   (a) C2 (b) C3
   (c) C4 (d) C5.
3. **The antibody produced in largest amount at the Peyer's patches is:**
   (a) IgA (b) IgE
   (c) IgM (d) IgG.

Bacteriology

4. **Ascoli's thermoprecipitation test helps in confirming the laboratory diagnosis of:**
   (a) Anthrax (b) Tetanus
   (c) Gas gangrene (d) Bartonella.
5. **Weil's disease is caused by:**
   (a) Treponema (b) Leptospira icterohemorrhagica
   (c) Borrelia recurrentis.
6. **TRIC agent includes which one of the following:**
   (a) Chlamydia trachomatis A to K (b) Chlamydia lymphogranulomatis

(c) Chlamydia psittacosis (d) All of the above.

7. **Drug resistance in mycobacterium tuberculosis is due to:**
   (a) Conjugation (b) Transduction
   (c) Mutation (d) None of the above.

8. **The specific micro-organism suspected to cause food poisoning on the basis of short incubation period (6-8 hours) are all of the following, except:**
   (a) Staphylococcus aureus (b) B. cereus
   (c) E. coli (d) C. botulinum.

9. **Which of the following diseases does not have carriers?**
   (a) Amoebiasis (b) Tetanus
   (c) Diphtheria (d) HBV.

10. **Direct demonstration of spirochaetes may be done by all of the following, except:**
   (a) Dark field microscopy (b) Gram's stain
   (c) Fontana's stain (d) Levaditi's stain.

11. **Venkataraman-Ramakrishnan medium is a transport medium employed for the isolation of:**
   (a) Vibrio cholerae (b) Campylobacter jejuni
   (c) Helicobacter pylori (d) Yersinia enterocolitica.

12. **Rapid urease test performed at the bedside dependable test for the detection of which one of following:**
   (a) Proteus mirabilis (b) Helicobacter pylori
   (c) Stenotrophomonas maltophilia (d) Moraxella lacunata.

13. **Infection with pseudomonas organisms is frequently associated with which of the following:**
   (a) Pneumonia gangrenosum (b) Pyoderma gangrenosum
   (c) Ecthyma gangrenosum and an invasive form of otitis externa.

14. **Most immunogenic antigen in salmonella typhi is:**
   (a) O antigen (b) Vi antigen
   (c) H antigen (d) M antigen.

15. **Chlamydia can survive within the phagocyte because they:**
   (a) Inhibit fusion of phagosome and lysosome
   (b) Resist lysosomal enzymes
   (c) Prevent degranulation (d) Escape from phagosome.

16. **Most common cause of lower respiratory infection is which one of the following:**
   (a) Viruses (b) Streptococcus pneumoniae
   (c) Mycoplasma (d) H. Influenza B.

Virology

17. **Common cold is caused most often by:**
   (a) Adenovirus (b) Influenza virus
   (c) Respiratory syncytial virus (d) Rhinovirus.

18. A tzanck smear of a scraping obtained from a vesicle on the skin shows multinucleate giant cells. This is typical of:

(a) Herpes simplex virus-2 (b) Hepatitis B virus
(c) Coxsackie virus (d) Molluscum contagiosum.

19. Paul bunnell test is used in the diagnosis of:

(a) Chicken pox (b) Genital herpes
(c) Infectious mononucleosis (d) Acute gingivostomatitis.

20. Virus used in preparation of antirabies vaccine is:

(a) Street virus (b) Wild virus
(c) Fixed virus (d) Live attenuated virus.

21. All of the following viruses are transmitted congenitally, except:

(a) Adenovirus (b) Herpes simplex virus
(c) Hepatitis B virus (d) Cytomegalovirus.

22. Diseases that spread by feco-oral route are all of the following, except:

(a) Poliomyelitis (b) Salmonellosis
(c) Cholera (d) Hepatitis-B.

Mycology

23. Which site of body is most affected by aspergillosis?

(a) CNS (b) Skin
(c) Bone and joints (d) Lungs.

24. All of the following are dimorphic fungi, except:

(a) Paracoccidiodes brasilensis (b) Cryptococcus neoformans
(c) Histoplasma capsulatum (d) Blastomyces dermatidis.

Parasitology

25. Which one of the following parasites can cause anemia?

(a) Enterobius vermicularis (b) Hymenolepis nana
(c) Taenia saginata (d) Ankylostoma duodenale.

26. Crescent shaped intra erythrocytic gametocytes identify infection caused by:

(a) P. vivax (b) P. falciparum
(c) P. ovale (d) P. malariae.

27. Most human infections by babesia follow bite by:

(a) Mites (b) Lice
(c) Ticks (d) Mango flies.

28. Sabin-Feldman dye test is employed in the diagnosis of which one of the following?

(a) Kala-azar (b) Toxoplasmosis
(c) Onchocerciasis (d) Cerebral malaria.

29. The promastigote form of leishmania donovani is seen in:

(a) Bone marrow aspirates (b) Splenic puncture aspirates
(c) Lymph node aspirates (d) Culture in NNN medium.

ANSWERS TO FMGE MARCH 2013

1. Ans. (c) T-cells

[*Ref.:* Ananthnarayan, 8th ed., page no. 162, 168]

- Delayed hypersensitivity (Type IV) can be passively transferred by Transfer factor (T cells).
- Immediate hypersensitivity (Type I, II, III) can be passively transferred by Serum therapy (Antibodies).

2. Ans. (b) C3

[*Ref.:* Ananthnarayan, 8th ed., page no. 118]

- C3 is the central component of all complement pathways.
- All the three complement pathways (classical, alternate and lectin pathways) differ from each other in the process of formation of C3.
- Once C3 is formed, the remaining pathway is common to all.

3. Ans. (a) IgA

[*Ref.:* Ananthnarayan, 8th ed., page no. 99]

- GIT mucosal secretions (e.g., at the Peyer's patches) are rich in secretory type of IgA antibodies.

4. Ans. (a) Anthrax

[*Ref.:* Ananthnarayan, 8th ed., page no. 244]

- Ascoli's thermoprecipitation test is done for – Anthrax.
- Elek's gel precipitation test is done for – toxigenicity testing for diphtheria.

5. Ans. (b) Leptospira icterohemorrhagica

[*Ref.:* Ananthnarayan, 8th ed., page no. 383]

- Weil's disease or hepatorenal hemorrhagic syndrome is caused by Leptospira icterohemorrhagica, transmitted by exposure to rodents.

6. Ans. (a) Chlamydia trachomatis A to K

[*Ref.:* Ananthnarayan, 8th ed., page no. 417]

Chlamydia trachomatis has two biovars:

- ***TRIC biovar agent includes:*** Trachoma serotypes (A, B, Ba, C) and inclusion conjunctivitis serotypes (D to K).
- ***LGV biovar includes:*** Serotype causing LGV, i.e., L1, L2, L3.

7. Ans. (c) Mutation

[*Ref.:* Ananthnarayan, 8th ed., page no. 358]

Drug resistance in Mycobacterium is due to to mutation.

Drug Resistance – Genes involved:

- INH – Kat G gene, Inh A gene, ahpC
- R – rpoB gene (RNA polymerase B)
- Z – Pnc A (Pyrazinamidase)
- E – Emb A, B, C (Arabinosyl transferase)
- S – Ribosomal protein subunit 12 (rpSL).

MRDTB	Resistant to INH and Rifampicin +/ Resistant to other 1st line drug 3.7% of new cases are MDRTB Level higher in previously treated cases (20%) 60% of total MDRTB resides in BRICS countries – Brazil, Russia, India, China, South Africa.
XDRTB	MDRTB + Resistant to quinolone + Resistant to aminoglycoside (amikacin/capreomycin/kanamycin) 9% of MDR TB are XDR TB.

8. Ans. (c) E. coli

[*Ref.:* Ananthnarayan, 8th ed., page no. 198]

Agents causing food poisoning with short incubation period (6-8 hours).

- Staphylococcus aureus
- B. cereus
- Clostridium botulinum.

9. Ans. (b) Tetanus

[*Ref.:* Ananthnarayan, 8th ed., page no. 258-59]

- Clostridium tetani is non-invasive, no man to man transmission, there is no carrier.

10. Ans. (b) Gram's stain

[*Ref.:* Ananthnarayan, 8th ed., page no. 371]

- Spirochetes are spirally coiled and hair like extremely thin.
- They are so thin that, they cannot be visualized by gram stain under light microscope.
- They are visualized by *dark field, fluorescent microscope or sliver staining methods (to increase the thickness) such as Levaditi stain and Fontana stain.*

11. Ans. (a) Vibrio cholerae

[*Ref.:* Ananthnarayan, 8th ed., page no. 303]

- Transport medium for Vibrio cholera – VR (Venkataraman-Ramakrishnan) medium, Carry Blair media and autoclaved sea water.

12. Ans. (b) Helicobacter pylori

[*Ref.:* Ananthnarayan, 8th ed., page no. 400]

- Rapid urease test (urea breath test) is a non-invasive method done for H. pylori.
- Biopsy urease test is – invasive method done for H. pylori.

13. Ans. (c) Ecthyma gangrenosum and an invasive form of otitis externa

[*Ref.:* Ananthnarayan, 8th ed., page no. 316]

- Pseudomonas causes – Ecthyma gangrenosum and malignant otitis externa.

14. Ans. (c) H antigen

[*Ref.:* Ananthnarayan, 8th ed., page no. 289]

H and O antigens of Salmonella typhi:

- ***H antigen → Flagellar antigen***
  - Heat labile, alcohol labile
  - Formaldehyde stable
  - Stronger immunogenic
  - H antibody appears late, goes late
  - Reacts to H antibody – forms large loosed fluffy clumps.

- *O Ag → Somatic polysaccharide*
    - Heat stable
    - Formaldehyde labile
    - Less immunogenic
    - O antibody appears early, goes early – indicates recent infection
    - Reacts to O antibody – forms granular chalky clumps.

15. Ans. (a) Inhibit fusion of phagosome and lysosome

[*Ref.:* Ananthnarayan, 8th ed., page no. 416]

- Chlamydia can survive within the phagocyte by inhibit fusion of phagosome and lysosome.

16. Ans. (b) Streptococcus pneumoniae

[*Ref.:* Ananthnarayan, 8th ed., page no. 221]

- *Streptococcus pneumoniae* is the most common cause of lower respiratory infection such as pneumonia.

17. Ans. (d) Rhinovirus

[*Ref.:* Ananthnarayan, 8th ed., page no. 491]

- Respiratory syncytial virus – Most common cause of brochiolitis in infants, coryza.
- Rhinovirus – Most common cause of common cold.
- Parainfluenza – Most common casue of croup (acute laryngo-tracheo-bronchioltis).

18. Ans. (a) Herpes Simplex virus-2

[*Ref.:* Ananthnarayan, 8th ed., page no. 38]

- Histroy of Tzanck smear of a scraping obtained from a vesicle on the skin shows multinucleate giant cells is suggestive of ...... Herpses simplex infection.

19. Ans. (c) Infectious mononucleosis

[Ref.: Ananthnarayan, 8th ed., page no. 38]

Paul Bunnell test is a heterophile agglutination test used as a screening test for the diagnosis of infectious mononucleosis and if found positive then it should be a confirmed by differential absorption test.

20. Ans. (c) Fixed Virus

[*Ref.:* Ananthnarayan, 8th ed., page no. 38]

- Street virus or Wild virus causes rabies naturally in man or animal.
- Fixed virus are prepared by serial subculture of wild virus and these can be used for vaccine preparation.

21. Ans. (a) Adenovirus

[*Ref.:* Ananthnarayan, 8th ed., page no. 38]

- Viruses are transmitted congenitally and are teratogenic – Herpes, Varicella, Rubella, CMV, Parvovirus
- Viruses transfer through placenta but not teratogenic – Coxsackie B, Hepatitis B, C, HIV, Measles, Mumps.

22. Ans. (d) Hepatitis-B

[*Ref.:* Ananthnarayan, 8th ed., page no. 38]

- Hepatitis-B is transmitted by blood and blood products, sexual mode and vertical mode.

23. Ans. (d) Lungs

[*Ref.:* Ananthnarayan, 8th ed., page no. 38]

- Pulmonary aspergillosis is the most common form of infection due to aspergillus and manifested as – bronchial asthma, ABPA, invasive aspergillosis and aspergilloma.

24. Ans. (b) Cryptococcus neoformans

[*Ref.:* Ananthnarayan, 8th ed., page no. 38]

Dimorphic fungi – Exist as mycelial forms at 25°C and as yeast forms at 37°C.

- Histoplasma capsulatum
- Blastomyces dermatitidis
- Coccidioides immitis
- Paracoccidioides brasiliensis
- Penicillium marneffi
- Sporothrix schenckii.

25. Ans. (d) Ankylostoma duodenale

[*Ref.:* Paniker's Parasitology, 7th ed., page no. 186]

Parasites Causing Anemia

- ***Hookworm:*** Iron deficiency anemia (thrives on Plasma) – Necator – 0.03 ml/day, Acylostoma-0.2 ml/day.
- ***Babesia:*** Hemolytic anemia.
- ***Plasmodium spp.:*** Autoimmune hemolytic anemia.
- ***Trichuris trichiura:*** Iron deficiency anemia.

26. Ans. (b) P falciparum

[*Ref.:* Paniker's Parasitology, 7th ed., page no. 71]

- P. falciparum has crescent shaped gametocyte.
- Non-falciparum plasmodium species has round gametocyte.

27. Ans. (c) Ticks

[*Ref.:* Paniker's Parasitology, 7th ed., page no. 84]

- Tick serves as the vector for Babesia.

28. Ans. (b) Toxoplasmosis

[*Ref.:* Paniker's Parasitology, 7th ed., page no. 92]

- Sabin-Feldman dye test is the gold standard method used in the diagnosis of toxoplasmosis.

29. Ans. (d) Culture in NNN medium

[*Ref.:* Paniker's Parasitology, 7th ed., page no. 57]

- Culture in NNN media – Promastigote form of Leishmania donovani seen.
- Smear microscopy – LD bodies containing amastigotes form seen.

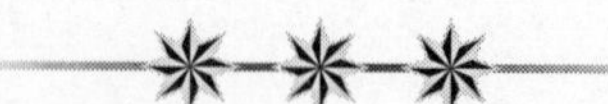

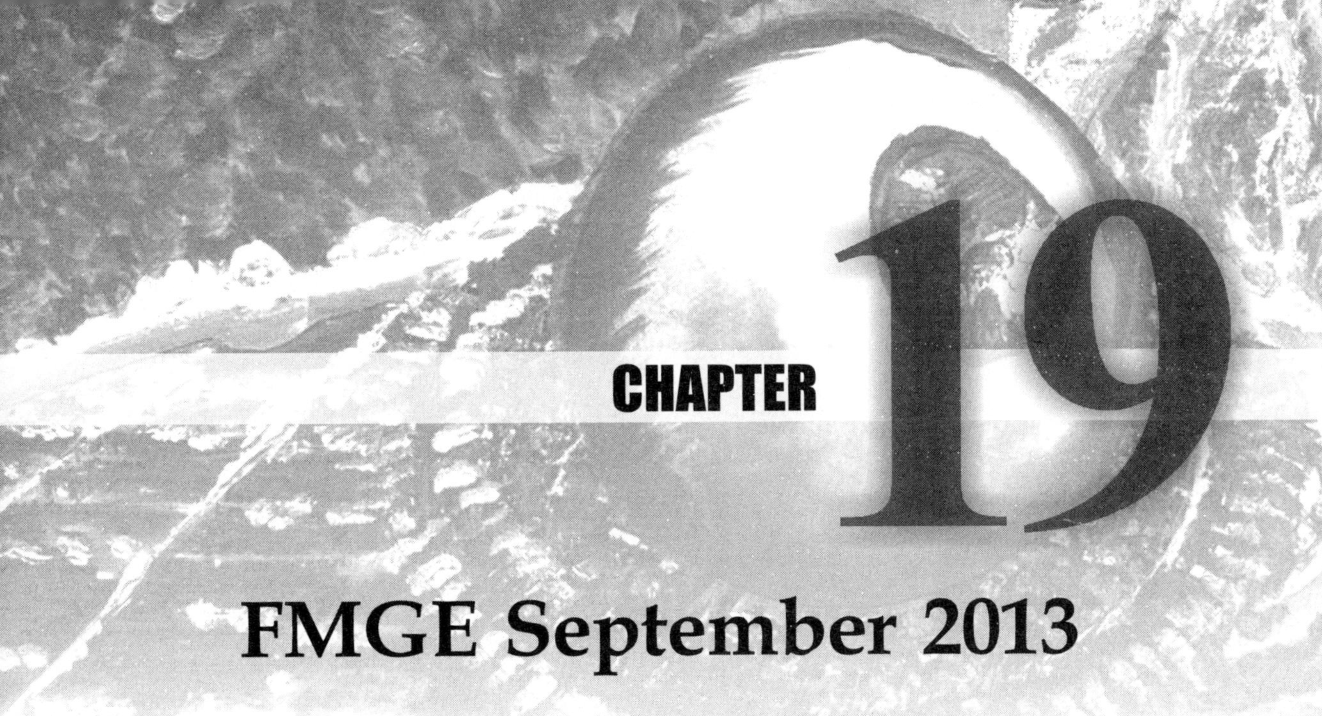

CHAPTER 19

FMGE September 2013

1. Which of the following is the primary opsonin in the complement system?

(a) C19
(b) C3b
(c) C5
(d) C5a.

2. Lyme disease is caused by which one of the following?

(a) Borrelia vincentii
(b) Borrelia recurrentis
(c) Borrelia hermsii
(d) Borrelia burgdorferi.

3. Q fever is caused by which one of the following?

(a) Ehrlichia sennetsu
(b) Coxiella burnetti
(c) Rickettsia akari
(d) Rochalimaea Quintana.

4. The bacteria most commonly associated with toxic shock syndrome is:

(a) Staphylococcus aureus
(b) Clostridium difficle
(c) Enterococcus faecium
(d) Salmonella enteridis.

5. A young man after consuming food in a party complaint of vomiting and diarrhea within 1 to 5 hours. The diagnosis is food poisoning due to:

(a) Staphylococus aureus
(b) Clostridium perfingens
(c) Streptococcus
(d) Clostridium botulinum.

6. All the following medically important gram negative bacilli are anaerobic, except:

(a) Bacteriodes
(b) Prevotella
(c) Fusobacterium
(d) Burkholderia.

7. Orchitis without epididymitis is seen in:

(a) Gonorrhoea
(b) TB
(c) Mumps
(d) Chlamydia infection.

8. Rabies virus isolated from natural human or animal infection is termed:

(a) Street virus
(b) Wild virus
(c) Fixed virus
(d) Free virus.

9. The most virulent plasmodium species causing malaria is:

(a) Plasmodium vivax
(b) Plasmodium falciparum
(c) Plasmodium ovale
(d) Plasmodium malariae.

10. The common name of Paragonimus westermani is:

(a) Cat liver fluke
(b) Oriental lung fluke
(c) Sheep liver fluke
(d) Vesical blood fluke.

11. Which of the following infestation leads to malabsorption:

(a) Giardia lamblia
(b) Ascaris lumbricoides
(c) Necator anericanus
(d) Ancylostoma duodenale.

ANSWERS TO FMGE SEPTEMBER 2013

1. Ans. (b) C3b

[*Ref.:* Ananthnarayan, 8th ed., page no. 111]

Opsonization: Enhanced phagocytosis by coating the microbial surfaces by opsonins, e.g., of most important opsonins – C3b and Fc (IgG), C4b, and iC3b.

2. Ans. (d) Borrelia burgdorferi

[*Ref.:* Ananthnarayan, 8th ed., page no. 379]

- Borrelia burgdorferi is the causative agent of Lyme's disease, transmitted by tick.
- Borrelia recurrentis is the causative agent of relapsing fever.

3. Ans. (b) Coxiella burnetti

[*Ref.:* Ananthnarayan, 8th ed., page no. 410]

- Q fever is caused by Coxiella burnetti, transmitted by inhalational route.

4. Ans. (a) Staphylococcus aureus

[*Ref.:* Ananthnarayan, 8th ed., page no. 199]

- Staphylococcus aureus is the most common cause of toxic shock syndrome, however it can also be caused by Streptococcus pyogenes.

5. Ans. (a) Staphylococus aureus

[*Ref.:* Ananthnarayan, 8th ed., page no. 198]

Agents causing food poisoning with short incubation period (6-8 hours).

- Staphylococcus aureus, B. Cereus and Clostridium botulinum.

6. Ans. (d) Burkholderia

[*Ref.:* Ananthnarayan, 8th ed., page no. 317]

- Burkholderia is obligate oxidase positive aerobic non fermenting gram negative bacilli.

7. Ans. (c) Mumps

[*Ref.:* Ananthnarayan, 8th ed., page no. 38]

Complication of Mumps:

- Epididymo-Orchitis (unilateral > bilateral) – seen in 1/3rd of post pubertal male patients.
- Aseptic meningitis and Pancreatitis leads to diabetes.

8. Ans. (a) Street virus

[*Ref.:* Ananthnarayan, 8th ed., page no. 38]

- Street virus or Wild virus causes rabies naturally in man or animal.
- Fixed virus are prepared by serial subculture of wild virus and these can be used for vaccine preparation.

9. Ans. (b) Plasmodium falciparum

[*Ref.:* Paniker's Parasitology, 7th ed., page no. 69]

- Plasmodium falciparum is the most virulent species among all the Plasmodium spp.

10. Ans. (b) Oriental lung fluke

[*Ref.:* Paniker's Parasitology, 7th ed., page no. 157]

Trematodes include:

- Schistosoma (blood fluke).
- Fasciola hepatica (liver fluke), Fasciolopsis buski (intestinal fluke).
- Paragonimus westermani (oriental lung fluke).
- Clonorchis (chinese liver fluke), Opisthorchis (bile duct fluke).

11. Ans. (a) Giardia lamblia

[*Ref.:* Paniker's Parasitology, 7th ed., page no. 32]

Pathogenesis of Giardia:

- It causes abnormalities of villous structure and causes malabsorption (lipids and lipid soluble vitamins).
- ***Malabsorption*** – there could be various types which include:
  - Malabsorption of fat (steatorrhea) – leads to foul smelling profuse frothy diarrhoea.
  - Disaccharidase deficiencies (lactate, xylose) – leading to lactose intolerance.
  - Malabsorption of vitamin B_{12} and folic acid and protein loosing enteropathy.

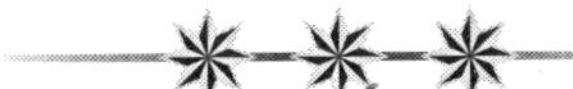